READY RECKONER

ANATOMY

Questions and Answers

Compiled by

VARSHA MOKHASI

Professor and HOD, Department of Anatomy

Vydehi Institute of Medical Sciences and Research Centre

Bengaluru

Peepee Publishers and Distributors Private Limited®

READY RECKONER
ANATOMY

Published by
Pawaninder P. Vij and Anupam Vij

Peepee Publishers and Distributors Private Limited
Head Office: 160, Shakti Vihar, Pitam Pura, Delhi-110 034 (India)

Correspondence Address:
7/31, First Floor, Ansari Road, Daryaganj
New Delhi-110 002 (India)

Ph: 41512412, 9811156083

e-mail: peepee160@yahoo.co.in

e-mail: peepee160@gmail.com

www.peepeepub.com

join us on facebook.com/pp.publishers

First Edition: 2024

ISBN: 978-81-9720-728-0

PREFACE

This book should help the students for their exam preparations as it is designed with questions and answers. This pattern also makes the concepts clear for their understanding. It took me a lot of time as we were busy with my personal and professional demands. Each chapter goes by question and answers covering the entire chapter. The language is kept very simple which will help them to remember and reproduce in the examination.

I thank my daughter Meghana Mokhasi, a qualified medical illustrator, for helping with a few illustrations and also technology. I thank Dr. Surendra Babu, my junior colleague for helping me with technology.

I also thank my family, institution and department colleagues, for great direct and indirect help during compilation of the book.

I thank Peepee Publishers for giving me an opportunity and bearing with my delays in submissions. This opportunity gave me a great learning experience.

Dr. Varsha Mokhasi

CONTENTS

1 CHAPTER

ANATOMICAL TERMINOLOGY

Objectives:
1. To define anatomical position.
2. To define anatomical planes.
3. To define terms and terminology.

1. a. Define anatomical position

b. What are the other positions of body?

Ans. a. Anatomical position: (Fig. 1.1)

It is the standard reference position of the body used to describe the location and inter-relationship of various parts and organs of the body. The body is in *anatomical position* when:

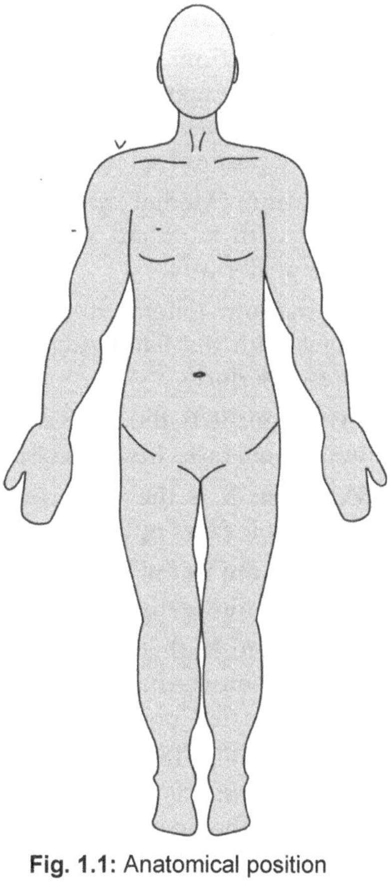

Fig. 1.1: Anatomical position

- Body is in upright standing position.
- Eyes are looking straight forward.
- Upper limbs are hanging by the sides and palms are facing forward with the fingers straight and together.
- Lower limbs are parallel and the toes are pointing forward.

b. Other positions of the body:
- Supine position.
- Prone position.
- Lithotomy position.

2. Define various anatomical planes.

Ans. The major imaginary planes that pass through the body in anatomical position are: (Fig. 1.2)

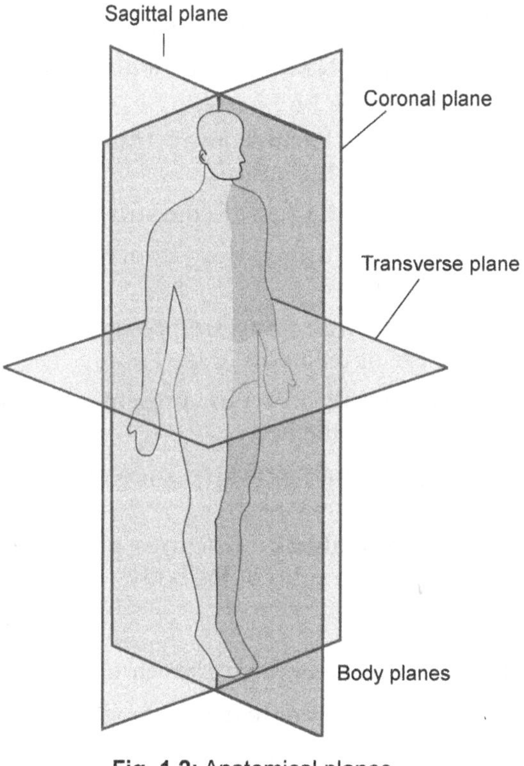

Fig. 1.2: Anatomical planes

- **Median plane:** It is a vertical plane that passes longitudinally through the midline of the body and dividing it into equal right and left halves.
- **Sagittal plane:** An imaginary vertical plane that is parallel to median plane and divides the body into right and left parts.
- **Coronal plane:** An imaginary vertical plane that is at right angle to the median plane and divides the body into anterior and posterior parts.
- Transverse plane.
- Horizontal plane.
- Oblique plane.

3. Enumerate and define the anatomical terms used to describe location and inter-relationship between structures.

Ans. Anatomical terms used to describe location and inter-relationship between structures are:

- **Anterior (Ventral):** Towards the front of the body.
- **Posterior (Dorsal):** Towards the back of the body.
- **Superior (Cephalic, Cranial):** Towards the head.
- **Inferior (Caudal):** Towards the feet.
- **Medial:** Nearer to the median plane of the body.
- **Lateral:** Further away from the median plane of the body.
- **Proximal:** Closer to the structure's origin.
- **Distal:** Further away from the structure's origin.
- **Unilateral:** Structure present only on one side of the body.
- **Bilateral:** Structure present on both the sides of the body.
- **Ipsilateral:** Structures present on the same side of the body.
- **Contralateral:** Structures present on the opposite sides of the body.

Examples:

- The sternum lies anterior to the heart.
- The heart lies superior to the diaphragm.
- The lungs lie lateral to the heart.
- The index finger lies lateral to little finger.
- The heart is deep to the sternum.
- The shoulder is proximal to the elbow.
- The wrist is distal to the elbow.
- Right leg and right arm are ipsilateral.
- Left forearm and right foot are contralateral.

4. Enumerate and define the anatomical terms used to describe movements.

Ans. Anatomical terms used to describe movements:

- **Flexion:** It is bending of part of the body in sagittal plane such that the two flexor surfaces come close to each other and the angle of the joint is decreased.
- **Extension:** The movement occurs in sagittal plane such that the angle of the joint increases.
- **Adduction:** The movement occurs in coronal plane such that the part of the body moves towards the median plane.
- **Abduction:** The movement occurs in coronal plane such that the part of the body moves away from the median plane.
- **Circumduction:** It is a combination of flexion, extension, abduction and adduction such that the distal end of the moving part moves in a circle.
- **Pronation:** Medial rotation of forearm along with the hand such that the palm faces posteriorly.
- **Supination:** Lateral rotation of forearm along with the hand such that the palm faces anteriorly.
- **Inversion:** It is the movement of foot in which sole faces inwards or medially.
- **Eversion:** It is the movement of foot in which sole faces outwards or laterally.
- **Protraction:** In this movement the part of the body moves forward.
- **Retraction:** In this movement the part of the body moves backward such that from the protracted position it moves back to the anatomical position.
- **Opposition:** It is the movement of thumb such that the tip of the thumb touches the tip of other digits.

2 CHAPTER

SKIN AND FASCIA

Objectives:
1. To define skin in detail.
2. To define and explain fascia in detail.

1. **Enumerate the:**
   a. **Functions of skin**
   b. **Layers of skin**
   c. **Layers of epidermis**
   d. **Appendages of skin**

Ans. a. **Functions of skin:**

- *Protection:* Protect the body from mechanical injury and pathogens.
- *Thermoregulation:* Helps in maintaining normal body temperature.
  - In summer, the excess heat is lost from the body by:
    - Secretion and evaporation of sweat from sweat glands.
    - Radiation from the dilated blood vessels.
- In winter, heat is conserved due to the presence of the subcutaneous fat and hair.
- *Prevents loss of body fluids.*
- *Acts as a sense organ:* Is provided with various types of sensory endings for the perception of sensations such as pain, touch, heat and cold.
- *Synthesizes Vitamin D.*

b. **Layers of skin: (Fig. 2.1)**

- Epidermis.
- Dermis.

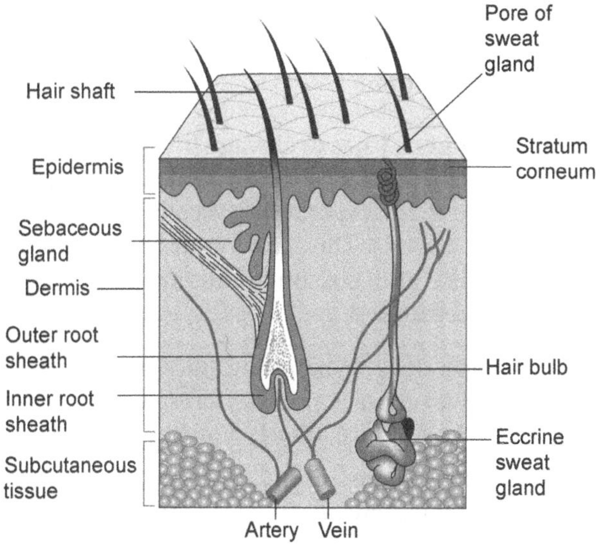

Fig. 2.1: Layers and structures of skin

c. **Layers of epidermis: (Fig. 2.2)**

- Stratum germinativum.
- Stratum spinosum.
- Stratum granulosum.
- Stratum lucidum.
- Stratum corneum.

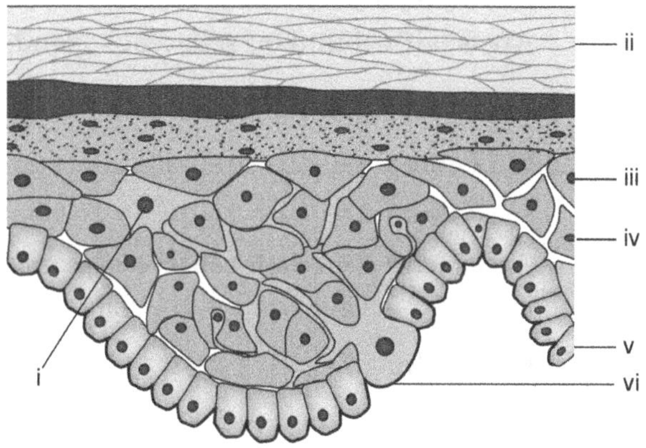

i. Langerhans cell
ii Horny cell layer
iii. Granular cell layer
iv. Squamous cell layer
v. Basal cell layer
vi. Melanocyte

Fig. 2.2: Layers of epidermis

Stratum lucidum is found only in thick skin, i.e., in sole and palm.

d. **Appendages of skin:**
- Hair.
- Nail.
- Sweat gland.
- Sebaceous gland.

2. **Define:**

a. **Langer's lines**

b. **Dermatome**

Ans. a. **Langer's lines or clevage lines** are the lines on the surface of skin which are caused due to the orientation of collagen fibers in the dermis. They run longitudinally in the limbs and circumferentially in the neck and trunk.

Incisions made along or parallel to the Langer's lines will severe fewer collagen fibers as a result the healing is faster and the scar formation is minimal.

b. **Dermatome (Fig. 2.3):** The area of skin supplied by a single segment of spinal nerve is called a dermatome. Knowledge of dermatomes is essential to carry out neurological examination.

Testing touch in a particular dermatome in conscious patient can be used to localize injury of a specific spinal nerve or specific spinal segment.

3. **Enumerate the:**

a. **Areas devoid of sebaceous glands**

b. **Areas with abundant sebaceous glands**

Ans. a. **Areas devoid of sebaceous glands:**
- Palm.
- Sole.

b. **Areas with abundant sebaceous glands:**
- Face.
- Scalp.
- Ears.
- Nostrils.

4. **How is the degree of burns calculated in extensive burns?**

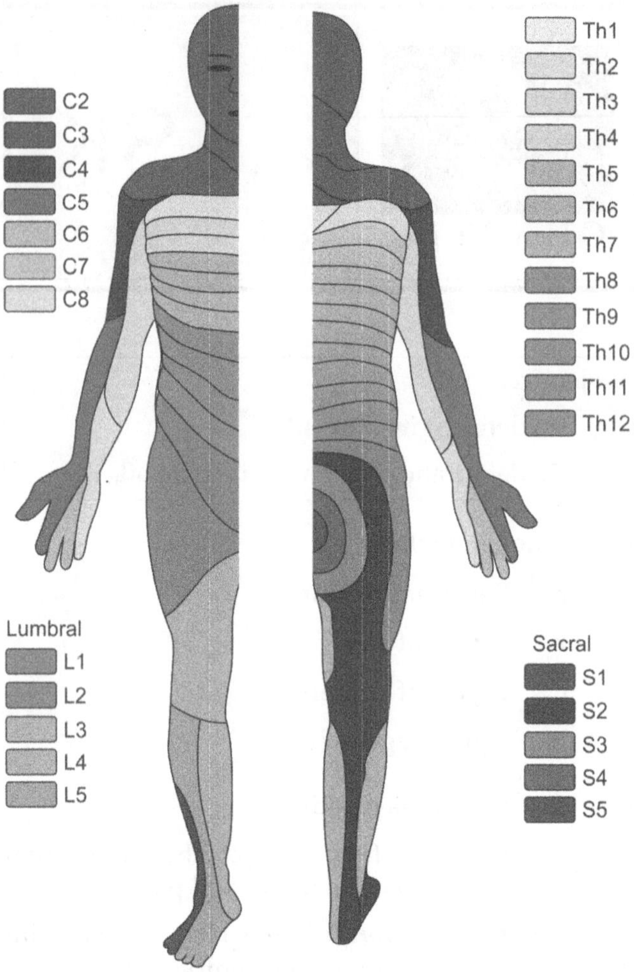

Fig. 2.3: Dermatome

Ans. It is assessed by calculating the percentage of the skin covered area affected. This follows the 'rule of nine' and is expressed as follows:
- Head and neck 9%
- Each upper limb 9%
- Front of the trunk 18%
- Back of the trunk 18%
- Each lower limb 18%
- Perineum 1%

5. **Define:**

a. **Superficial fascia and enumerate its contents**

b. **Deep fascia and name its modifications**

c. **Bursa and write its functional significance**

Ans. a. **Superficial fascia** is a layer of loose

connective tissue that connects the skin to the underlying deep fascia. Its contents are:

- Fat.
- Superficial blood vessels.
- Cutaneous nerves.
- Superficial lymphatics.
- Mammary gland in females.
- Remnants of panniculus carnosus (muscle in superficial fascia), e.g., platysma in neck, muscles of scalp and muscles of facial expression.

b. **Deep fascia** is a dense, inelastic fibrous layer that lies deep to superficial fascia and covers the deeper structures such as bones, muscles, nerves and blood vessels. It becomes continuous with the outermost covering layer of underlying structures, i.e., periosteum, perimysium, perineurium and adventitial layer of blood vessels.

Modifications of deep fascia are:

- ***Intermuscular septa (Fig. 2.4a):*** In limbs the deep fascia sends septa from its deep surface to the bone which separate the muscles into different compartments. They are between the groups of muscles.

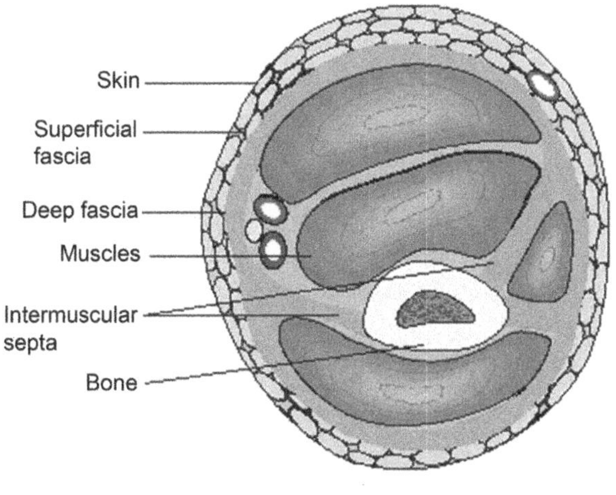

Fig. 2.4a: Intermuscular septa

- ***Retinaculum (Fig. 2.4b):*** Are present where tendons cross the joint. Flexor and extensor retinacula are present around the wrist and ankle joint.

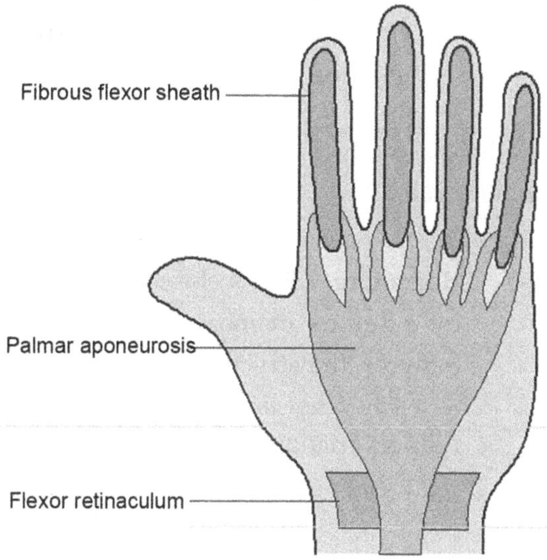

Fig. 2.4b: Modification of deep fascia (retinaculum, aponeurosis, fibrous flexor sheath)

- ***Fibrous flexor sheath:*** Thickened deep fascia of fingers and toes on the flexor surface. It retains the fexor tendon close to the joint and prevents its bow stringing.
- ***Aponeuroses:*** Deep fascia of palm and sole are thickened to form palmar and plantar aponeuroses respectively. They protect the underlying structures.
- ***Ligament (Fig. 2.4c):*** Thickenings of deep fascia which connect bones at

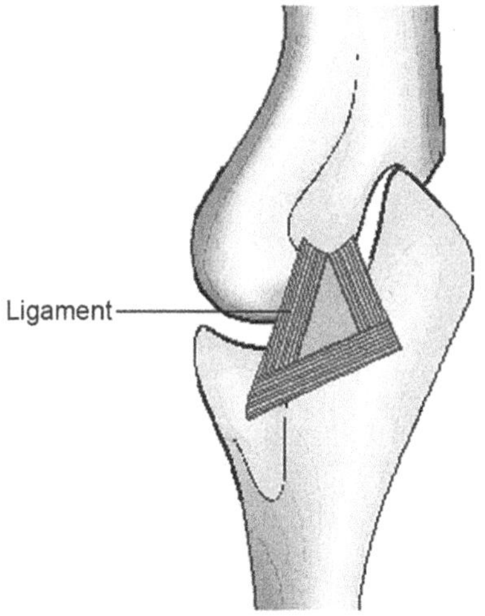

Fig. 2.4c: Ligament

joints. They hold ends of the bones close to each other during movements and thus provide stability to the joints.

Sites where deep fascia is absent: Face and anterior abdominal wall.

c. **Bursa (Fig. 2.5)** is a closed serous sac lined by a serous membrane. They are found between the structures that move relative to each other in close apposition. They reduces friction and allow free movement between the apposed surfaces, e.g., subcutaneous, subtendinous, subscapular, intertendinous etc. Infection of bursa is called *bursitis*.

Adventitious bursae: Bursae that are not normally present but develop over bony surfaces which are subjected to frequent friction and pressure, e.g.:

a. ***Tailor's ankle:*** Appears in tailors above the lateral malleolus.

b. ***Porter's shoulder:*** In porters, between upper surface of clavicle and skin.

c. ***Weaver's bottom:*** Between gluteus maximus and ischial tuberosity.

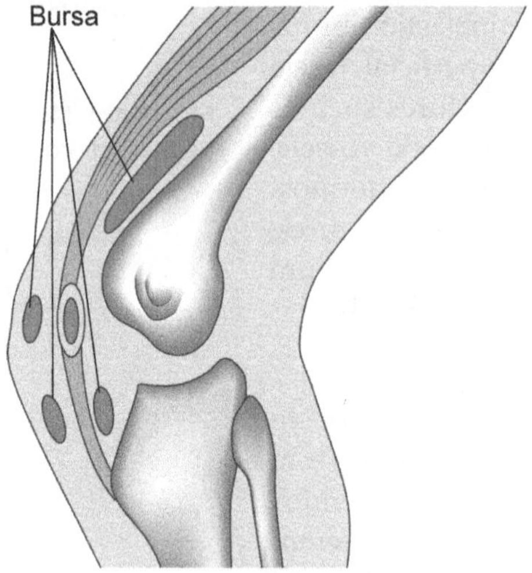

Fig. 2.5: Bursa

3 CHAPTER BONE

> **Objectives:**
> 1. To explain bone with classification, functions and blood supply.
> 2. To explain types of epiphysis with examples.

1. Enumerate the functions of bone.

Ans. Functions of bone:

- Form skeletal framework of the body and give shape to the body.
- Protect vital organs such as brain, heart and lungs.
- Store mineral salts, e.g., calcium and phosphorus.
- Is the site of blood cell production.
- Provide surface for attachment of muscles, thereby help in producing movements.

> Total number of bones in adults – 206.

2. Classify bones according to:

a. **Shape**

b. **Structure**

c. **Ossification**

Ans. CLASSIFICATION OF BONES

a. **According to the shape:**

- *Long bones:*
  - Typical long bones, e.g., Humerus, femur, radius, ulna, tibia, fibula.
  - Miniature long bones, e.g., Metacarpals, metatarsals and phalanges.
  - Modified long bones, e.g., Clavicle and body of vertebrae.
- *Short bones:* Carpals and tarsals.
- *Flat bones:* Frontal, parietal, ribs, sternum.
- *Irregular bones:* Hip bone, vertebrae, sphenoid, maxilla, ethmoid.
- *Pneumatic bones (contain air filled cavities):* Maxilla, sphenoid, ethmoid, frontal.
- *Sesamoid bones:* Patella, pisiform, fabella.

> **Supernumerary bones/accessory bones:** These are the bones that are not normally present. They may be formed due to:
> - Appearance of extra centres of ossification, e.g., sutural bones in skull.
> - Non-union of an epiphysis, e.g., ostrigonum–the posterior tubercle of talus fails to fuse with the rest of the bone.

b. **According to the structure:**

- *Compact bone:* For example, shaft of the long bones.
- *Cancellous bone (spongy or trabecular):* For example, ends of long bones.

c. **According to the ossification:**

- *Membranous bones:* Bones are formed by intramembranous ossification. Bones are formed by ossification of the mesenchymal tissue without the intervention of cartilage model, e.g., bones of vault of skull (parietal, frontal and occipital) and bones of face.
- *Cartilaginous bones:* Bones are formed by endochondral ossification. The bone is preformed as a cartilage model, the cartilage model is then replaced by bone following ossification, e.g.,

Bones of limbs (humerus, femur, radius, ulna, fibula, tibia), bones of base of skull, vertebrae, ribs, sternum.

Membranocartilaginous bones: Some bones partly develop in mesenchyme (membranous ossification) and partly in cartilage (endochondral ossification), e.g., mandible, clavicle, occipital the temporal.

3. **Enumerate:**
   a. **Features of a long bone**
   b. **Characteristic features of sesamoid bone**
   c. **Functions of sesamoid bone**

Ans. a. **Features of a long bone:**
- Has an elongated tubular shaft (diaphysis) and two expanded ends (epiphysis).
- Contains medullary cavity (except clavicle) filled with bone marrow.
- Ossify by endochondral ossification (except clavicle).
- Are weight bearing bones.
- Lie vertically in the body (except clavicle).

b. **Sesamoid bones** are the bones that are embedded in the tendons, e.g., patella in the tendon of quadriceps femoris and pisiform in the tendon of flexor carpi ulnaris.

They have the following *characteristic features:*
- They develop in the tendons after birth.
- They are found where the tendon crosses the end of long bone of limbs.
- They are not covered by periosteum.
- Their surface that comes in contact with the bone is covered by hyaline cartilage.

c. **Functions of sesamoid bone:**
- To minimize friction.
- To alter the direction of pull of muscle.

4. **Describe briefly the following term:**
   a. **Epiphysis**
   b. **Diaphysis**
   c. **Metaphysis**
   d. **Epiphyseal plate**
   e. **Primary centre of ossification**
   f. **Secondary centre of ossification**
   g. **Growing end of the long bone**

Ans. a. **Epiphysis:** The expanded end of long bone that ossifies from the secondary centre of ossification.

Epiphyses are made of spongy bone covered by a thin layer of compact bone.

b. **Diaphysis:** The elongated, cylindrical shaft of long bone that ossifies from the primary centre of ossification. It is made up of compact bone and encloses a tubular cavity called marrow cavity.

c. **Metaphysis:** It is part of the diaphysis that is adjacent to the epiphyseal plate. This is the most active site of bone formation in the developing bone. It has rich blood supply.

Metaphysis is the common site of osteomyelitis in children because metaphysis is supplied by end arteries that form hair-pin bends and the bacteria or emboli can be easily trapped in the bends of arteries causing infarction.

d. **Epiphyseal plate:** It is a thin plate of hyaline cartilage placed between the diaphysis and epiphysis. The continuous proliferation of cartilage cells in the epiphyseal plate is responsible for the growth of developing bone in length. The epiphyseal plate disappears when the growth in the length of bone stops. Following are the zones of epiphyseal plate:
- Zone of resting cartilage.
- Zone of proliferating cartilage.
- Zone of hypertrophied cartilage.
- Zone of calcification.
- Zone of ossification.

e. **Primary centre of ossification:** The site in the mid region of cartilage where ossification begins first and forms the main part of the bone is called primary centre of ossification. In case of long bones it forms the shaft (diaphysis). It usually appears before birth.

f. **Secondary centre of ossification:** The secondary centre of ossification usually appears after birth at the ends of the developing long bone. They form the epiphyses of the long bones.

In case of femur, the secondary centre of ossification for the lower end appears just before birth.

g. **Growing end of the long bone:** It is that end of the long bone whose epiphysis fuses with the diaphysis later than the other end (it continues to grow in length a little longer). The growing end of the long bone is opposite to the direction of the nutrient foramen (exception to the fibula where the nutrient foramen is directed towards the growing end).

The growing end in upper limb bones is away from the elbow, i.e., upper end of humerus and lower end of radius and ulna. In lower limb bones the growing end is towards the knee, i.e., lower end of femur and upper end of tibia and fibula.

5. **Enumerate the types of epiphyses and give one example of each.**

Ans. TYPES OF EPIPHYSES

a. **Pressure epiphysis: (Fig. 3.1a)**
   - Is present at the end of the long bone.
   - Is articular in nature.
   - Takes part in transmission of weight.
   - For example, head of humerus and femur, lower end of radius.

b. **Traction epiphysis:**
   - Is produced due to the pull of the muscle and therefore provide attachment to the muscle/s.
   - Is non-articular.
   - Is not involved in transmission of weight.
   - For example, greater and lesser tubercles of humerus, greater and lesser trochanters of femur and mastoid process of temporal bone.

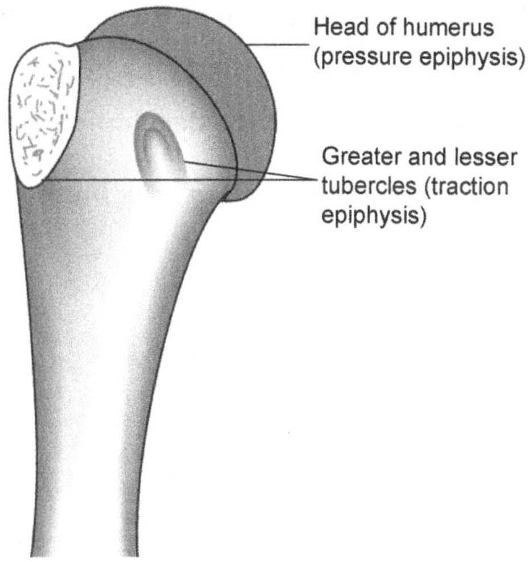

Fig. 3.1a: Pressure and traction epiphysis

c. **Atavistic epiphysis: (Fig. 3.1b)**
   - Is phylogenetically an independent bone in lower animals but in humans is part of another bone.
   - For example, coracoid process of scapula, posterior tubercle of talus.

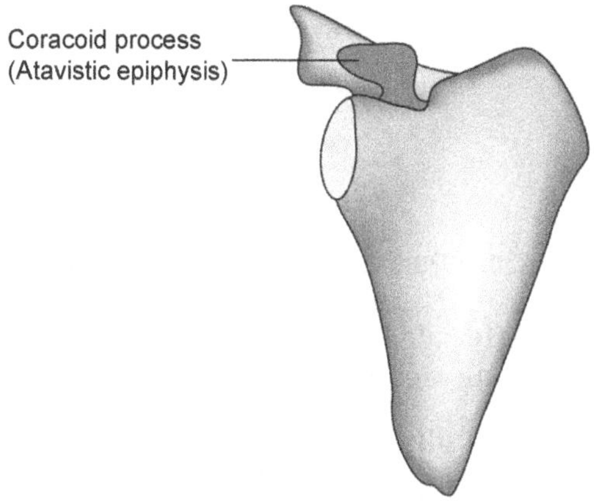

Fig. 3.1b: Atavistic epiphysis

d. **Aberrant epiphysis:**
   - Is not always present but may be present in some individuals.
   - For example, epiphysis at the head of first metacarpal and base of other metacarpals (normally metacarpals have only one epiphysis, i.e., base of 1st metacarpal and heads of other metacarpals).

Pressure epiphysis ossifies earlier than the traction epiphysis, i.e., secondary centre of ossification appear earlier in pressure epiphysis than in traction epiphysis.

6. **Draw labelled diagram of the following:**
   a. **Parts of a developing long bone**
   b. **Arterial supply of a developing long bone**

Ans. a. Parts of a developing long bone: (Fig. 3.2)

- Diaphysis.
- Metaphysis.
- Epiphyseal plate.
- Epiphysis.

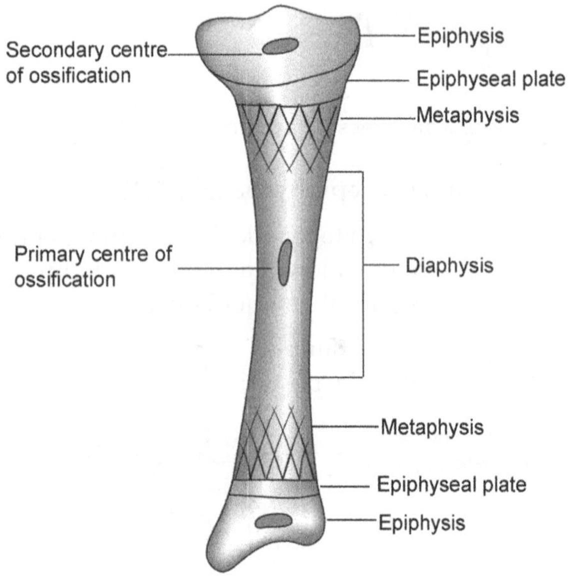

Fig. 3.2: Parts of a developing long bone

b. Arterial supply of a developing long bone are: (Fig. 3.3)

- Nutrient artery.
- Periosteal arteries.
- Metaphyseal arteries.
- Epiphyseal arteries.

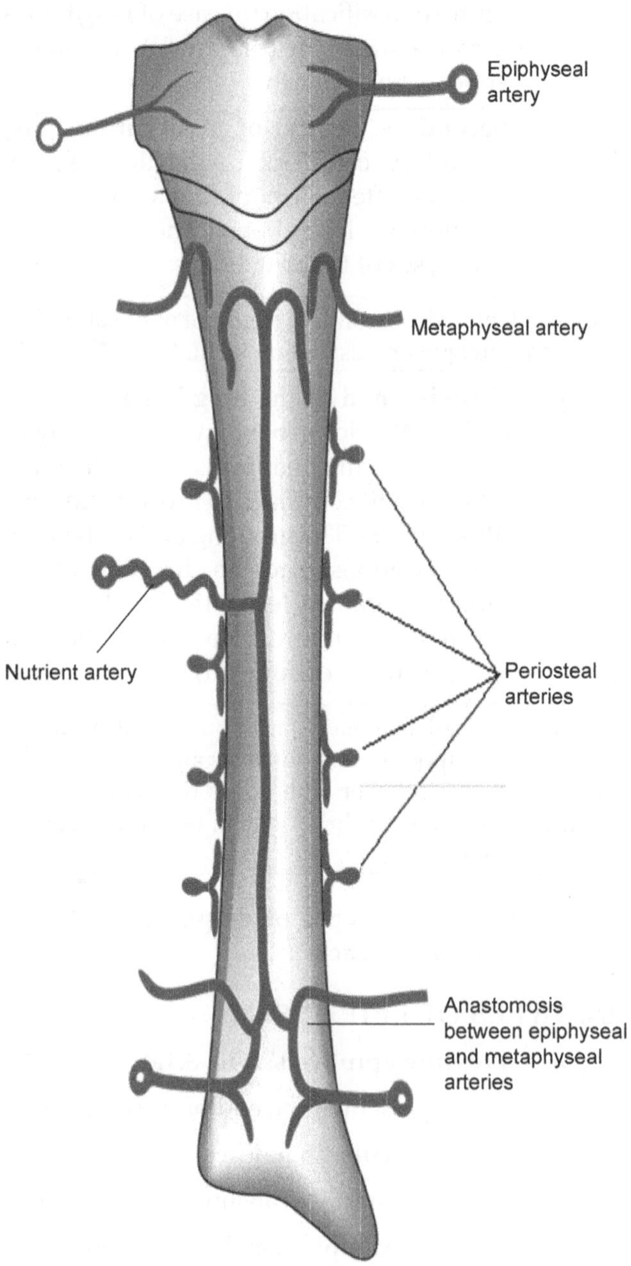

Fig. 3.3: Arterial supply of a developing long bone

4 CHAPTER JOINTS

Objectives:
1. To describe joints under following headings:
   a. Definition b. Functions c. Classifications.
2. To describe types of cartilaginous joints.
3. To understand synovial joints.

1. Define joint.

Ans. Joint (articulation) is a point of contact between two or more bones.

2. What are the functions of joints?

Ans. Functions of joints are:
- Allow movement.
- Allow growth.
- Allow moulding of head during childbirth.
- Allow transmission of forces.

3. Classify joints on the basis of structure and function.

Ans. Joints can be classified on the basis of function or structure:
- ***Functional classification:*** Based on amount of movement possible at the joint.
  - *Synarthroses*–Immovable–common in axial skeleton.
  - *Amphiarthroses*–Slightly movable–common in axial skeleton.
  - *Diarthroses*–Freely movable–common in appendicular skeleton.
- ***Structural classification*** is based on:
  - Material that binds the bones together.
  - Presence or absence of a joint cavity.

Structural classification includes:
- ***Fibrous joint:***
  - Bones are connected by fibrous connective tissue.
  - Do not have a joint cavity.
  - Most are immovable or only slightly movable.
- ***Cartilaginous joint:***
  - Bones are united by cartilage.
  - Most are slightly movable (amphiarthrotic).
  - Lack a joint cavity.
- ***Synovial joint:***
  - Joint cavity is present between the bones, and the joint is surrounded by articular capsule.
  - Most movable type of joint.
  - Most are 'simple' and have just two articulating surfaces.
  - Some are 'compound' with more than two articulating surfaces [e.g., elbow (humerus, radius and ulna) and knee (femur, tibia, fibula, patella) joints].

4. Name the different types of fibrous joints and give example of each.

Ans. Following are the three types of fibrous joints: (Fig. 4.1)

a. Sutures:
- Sutural joints are present between the bones which ossify in membrane.
- They are present between the bones of skull (e.g., coronal suture between frontal and parietal bones and sagittal suture between the two parietal bones).
- Bones are bound together by *sutural ligaments.*

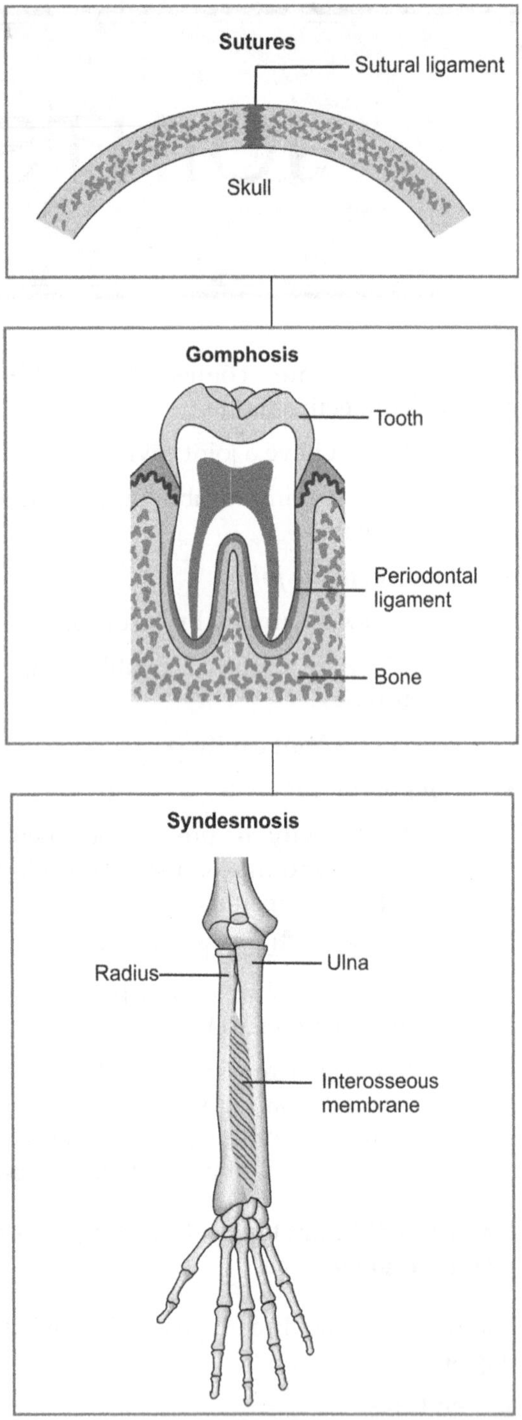

Fig. 4.1: Fibrous joints

- In adults, sutures allow almost no movement between the bones.

b. **Syndesmosis:**
- Bones are held together by the interosseous membrane or ligament.
- Slight movement is possible.
- For example, intermediate radioulnar and inferior tibiofibular joints.

c. **Gomphosis:**
- Cone shaped root of tooth fits into the socket of the jaw (like a peg in the socket).
- The tooth is attached to the alveolar socket by periodontal ligament.
- The joint is immovable.

5. What are the different types of cartilaginous joints? Give example of each.

Ans. There are two types of cartilaginous joints: (Fig. 4.2)

- **Primary cartilaginous joint (synchondrosis):**

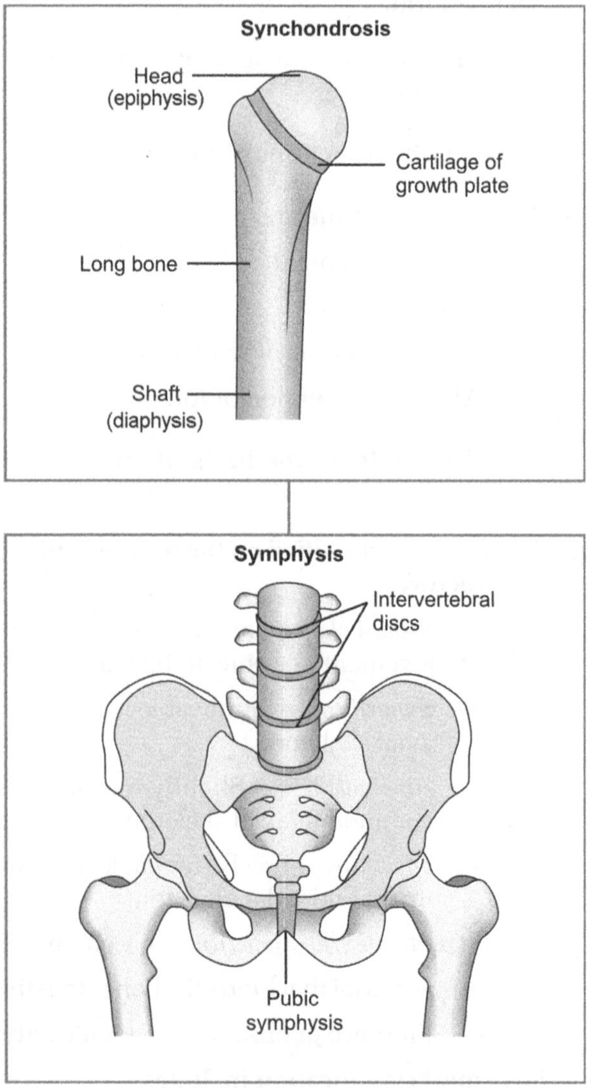

Fig. 4.2: Cartilaginous joints

- The articulating bones are connected via hyaline cartilage.
- The joints are immovable and temporary in nature, i.e., after certain age the cartilaginous plate is replaced by bone (synostosis).
- For example, between epiphysis and diaphysis (epiphyseal plate).

• **Secondary cartilaginous joint (symphysis):**
  - The articulating bones are connected via fibrocartilage.
  - They are slightly movable joints.
  - These are permanent joints and persist throughout life.
  - They are present in the median plane.
  - For example, between two vertebral bodies (intervertebral disc), pubic symphysis and manubriosternal joint.

6. **What are the characteristic features of a typical synovial joint? Draw a labelled diagram of a typical synovial joint.**

Ans. Following are the characteristic features of a typical synovial joint: (Fig. 4.3)

- Presence of synovial cavity.
- Joint is surrounded by fibrous articular capsule.
- The fibrous capsule is lined by synovial membrane (it produces synovial fluid which percolates into the joint cavity and lubricates the articular surfaces).
- Ends of the articulating bones are covered by articular cartilage (mostly hyaline cartilage).

The articular surfaces of bones which are formed by membranous ossification are covered by fibrocartilage, e.g., in temporomandibular and sternoclavicular joint.

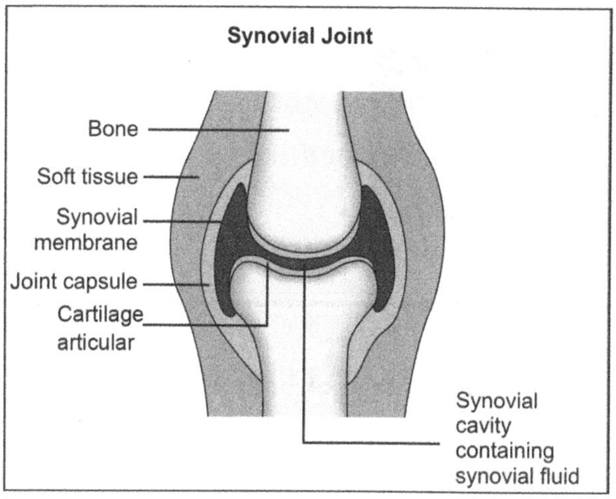

Fig. 4.3: Typical synovial joint

7. **Classify synovial joints and give example of each.**

Ans. Following are the different types of synovial joints according to the axis of movement and shape of articular surfaces.

- **Uniaxial joints:**
  - *Pivot joint:* Atlantoaxial and superior radioulnar joints.
  - *Hinge joint:* Elbow, ankle and interphalangeal joints.
- **Biaxial joints:**
  - *Ellipsoid joint:* Wrist and metacarpophalangeal joints.
  - *Condylar joint:* Knee joint, temporomandibular joint (bicondylar).
- **Multiaxial joints:**
  - *Ball and socket joint:* Shoulder and hip joint.
  - *Saddle joint:* 1st carpometacarpal and sternoclavicular joints.
- **Plane joint:** Intercarpal and intertarsal joints.

CHAPTER 5

MUSCLES

1. **What percentage of body mass is comprised muscle?**

Ans. Muscle comprises approximately 48% of the body mass.

2. **What is the basic property of muscular tissue?**

Ans. Contractility.

3. **What are the different types of muscles in the body?**

Ans. There are three types of muscles: (Fig. 5.1)

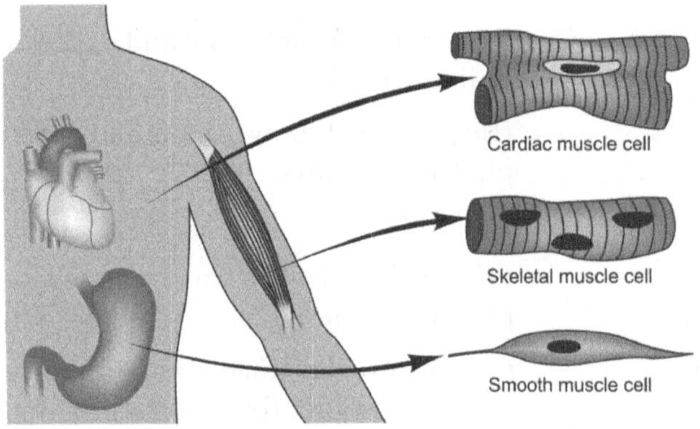

Fig. 5.1: Types of muscles

a. Skeletal/striated/voluntary muscle.

b. Smooth/visceral/involuntary muscle.

c. Cardiac muscle.

4. **Compare the three types of muscles in a tabulated form.**

Ans. See Table 5.1.

5. **Classify the skeletal muscle according to the arrangement of muscle fibers.**

Ans. Classification of skeletal muscle according to the arrangement of muscle fibers: (Fig. 5.2)

a. **When muscle fibers are parallel to each other:**
- ***Strap like:*** Sartorius, sternohyoid, sternothyroid.
- ***Quadrate:*** Pronator quadrates, quadrates lumborum.
- ***Fusiform:*** Biceps brachii, digastric.

b. **When muscle fibers are oblique:**
- ***Unipennate:*** Flexor pollicis longus, peroneus tertius.

Table 5.1: Comparison between the three types of muscles

Feature		*Skeletal muscle*	*Smooth muscle*	*Cardiac muscle*
Location		Attached to skeleton	In the wall of hollow viscera	In the heart
Structure of muscle fiber	Shape	Cylindrical, unbranched	Spindle shaped	Cylindrical, branched
	Nucleus	Multiple, located peripherally	Single and centrally placed	Single and centrally placed
	Striations	Prominent transverse striations	Transverse striations absent	Faint transverse striations
Action		Quick voluntary contraction	Slow and sustained involuntary contraction	Rhythmic involuntary contraction
Innervation		Somatic nervous system	Autonomic nervous system	Autonomic nervous system

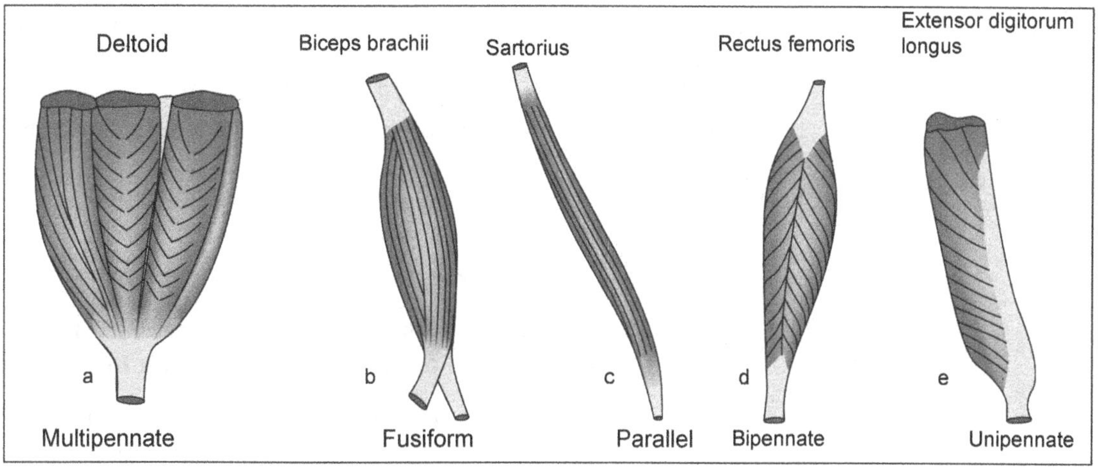

Fig. 5.2: Arrangement of skeletal muscle fibers

- *Bipennate:* Flexor hallucis longus, rectus femoris and dorsal interossei.
- *Multipennate:* Deltoid, subscapularis.

6. **What are the different types of muscles according to their action?**

Ans. a. **Prime movers:** Muscles that are responsible for the initiation and maintenance of desired movement are called prime movers, e.g., biceps and brachialis are prime movers for flexion of elbow joint.

b. **Antagonist:** Muscles that oppose the action of prime movers, e.g., triceps which extends the elbow joint is antagonistic to the biceps brachii which is responsible for flexion of elbow joint.

> A prime mover for a particular movement (triceps acts a prime mover for extension at elbow) may act as antagonist for opposite movement (flexion at elbow).

c. **Synergists:** Muscles that help in the action of prime movers (when prime mover is a long muscle and crosses more than one joint) by preventing the undesired movements at the intermediate joints, e.g., during flexion of fingers by the long flexors of digits, the wrist joint is fixed and extended by the extensors which act as synergist to the flexors (Flexion of fingers is efficient when the wrist is fixed and extended).

d. **Fixators:** They stabilize the proximal attachment of a muscle or joint so that the muscle can act more efficiently at the distal joint.

> A muscle that acts as a prime mover for one movement can act as an antagonist, fixator or synergist at other times.

7. **What are the different types of contractions a muscle can undergo?**

Ans. a. **Isometric contraction:** The muscle contracts and exerts force without alteration in the length or without any movement, e.g., flexors of the forearm trying to lift weight that is too heavy.

b. **Isotonic contraction:** The muscle contracts and shortens to produce movement, e.g., flexors of the forearm contract to lift a glass of water.

8. **Describe briefly the motor unit.**

Ans. **Motor Unit (Fig. 5.3):** All the muscle fibers innervated by a single α motor neuron constitutes a *'motor unit'*. Trunk muscles have few large motor units and can perform only gross movements, whereas extraocular muscles of eye and muscles of thumb have smaller motor units (a single motor neuron innervates 5–10 muscle fibers) and are capable of delicate and precise movements.

9. **What is motor point?**

Ans. It is the point of entrance of the nerve trunk into the muscle. Usually a nerve enters the deep surface of the muscle. Electrical stimulation of the muscle is most effective at the motor point.

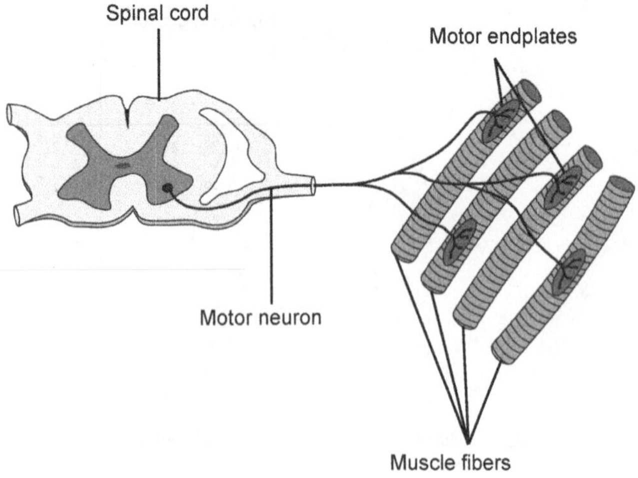

Fig. 5.3: Motor unit

10. **Describe the nerve supply of the skeletal muscle.**

Ans. Skeletal muscle is supplied by somatic nerves. The nerve to a skeletal muscle is a mixed nerve containing 60% motor and 40% sensory fibers.

a. **Motor supply:** Extrafusal fibers of the muscle which produce movements are innervated by motor neuron of the anterior horn of spinal cord or motor nuclei of cranial nerves in case of head and neck. Intrafusal fibers of the muscle spindle are innervated by the gamma neurons.

b. **Sensory supply:** Sensory nerve fibers innervate muscle spindles, tendons, ligaments and joint capsules to mediate proprioceptive impulses.

11. **Define:**
   a. **Muscle tone**
   b. **Myotome**

Ans. a. **Muscle tone:** Skeletal muscle fibers even in resting condition remain in a state of partial contraction. This is referred to as muscle tone.

b. **Myotome:** Muscle fibers supplied by a spinal nerve constitute a myotome.

Paralysis of muscle: When a muscle is unable to contract either due to injury to the motor nerve or spinal cord is called paralysis.

Hemiplegia: Muscles of one side of the body are paralysed.

Paraplegia: Muscles of both the lower limbs are paralysed.

Quadriplegia: All the four limbs are paralysed.

12. **List the differences between the upper motor neuron and lower motor neuron paralysis.**

Ans. Differences between upper motor neuron and lower motor neuron paralysis are: (Fig. 5.4)

Features	*Upper motor neuron (UMN) paralysis*	*Lower motor neuron (LMN) paralysis*
Paralysis type	Spastic	Flaccid
Muscle tone	Increased	Decreased
Muscle atrophy	Absent	Present
Tendon reflexes	Exaggerated	Diminished
Babinski's sign	Present	Absent
Affected side	Contralateral	Ipsilateral

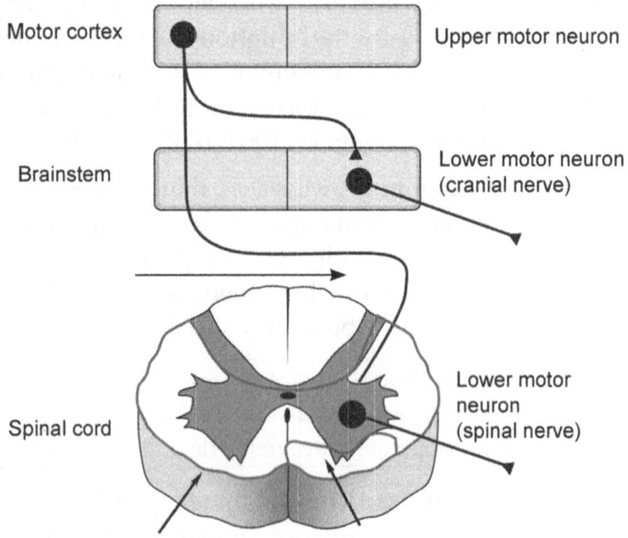

Fig. 5.4: Upper and lower motor neuron

- **Babinski's sign:** Dorsiflexion of great toe with fanning of lateral toes on scratching lateral aspect of plantar surface of foot (Normal: Plantar flexion of toes).

CHAPTER 6 CARDIOVASCULAR SYSTEM

1. **What are the components of the cardiovascular system?**

Ans. Cardiovascular system includes heart and blood vessels, i.e., arteries, veins and capillaries.

2. **What are the different types of circulation?**

Ans. a. **Systemic circulation (Fig. 6.1):** It is responsible for transporting oxygenated blood through arteries to the entire body and then returns deoxygenated blood to the heart via veins. The circulation of blood flow is as follows:

Left ventricle
↓ } Oxygenated blood
Aorta and its branches

↓

Capillaries (exchange of gases (O_2 and CO_2) and nutrients)

↓

Veins
↓ } Deoxygenated blood
Right atrium

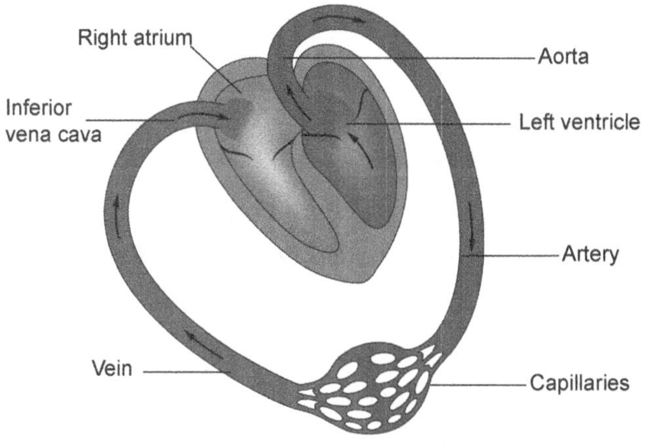

Fig. 6.1: Systemic circulation

b. **Pulmonary circulation (Fig. 6.2):** It consists of that part of circulatory system which pumps deoxygenated blood to the lungs and returns oxygenated blood to the heart. The circulation of blood flow is as follows:

Right ventricle
↓ } Deoxygenated blood
Pulmonary trunk and pulmonary arteries

↓

Lungs (exchange of CO_2 and O_2)

↓

Pulmonary veins
↓ } Oxygenated blood
Left atrium

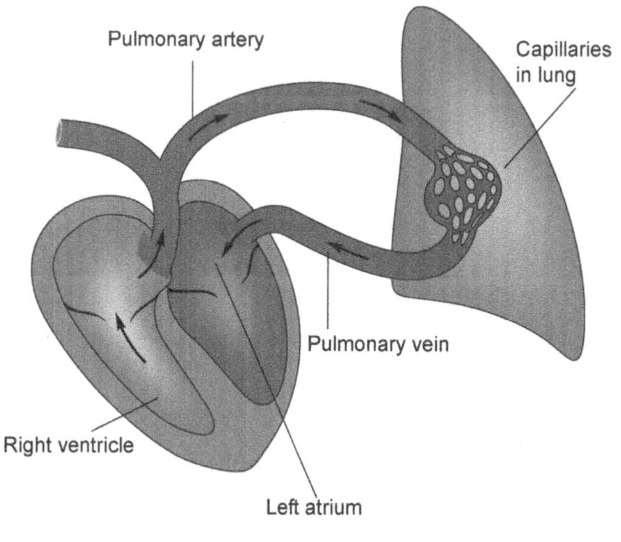

Fig. 6.2: Pulmonary circulation

c. **Portal circulation (Fig. 6.3):** It is part of systemic circulation. The blood passes through two sets of capillaries, the circulation begins with capillaries and ends with capillaries. The vessel between the two sets of capillaries is known as portal vein. Portal circulation is found at the following sites:

- Hepatic portal system–between intestines and liver.
- Renal portal system–in the kidney.
- Hypothalamo-hypophyseal system – between hypothalamus and hypophysis cerebri.
- Suprarenal portal system–between the cortex and medulla of adrenal gland.

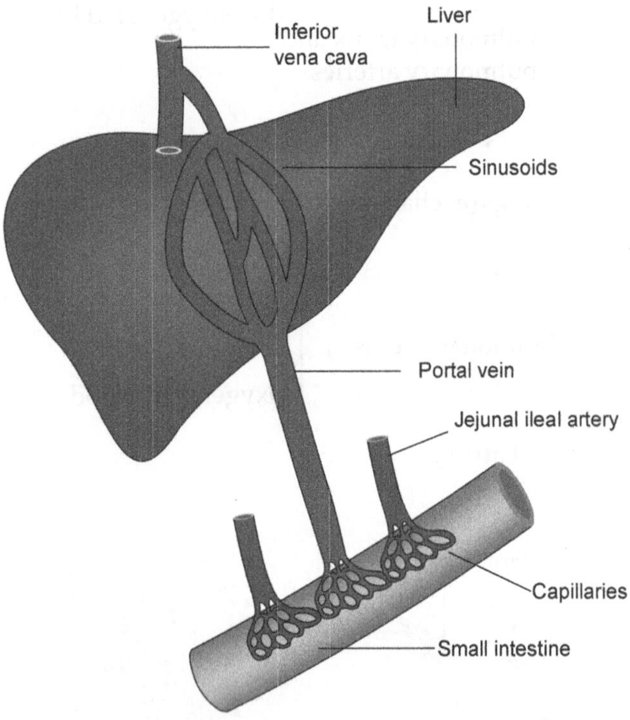

Fig. 6.3: Portal circulation

3. **Enumerate the:**
   a. **Types of arteries and write examples of each**
   b. **Avascular tissues or structures**
   c. **Structures/organs supplied by end arteries**
   d. **Types of capillaries with examples of each**
   e. **Sites where sinusoids are found**
   f. **Factors responsible for venous return**
   g. **Sites where arterial pulsation is felt**

Ans. a. **Types of arteries with examples of each:**

- *Elastic/conducting arteries,* e.g., aorta, pulmonary trunk.
- *Muscular/distributing arteries,* e.g., radial artery, femoral artery etc.

b. **Avascular tissues or structures:**

- Epithelium.
- Epidermis of skin.
- Hair.
- Nail.
- Cornea.
- Cartilage.

c. **Structures or organs supplied by end arteries:**

- Heart.
- Kidneys.
- Liver.
- Brain.
- Retina.

d. **Types of capillaries with examples of each:**

a. *Continuous capillaries,* e.g., in muscle, brain, connective tissue, skin, lung.

b. *Fenestrated capillaries,* e.g., in endocrine glands, intestinal villi, renal glomeruli.

e. **Sites where sinusoids are found:**

- Liver.
- Spleen.
- Bone marrow.
- Anterior pituitary gland.

f. **Factors responsible for venous return:**

- Contraction of muscles.
- Presence of valves in the veins.
- Negative intrathoracic pressure.
- Pulsation of arteries.

g. **Sites where arterial pulsations can be felt:**
- ***Carotid artery:*** Along the anterior border of sternocleidomastoid muscle at the level of cricoid cartilage.
- ***Brachial artery:*** In front of the elbow medial to the tendon of biceps brachii.
- ***Radial artery:*** Lateral side of front of forearm at wrist against the lowered of radi.
- ***Femoral artery:*** Below the inguinal ligament at midinguinal point
- ***Popliteal artery:*** In the popliteal fossa.
- ***Dorsalis pedis:*** On the dorsum of foot between the tendon of extensor hallucis longus and extensor digitorum longus.

4. **Describe in brief the structure and functions of the arteries, arterioles, capillaries venules and veins.**

Ans. See Table 6.1.

5. **Enumerate the differences between the arteries and veins.**

Ans. See Table 6.2.

Table 6.1: Structure and functions of blood vessels

	Structure	*Functions*
Arteries	The walls of arteries contain smooth muscle fibers that contract and relax under the control of the sympathetic nervous system.	• Transport blood away from the heart. • Transport oxygenated blood only (except in the case of the pulmonary arteries).
Arterioles	Arterioles are smaller branches (diameter <1 mm) of arteries that lead to capillaries. These are also under the control of the sympathetic nervous system, and constrict and dilate, to regulate blood flow (Also known as resistance vessels).	• Transport blood from arteries to capillaries. • Are the main regulators of blood flow and pressure.
Capillaries	There is network of capillaries in most of the organs and tissues of the body. They receive blood from the arterioles and are drained by venules. Capillary walls are only one cell thick (endothelium) (Also known as exchange vessels).	• Exchange of oxygen, carbon dioxide, water, salts, etc., between the blood and the surrounding body tissues.
Venules	Venules are the vessels that drain blood from capillaries and into veins. Many venules unite to form a vein.	• Drains blood from capillaries into veins.
Veins	The walls of veins are thinner and less elastic than the corresponding layers of arteries. They contain valves that aid in the return of blood to the heart by preventing blood from flowing in the reverse direction.	• Transport blood towards the heart. • Transport deoxygenated blood only (except in the case of the pulmonary vein).

Table 6.2: Differences between the arteries and veins

Arteries	*Veins*
• Transport blood away from the heart.	• Transport blood towards the heart.
• Carry Oxygenated Blood (except in the case of the Pulmonary Artery).	• Carry De-oxygenated Blood (except in the case of the Pulmonary Vein).
• Have relatively narrow lumen.	• Have relatively wide lumens.
• Have relatively more muscle/elastic tissue in the wall.	• Have relatively less muscle/elastic tissue in the wall.
• Transports blood under higher pressure (than veins).	• Transports blood under lower pressure (than arteries).
• Do not have valves.	• Have valves to prevent blood flowing in the reverse direction.

6. **Explain the following terms:**
   a. **End arteries**
   b. **Functional end arteries**
   c. **Anastomosis**
   d. **Collateral circulation**

Ans. a. End arteries: End arteries are those arteries that do not anastomose with their neighbouring arteries. In case of blockage of an end artery due to a thrombus, the part supplied by it undergoes ischemia and later avascular necrosis, e.g., in kidneys, brain and retina.

b. Functional end arteries: Functional end arteries are those arteries whose terminal branches do anastomose, but the anastomosis is not sufficient to maintain the blood supply to the part they supply in case of any blockage in the artery, e.g., coronary arteries.

c. Anastomosis: Anastomosis is defined as communication between the neighbouring blood vessels. It is of two types:

- *Arterial anastomosis:* The branches of an artery are connected to the branches of another neighbouring artery. The anastomosis provide collateral channel for circulation when one of the arteries is blocked, e.g., labial branches of facial arteries, intercostal arteries, uterine and ovarian arteries, arterial arcades in the mesentery of intestine, etc.
- *Arteriovenous anastomosis:* The direct connection between the arteries and veins without the intervention of capillaries is termed arteriovenous anastomosis. Their function is to regulate temperature and regional blood flow. They are found in the lip, ear, nose, nasal mucosa, kidney, intestine etc.

> Anuria often occurs after accidents because arteriovenous anastomosis in the organs such as kidney and intestine open up following massive haemorrhage. They allow the blood to bypass organs like kidney and intestine and make it available to the vital organs like heart and lungs.

d. Collateral circulation: Collateral circulation is possible when an area of tissue or an organ has a number of different pathways for blood to reach it. This is as a result of anastomosis formed between adjacent blood vessels. In this process small arteries connect two larger arteries or different parts of the same artery and serve alternate route of blood supply.

CHAPTER 7

LYMPHATIC SYSTEM

1. What are the functions of lymphatic system?

Ans. The functions of lymphatic system are:

- Protects the body from the disease causing agents.
- Transports interstitial fluid formed as a blood filterate back to blood and thus help in maintaining fluid balance.
- Serves as the route by which absorbed fat from the small intestine is transported to the blood.

> - **Spread of cancer**–Lymphatics is the major route by which carcinoma metastatises.
>   - Knowledge of lymphatic drainage of organs commonly involved in cancer is helpful in:
>   - Diagnosis of primary site of cancer.
>   - Prognosis and classifying the stage of cancer.

2. Enumerate the components of the lymphatic system.

Ans. Components of the lymphatic system are:

- Circulating lymphocytes.
- Lymph vessels.
- **Central (primary) lymphoid organs:** Bone marrow and thymus.
- **Peripheral (secondary) lymphoid organs:** Lymph nodes, spleen, tonsils, mucosa associated lymphoid tissue.

3. With the help of flowchart explain the general plan of lymphatic system.

Ans. See the following Flowchart.

Intercellular space containing interstitial fluid
⇩
Lymph capillaries
⇩
Larger lymph vessels
⇩
Afferent lymph vessels to lymph nodes
⇩
Lymph nodes
⇩
Efferent lymph vessels from lymph nodes
⇩
Lymph ducts or trunks (lumbar, intestinal, bronchomediastinal, subclavian and jugular on either side)
⇩
Two large ducts are formed

Right side	Left side
⇩	⇩
Right lymphatic duct (right side)	Thoracic duct (left side)
⇩	⇩
Drain into the junction of Right internal jugular and right subclavian veins	Drain into the junction of Left internal jugular vein and left subclavian vein

Flowchart

General Plan of Lymphatic System: (Fig. 7.1)

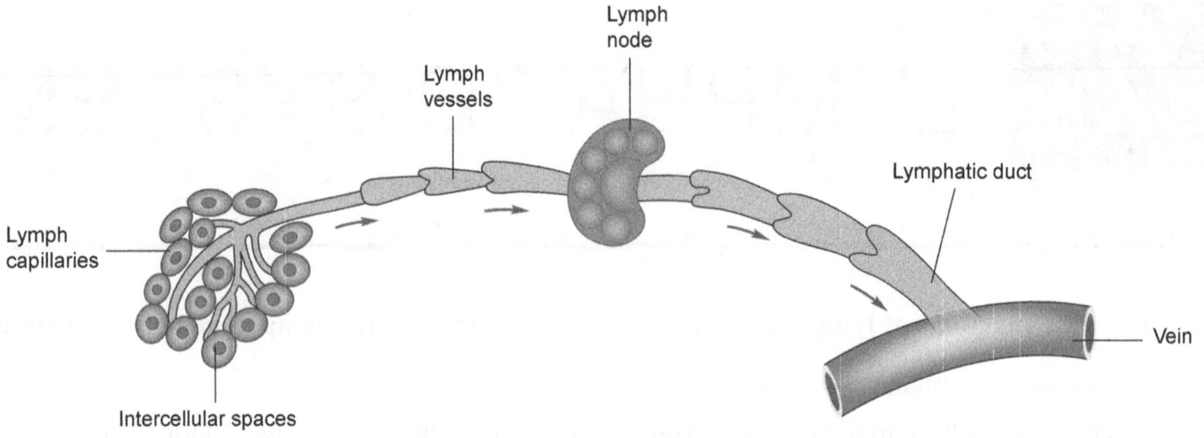

Fig. 7.1: General plan of lymphatic system

3. **Enumerate the:**
   a. **Factors that help in lymph flow**
   b. **Tissues/organs where lymph capillaries are absent**
   c. **Primary lymphoid organs**
   d. **Secondary lymphoid organs**
   e. **Areas drained by thoracic duct**
   f. **Areas drained by right lymphatic duct**
   g. **Types of lymphocytes and their functions**

Ans.

a. **Factors that help in lymph flow:**
   - Tissue fluid pressure.
   - Contraction of surrounding muscles.
   - Pulsations of adjacent arteries.
   - Negative intrathoracic pressure.
   - Presence of valves which prevent backflow.

b. **Lymphatic capillaries are absent in:**
   - All avascular structures, i.e., epidermis, cornea, nail, hair and cartilage.
   - Spleen and bone marrow.
   - Alveoli and respiratory bronchiole.
   - Brain and spinal cord.

> - Lymph capillaries are numerous in:
>   - Dermis of skin.
>   - Serous surfaces.
>   - Mucous membrane.

c. **Primary lymphoid organs are:**
   - Bone marrow.
   - Thymus.

d. **Secondary lymphoid organs are:**
   - Lymph node.
   - Spleen.
   - Tonsil.
   - Mucosa associated lymphoid tissue:
     - Gut associated lymphoid tissue.
     - Bronchii associated lymphoid tissue.

> Antigens in the tissues stimulate an immune response first in the lymph nodes, whereas those present in the blood initiate an immune response in spleen.

e. **Areas/regions drained by thoracic duct:**
   - Lower limbs.
   - Abdomen.
   - Left thoracic region.
   - Left upper limb.
   - Left side of head and neck.

f. **Areas/regions drained by right lymphatic duct:**
   - Right upper extremity.
   - Right thoracic region.
   - Right side of head and neck.

g. **Types of lymphocytes and their functions:**
   - *B lymphocytes:*
     - Are derived from precursor cells.

in bone marrow and they also mature within the bone marrow.
   - Mature cells migrate to secondary lymphoid organs.
   - On being exposed to antigens they proliferate and produce antibody producing cells–plasma cells and memory cells.
   - Are responsible for antibody mediated (humoral) response.
- ***T lymphocytes:***
   - Immunologically immature T lymphocytes migrate from bone marrow to thymus.
   - Immature T lymphocytes proliferate and acquire variety of surface markers and become immunologically competent cells in the thymus.
   - *Types of T lymphcytes:*
     - T helper cells.
     - Cytotoxic T cells.
     - Suppressor T cells.
   - Are responsible for cell mediated immunity.

> - T lymphocytes with ability to react to body's own normal constituents (self antigens) are destroyed and removed in the thymus.
> - One of the main causes of acquired immunodeficiency syndrome (AIDS) is destruction of T-helper lymphocytes by HIV virus.
> - T- killer cells are responsible for transplant rejection.

4. Explain the following briefly:

a. Lymphangitis

b. Lymphadenitis

c. Elephantiasis

Ans.

a. Lymphangitis:
- Is the inflammation of the lymphatic vessels.
- Is caused by inflammatory conditions of the skin caused by bacterial infections.
- Thin red lines may be observed running along the course of the lymphatic vessels in the affected area.
- Is accompanied by painful enlargement of the nearby lymph nodes.

b. Lymphadenitis:
- Occurs when the lymph nodes become overwhelmed by bacteria, virus, fungi, cancer cells, or inflammation.
- The swollen LNs are usually found near the site of an underlying infection, tumor, or inflammation.

c. Elephantiasis:
- Massive swelling and enlargement of the limbs resembling elephant's leg.
- Adult worms of filariasis are lodged in the lymph vessels of leg and foot which causes blokage of lymph flow and as a result fluid accumulates in interstitial spaces leading to oedema.

8

CHAPTER

NERVOUS SYSTEM

1. **Enumerate the:**
   a. **Functions of nervous system**
   b. **Parts of nervous system**
   c. **Types of neurons with examples**
   d. **Types of neuroglia and their function**

Ans.

a. **Functions of nervous system:**
   - Gathers information both from the outside world and from inside the body–SENSORY FUNCTION.
   - Transmits the information to the processing area of the brain and spinal cord–TRANSMISSION.
   - Processes the information to determine the best response INTEGRATIVE FUNCTION.
   - Sends information to muscles, glands and organs (effectors) for muscular contraction and glandular secretion–MOTOR FUNCTION.

b. **Parts of nervous system:**

   Nervous system is divided into:
   - ***Central nervous system (CNS):*** Consists of:
     - Brain; and
     - Spinal cord.
   - ***Peripheral nervous system (PNS):*** Consists of:
     - 12 pairs of cranial nerves.
     - 31 pairs of spinal nerves.

c. **Types of neurons: *(Fig. 8.1 and Fig. 8.2)***
   - ***According to the shape:***
     - *Unipolar (pseudounipolar) neuron:* Single process from the cell body which divides to form dendrite and axon, e.g., dorsal root ganglion cells of the spinal cord.
     - *Bipolar neuron:* Two processes arise from the cell body, one on each pole. One of them is dendrite, the other axon, e.g., bipolar neurons in the retina, olfactory epithelium and vestibulocochlear ganglia.
     - *Multipolar neuron:* Several dendrites and one axon arise from the cell body, e.g., pyramidal cells of cerebral cortex, motor neurons of anterior horn of spinal cord.
   - ***According to the functions:***
     - *Sensory or afferent neuron:* Neurons that transmit impulses from a sensory receptor to the CNS, e.g., dorsal root ganglion cells of spinal cord.

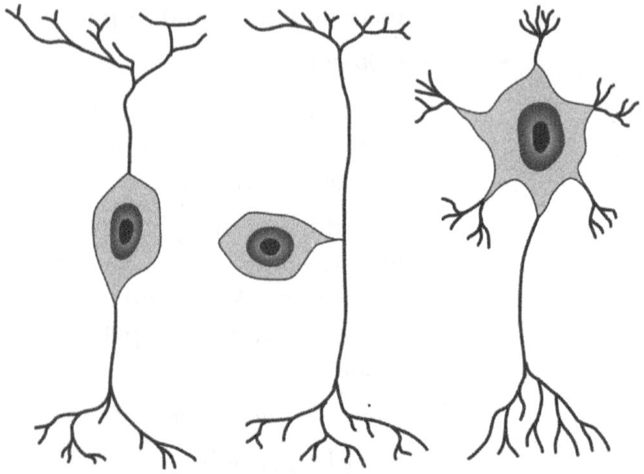

Fig. 8.1: Types of neurous

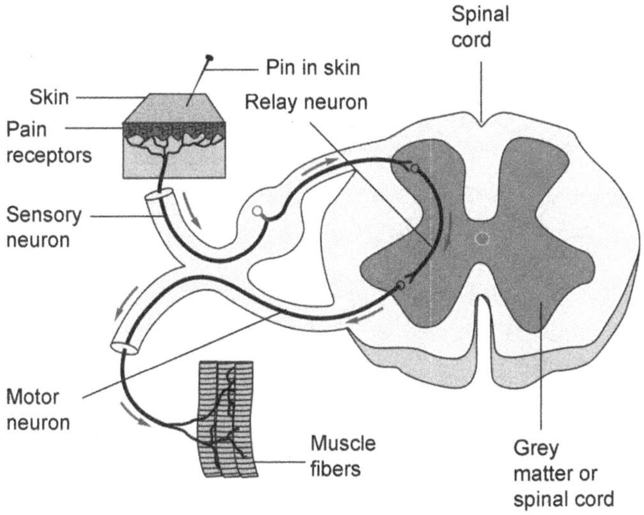

Fig. 8.2: Sensory and motor neurons

- *Motor or efferent neurons:* Neurons that transmit impulses from the CNS to an effector organ (muscle or gland), e.g., pyramidal cells of cerebral cortex.

d. **Types of neuroglia:**

- *Neuroglia in CNS:*
  - *Astrocytes:* Are star shaped with many processes whose ends called foot processes cover the capillaries to form blood brain barrier. Astrocytes are of two types:
    - Protoplasmic astrocytes.
    - Fibrous astrocytes.
  - *Oligodendrocytes:* Are smaller than astrocytes with fewer processes. Form myelin around the axons in CNS.
  - *Microglia:* Are the smallest glial cells. They phagocytize pathogens and cell debris within the CNS.
  - *Ependymal cells:* They line the ventricles of brain and central canal of spinal cord produce cerebrospinal fluid.
- *Neuroglia in PNS:*
  - *Schwann cells:* Surround the axons of peripheral nerves and form myelin sheath around these nerve fibers.
  - *Satellite (capsular) cells:* They surround the cell bodies of neurons in the autonomic and sensory ganglia and provide support to them.

All neuroglial cells develop from neural crest except microglia which develop from mesoderm.

2. **Draw labeled diagram of the following:**

a. **Typical neuron**
b. **Neuroglial cells**
c. **Typical spinal nerve**
d. **Reflex arc**

Ans.

a. **Typical neuron (Fig. 8.3).**
b. **Neuroglial cells (Fig. 8.4).**
c. **Typical spinal nerve (Fig. 8.5).**
d. **Refex arc (Fig. 8.6).**

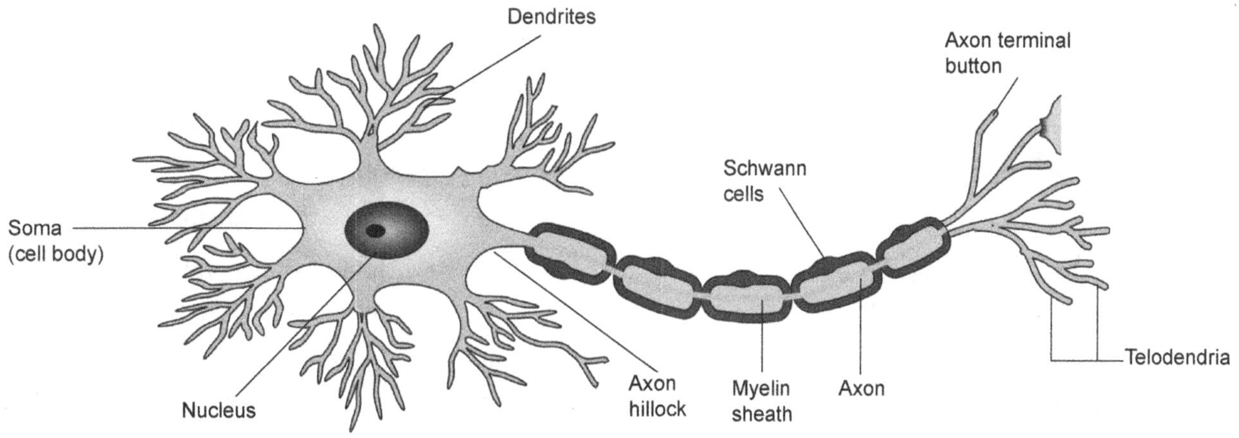

Fig. 8.3: Typical neuron

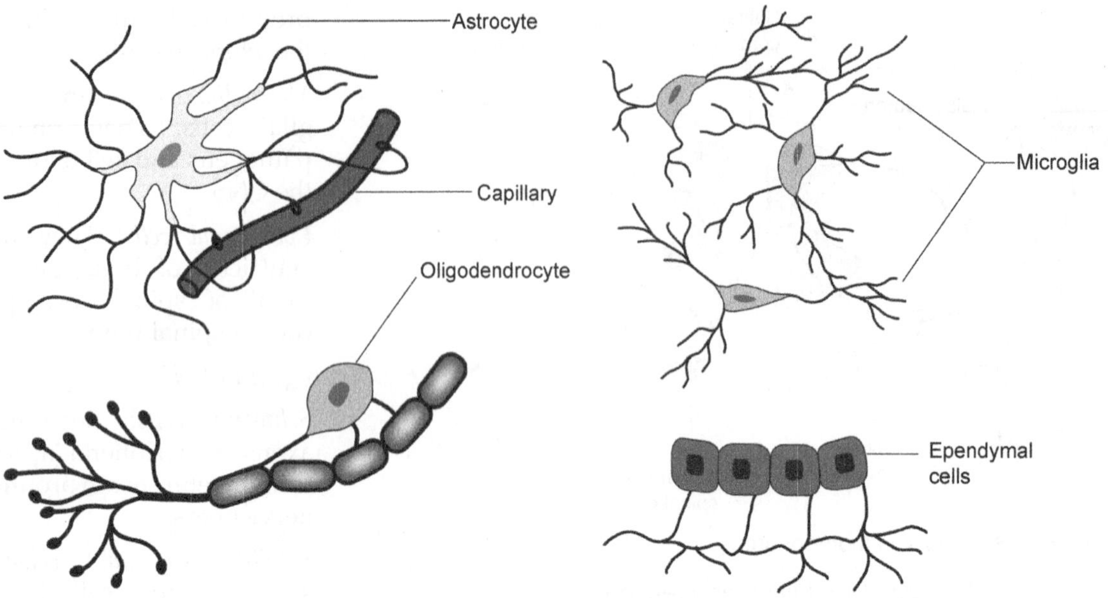

Fig. 8.4: Neuroglial cells

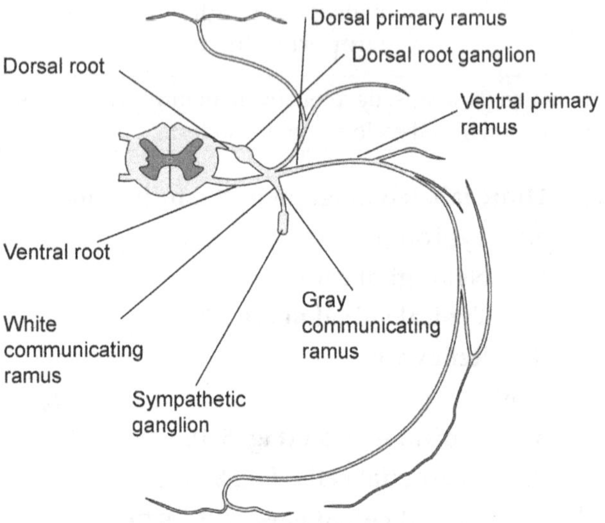

Fig. 8.5: Typical spinal nerve

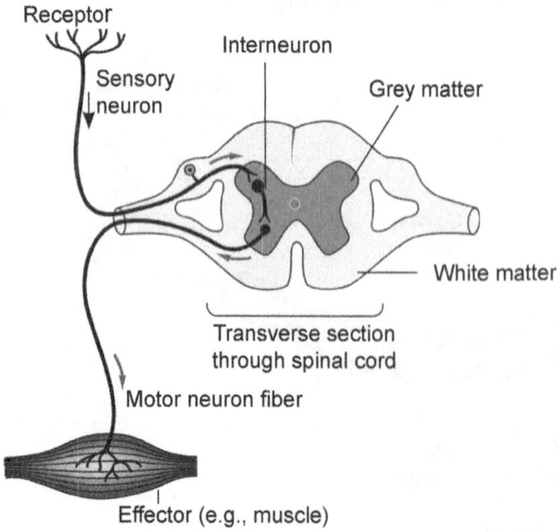

Fig. 8.6: Reflex arc

3. **Define the following:**
   a. **Neurilemmal sheath**
   b. **Myelin sheath**

Ans.

a. **Neurilemmal sheath:** It is the outer cell membrane of Schwann cells. Beneath the membrane lies a thin layer of cytoplasm of Schwann cell and its nucleus. It is present only in the PNS.

b. **Myelin sheath:** It is a laminated sheath made up of lipoproteins. Its outer surface is encased in neurilemmal sheath. It is interrupted at the nodes of Ranvier. In case of peripheral nerves the myelin sheath is formed by the Schwann cells and in the central nervous system the sheath is derived from oligodendrocytes. Its functions are:
   - Protect and insulate the nerve fibers.
   - Increase the rate of conduction of nerve impulse (saltatory conduction).

All myelinated and non-myelinated nerve fibers in PNS are surrounded by the neurilemmal sheath but only myelinated fibers are surrounded by myelin sheath. Axons less than 2 μm in diameter are unmyelinated.

4. **When does myelination begins?**

Ans. Myelination begins as early as fourth month of fetal life.

5. **Name the areas of a peripheral nerve where myelin sheath is absent.**

Ans. The following sites are devoid of myelin sheath:

- Nodes of Ranvier (gaps of exposed axon between the adjacent Schwann cells).
- Proximal part of the axon, close to the cell body.
- Near the termination of axon before it divides.

6. **Can a non-myelinated nerve regenerate?**

Ans. A non-myelinated nerve possesses neurilemmal sheath which is essential for regeneration, therefore, it can regenerate.

7. **Define the following:**

   a. **Nerve**

   b. **Fiber tract**

   c. **Ganglion**

   d. **Nucleus**

Ans.

   a. **Nerve:** Is a collection of axons *outside* the CNS.

   b. **Fiber tract:** Is a collection of axons *within* the CNS.

   c. **Ganglion:** Is a collection of nerve cell *bodies* outside the CNS.

   d. **Nucleus:** Is a collection of nerve cell *bodies* within the CNS.

8. **Define synapse and give morphological classification.**

Ans. The junction between two neurons across which the nerve impulse passes from one neuron to another is called synapse (Fig. 8.7).

- There is no physical contact between the two neurons.
- Presynaptic axon ends in a bulb-like structure (boutons terminaux).

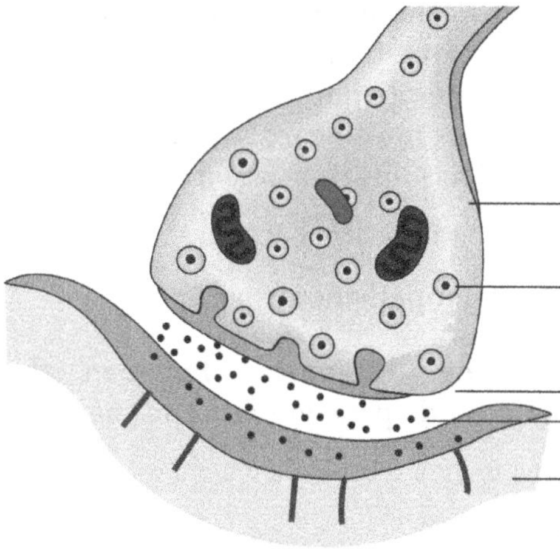

Fig. 8.7: Synapse

- There is a space, the synaptic cleft, between the presynaptic and the postsynaptic neuron 20–30 nm.
- The end bulb contains synaptic vesicles that release neurotransmitters and postsynaptic neuron contains receptors for the neurotransmitter.
- These can either stimulate or inhibit the postsynaptic neuron.

Morphological classification of synapses:

- Axo-dendritic (most common).
- Axo-somatic.
- Axo-axonic.
- Dendro-dendritic.
- Dendro-somatic.
- Dendro-axonic.

9. **What are the functional parts of nervous system?**

Ans. Following are the functional parts of nervous system:

   a. **Somatic nervous system:** It innervates the somatic structures of the body (head and neck, limbs, trunk). It is concerned with receiving and modifying conscious and unconscious sensory impulses from the body wall and sending motor impulses for control of skeletal muscles. It responds to external environment.

   b. **Autonomic nervous system:** It innervates

the viscera, blood vessels and glands. It maintains the internal environment of the body and is involved in regulation of body temperature, blood pressure respiratory, rate, heart rate and gastrointestinal motility. It has two components:

- Sympathetic system.
- Parasympathetic system.

10. Enumerate the differences between the sympathetic and parasympathetic nervous system.

Ans. See Table 8.1.

11. What is the action of sympathetic and parasympathetic nervous system on various tissues/organs?

Ans. Action of sympathetic and parasympathetic nervous system (See Table 8.2).

12. Write anatomical basis of referred pain.

Ans. The pain arising from the diseased viscera is referred to the skin which is innervated by the same spinal segment/s that supply the diseased viscera, e.g., gallbladder pain is referred to right shoulder tip and pain in appendicitis is referred to umbilicus (Fig. 8.8).

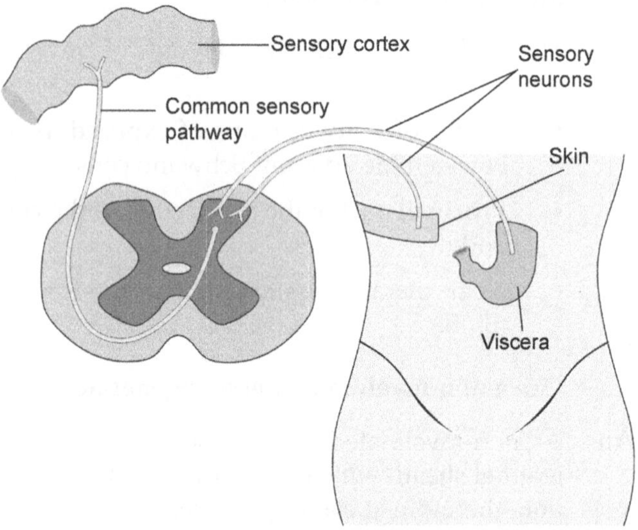

Fig. 8.8: Referred pain

Table 8.1: Difference between sympathetic and parasympathetic nervous system

	Sympathetic nervous system	*Parasympathetic nervous system*
Origin of nerves	Thoracolumbar	Craniosacral
Length of pre-ganglionic fibers	Long	Short
Length of post-ganglionic fibers	Short	Long
Position of ganglion	Away from the organ	Near the organ
Neurotransmitter	Acetylcholine and Epinephrine and Nor-epinephrine	Acetylcholine

Table 8.2: Action of sympathetic and parasympathetic nervous system

Sympathetic nervous system	*Parasympathetic nervous system*
Is involved in fight, fright or flight reactions	Conserves body energy
Involved in 'E' activities–exercise, emergency, excitement, embarrassment	Involved in 'D' activities–Digestion, defecation, diuresis
Increases heart rate Raises blood pressure Dilates pupil Suppresses peristaltic movements Sphincters of GIT are closed Increase sweat secretion Constriction of blood vessels Blood vessels of skeletal muscles heart and brain dilate	Blood pressure decreased Heart rate decreased Respiratory rate decreased Pupils are constricted Stimulates peristaltic movements of GIT

9 CHAPTER PECTORAL REGION

1. **Draw a labeled diagram showing cutaneous innervation of:**
   a. **Pectoral region**
   b. **Upper limb proper**

Ans.
   a. **Pectoral region (Fig. 9.1a).**
   b. **Upper limb proper (Fig. 9.1b).**

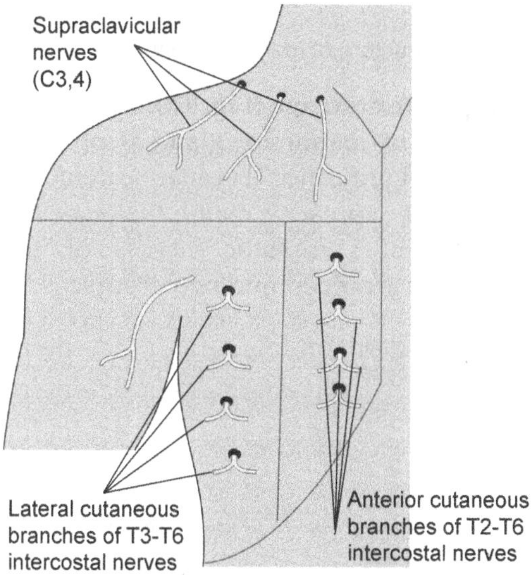

Fig. 9.1a: Cutaneous innervations of pectoral region

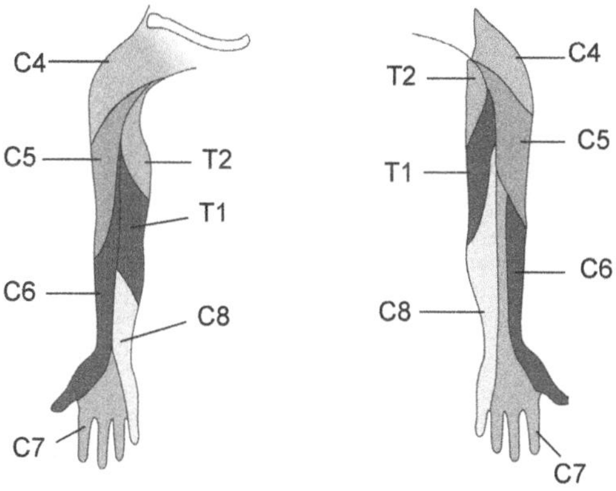

Fig. 9.1b: Cutaneous innervations of upper limb proper

Cutaneous Nerves of the Upper Limb:

- Most cutaneous nerves of the upper limb are derived from the brachial plexus formed by the anterior rami of C5-T1 spinal nerve.
- The cutaneous nerves to the shoulder are derived from the cervical plexus – formed by anterior rami of the C1-4.
- C3 and C4 nerves supply the region at the base of the neck extending laterally over the shoulder.
- C5 nerve supplies the arm laterally.
- C6 nerve supplies the forearm laterally and the thumb.
- C7 supplies the middle and ring fingers and middle of the posterior surface of the limb.
- C8 nerve supplies the little finger, the medial side of the hand and the forearm.
- T1 supplies the middle of the forearm to the axilla.
- T2 supplies a small part of the arm and the skin of the axilla.

2. **Enumerate the contents of superficial fascia of pectoral region.**

Ans. Contents of superficial fascid of pectoral region:
   a. *Cutaneous nerves:* Medial, intermediate, lateral supraclavicular nerves (C3, C4), anterior and lateral cutaneous branches of 2nd to 6th intercostal nerves.
   b. Cutaneous branches from internal thoracic and posterior intercostal arteries.
   c. Platysma muscle.
   d. Mammary gland.

3. **Describe mammary gland under the following headings:**
   a. **Extent**
   b. **Deep relations**

c. **Structure**
d. **Arterial supply**
e. **Lymphatic drainage**
f. **Applied anatomy**

Ans. Mammary gland is a modified sweat gland situated in the superficial fascia of pectoral region. A small extension called axillary tail of Spence pierces deep fascia and lies in the axilla.

a. **Extent:** Vertically from 2nd to 6th rib and horizontally from lateral border of the sternum to the mid-axillary line.

b. **Deep relations:** From superficial to deep are:
- Loose areolar tissue (retromammary space).
- Deep fascia (pectoral fascia).
- Three muscles – pectoralis major, serratus anterior and external oblique (abdominis).

c. **Structure:** Is made up of the following two components: (Fig. 9.2)
- ***Parenchyma (glandular tissue):*** Is made up of 15 to 20 radially arranged pyramidal lobes. Each lobe has a cluster of alveoli which is drained by a lactiferous duct. Lactiferous ducts open on the nipple and just before termination each duct is dilated to form lactiferous sinus.
- ***Stroma (fibrofatty tissue):*** The fibrous septa (suspensory or Cooper's ligament) anchor the skin overlying the gland and the gland to the pectoral fascia. Fatty tissue forms the main bulk of the gland but is absent beneath the areola and nipple.

d. **Arterial supply:** Following arteries supply the gland:
- Perforating branches of internal thoracic artery.
- Branches of axillary artery (superior thoracic, thoracoacromial and lateral thoracic).
- Lateral branches of 2nd, 3rd and 4th posterior intercostal arteries.

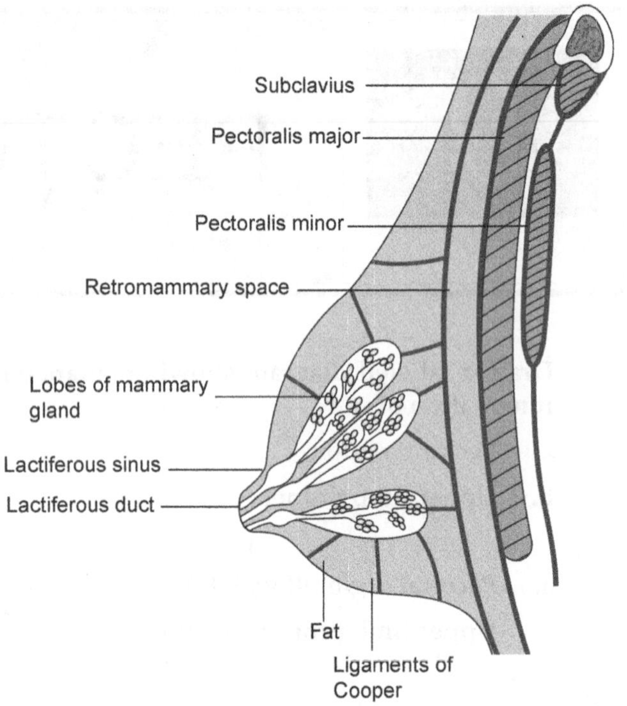

Fig. 9.2: Structure of mammary gland

e. **Lymphatic drainage (Fig. 9.3):** Lymphatic drainage of mammary gland is of great clinical significance because carcinoma of breast spreads mainly along the lymphatics. Lymphatic vessels of the breast are arranged into two groups:

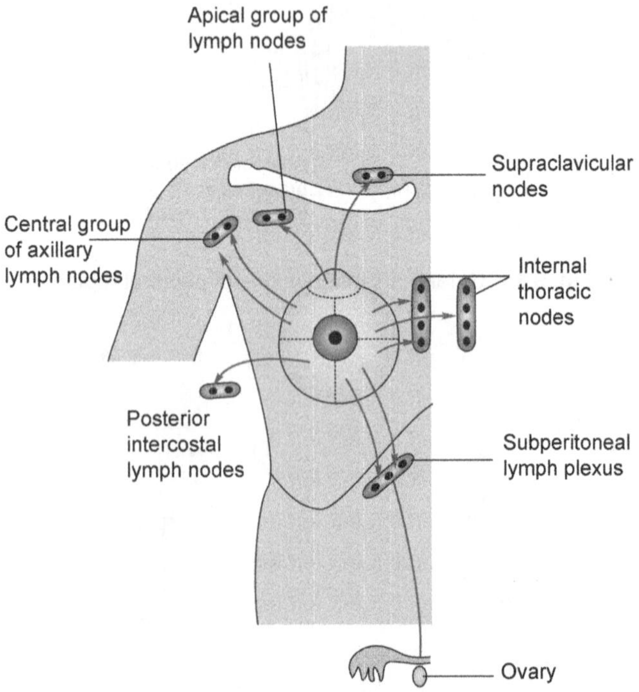

Fig. 9.3: Lymphatic drainage of mammary gland

- Superficial lymphatic vessels drain the lymph from the overlying skin except nipple and areola.
- Deep lymphatic vessels drain the parenchyma along with nipple and areola.

Lymph from the mammary gland is drained into the following groups of lymph nodes:

- 75% of the lymph drains into axillary lymph nodes.
- 20% of the lymph drains into internal mammary (parasternal) lymph nodes.
- 5% of the lymph drains into posterior intercostals lymph nodes.
- Lymph from superior quadrants drains into supraclavicular lymph nodes.
- Lymph vessels from inferomedial quadrant communicate with the subperitoneal lymph plexus.

f. **Applied anatomy:**

- Obstruction of superficial lymph vessels leads to stagnation of lymph resulting in odema of skin (peau d'orange appearance – like the skin of orange).
- Cancer cells may infilterate the suspensory ligaments resulting in fixation of breast to pectoral fascia and retraction or puckering of skin.
- Infiltration of lactiferous ducts by cancer cells leads to fibrosis of lactiferous ducts which causes retraction of nipple.
- As lactiferous ducts run radially, incisions into the breast are usually made radially to prevent damage to the lactiferous ducts.
- Cancer may spread from one breast to the other because of the communication between the superficial lymphatics across the midline.
- Lymph vessels from inferomedial quadrant communicate with subperitoneal lymph plexus. Cancer cells, therefore, may spread to the liver, may drop into the pelvis and produce secondary tumour in the ovary (Krukenberg's tumor).
- Besides lymphatics cancer may spread via the veins. Intercostal veins draining mammary gland communicate with the internal vertebral venous plexus. Cancer from breast, therefore, may spread via this communication to the vertebrae and to the brain.

4. **Enumerate the muscles of pectoral region and write their action and nerve supply.**

Ans. Muscles of pectoral region:

Muscle		*Nerve supply*
a.	Pectoralis major	Medial and lateral pectoral nerves
b.	Pectoralis minor	Medial and lateral pectoral nerves
c.	Subclavius	Nerve to subclavius
d.	Serratus anterior	Long thoracic nerve

5. **Write origin, insertion, action and nerve supply of:**
   a. **Pectoralis major**
   b. **Serratus anterior**

Ans. a. **Pectoralis major**

Origin:

- Anterior surface of medial ½ of the clavicle.
- Anterior surface of sternum up to the 6th costal cartilage.
- 2nd to 6th costal cartilages.
- Aponeurosis of external oblique abdominis muscle.

Insertion: Lateral lip of bicipital groove of humerus.

Action:

- When both clavicular and sternocostal parts act – adduction and medial rotation of the arm.
- Action of only clavicular part–Flexion of the arm.
- Action of only sternocostal part – Extention of flexed arm.
- When the arm is fixed – Helps in climbing.

Nerve Supply: Medial and lateral pectoral nerves.

b. **Serratus anterior**

Origin: Outer surface of upper eight ribs and fascia covering the intervening intercostal muscles.

Insertion: Costal surface of the medial border of scapula.

Action:

- Protraction of upper limb, i.e., pulling the scapula forwards around the chest wall during pushing and punching actions.
- Rotate the scapula (along with trapezius) so that glenoid cavity faces upwards and thereby helping in overhead abduction.

Nerve Supply: Long thoracic nerve (C5,6,7).

6. **Describe briefly:**
   a. **Winging of scapula**
   b. **Clavipectoral fascia**

Ans.

a. **Winging of scapula:** Paralysis of serratus anterior muscle due to injury to long thoracic nerve produces 'Winging of scapula' in which the medial border and inferior angle of scapula become unduly prominent specially when the patient tries to do pushing and punching actions.

b. **Clavipectoral fascia (Fig. 9.4a and Fig. 9.4b):** Clavipectoral fascia is a fibrous sheet present deep to the clavicular part of the pectoralis major muscle.

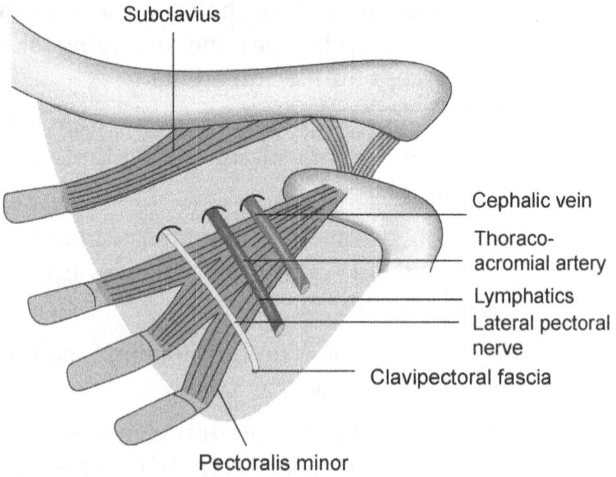

Fig. 9.4a: Clavipectoral fascia

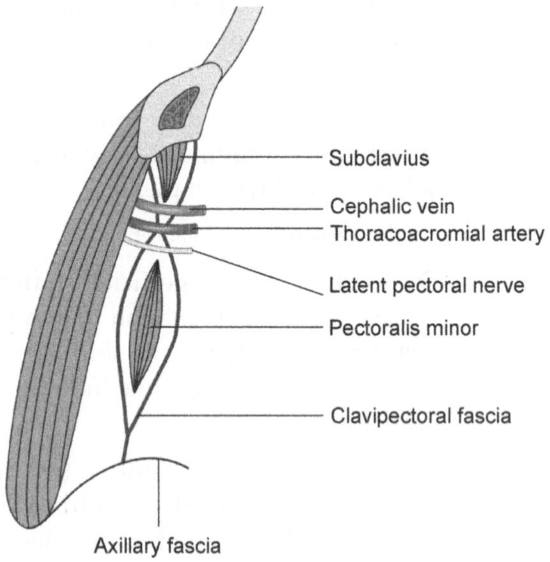

Fig. 9.4b: Clavipectoral fascia (Sagittal section)

Extent: From clavicle above to the axillary fascia below.

Muscles enclosed: Subclavius and pectoralis minor.

Structures piercing:

- Lateral pectoral nerve.
- Cephalic vein.
- Thoracoacromial vessels.
- Lymphatics from mammary gland to the apical group of axillary lymph nodes.

10 CHAPTER AXILLA

1. **Describe briefly the boundaries of axilla.**

Ans. Axilla is a four sided pyramidal space situated between the upper part of the arm and upper part of lateral thoracic wall.

Boundaries: (Fig. 10.1)

a. *Apex:* Is directed upwards and medially and is formed by cervicoaxillary canal via which it communicates with the posterior triangle of neck.

b. *Base:* Skin and fascia.

c. *Anterior wall:* Is formed by pectoralis major, clavipectoral fascia enclosing pectoralis minor and subclavius muscles.

d. *Posterior wall:* Is formed by subscapularis, teres major and latissimus dorsi.

e. *Medial wall:* Is formed by upper four ribs and intercostal muscles, upper part of serratus anterior.

f. *Lateral wall:* Is formed by upper part of humerus (intertubercular sulcus) and short head of biceps brachii and coracobrachialis muscle.

2. **Enumerate the:**

a. **Boundaries and structures passing through cervicoaxillary canal**

b. **Contents of axilla**

Ans.

a. **Boundaries of cervicoaxillary canal:**

- *Anteriorly:* Clavicle.
- *Medially:* Outer border of 1st rib.
- *Posteriorly:* Superior border of scapula.

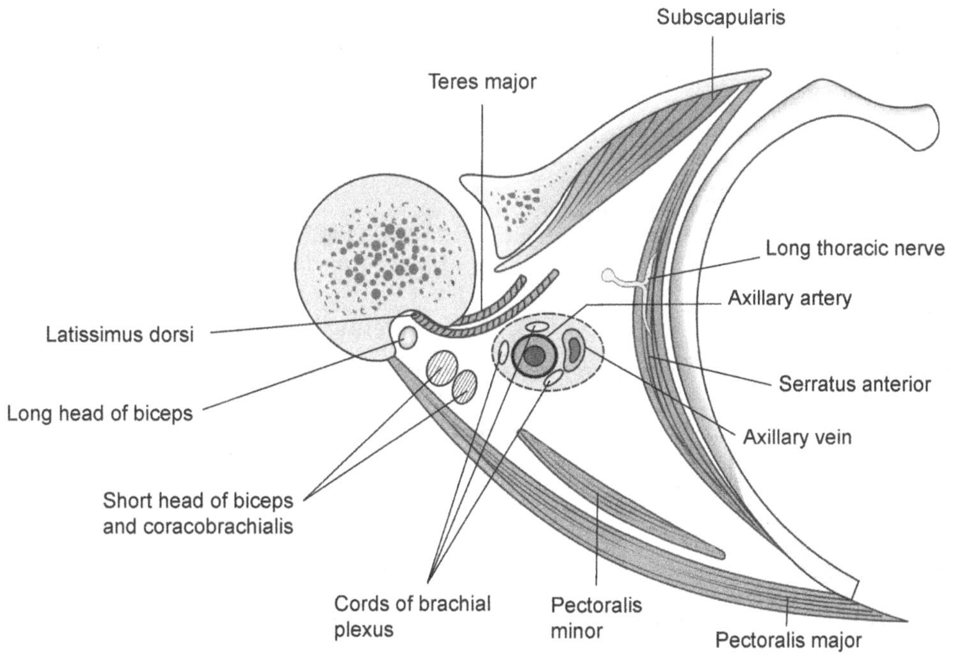

Fig. 10.1: Boundaries and contents of axilla

- ***Structures passing through the cervicoaxillary canal:***
  - Axillary vessels; and
  - Brachial plexus.

b. **Contents of axilla:**
- Axillary artery and its branches.
- Axillary vein and its tributaries.
- Axillary lymph nodes.
- Axillary tail of mammary gland (tail of Spence).
- Cords of brachial plexus.
- Long thoracic nerve.
- Intercostobrachial nerve.
- Axillary fat and areolar tissue.

3. **Describe brachial plexus under the following headings:**
   a. **Location**
   b. **Formation**
   c. **Components**

Ans.

a. **Location:** Brachial plexus is divided into two parts:
- Supraclavicular (in the posterior triangle of neck) – Contains roots and trunks of brachial plexus.
- Infraclavicular (in the axilla) – Contains cords.
  - * Divisions are located behind the clavicle.

b. **Formation:** Is formed by the ventral ramii of C5-C8 and T1 spinal nerves.

Prefixed plexus: If there is contribution from C4 spinal nerve.

Postfixed plexus: If there is contribution from T2 spinal nerve.

c. **Components:**
- ***Roots***: Ventral ramii of C5-C8 and T1 spinal nerves.
- ***Trunks***: Three.
  - *Upper trunk*–C5 and C6 roots join.
  - *Middle trunk*–C7 root.
  - *Lower trunk*–C8 and T1 roots join.
- ***Divisions:*** Each trunk divides into anterior (ventral) and posterior (dorsal) divisions.
- ***Cords:*** Three
  - *Lateral cord*–Anterior divisions of upper and middle trunk join.
  - *Medial cord*–Anterior division of lower trunk.
  - *Posterior cord*–Posterior divisions of all the three trunks join.

4. **Draw a labeled diagram showing all the components of brachial plexus.**

Ans. Components of brachial plexus: (Fig. 10.2)

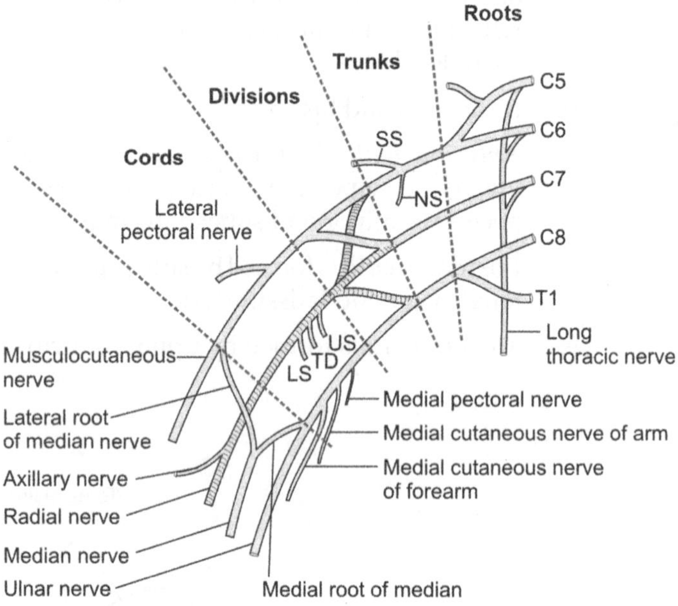

Fig. 10.2: Brachial plexus
DS – Dorsal scapular nerve; SS – Suprascapular nerve

5. **Enumerate the branches from roots and trunks of brachial plexus.**

Ans. From the roots:
- Dorsal scapular nerve (C5).
- Long thoracic nerve (C5, C6, C7).

From the upper trunk:
- Suprascapular nerve (C5, C6).
- Nerve to subclavius (C5, C6).

6. **Enumerate:**
   a. **Branches from the three cords of brachial plexus**
   b. **Structures supplied by the branches of brachial plexus**

Ans.

a. **Branches of lateral cord – Three**
- Lateral pectoral nerve (C5-7).
- Lateral root of median nerve (C5-7).
- Musculocutaneous nerve (C5-7).

Branches of medial cord – Five
- Medial pectoral nerve (C8,T1).
- Medial cutaneous nerve of arm (C8,T1).
- Medial cutaneous nerve of forearm (C8,T1).
- Medial root of median nerve (C8,T1).
- Ulnar nerve (C8,T1).

Branches of posterior cord – Five
- Upper subscapular nerve (C5,C6).
- Lower subscapular nerve (C5,C6).
- Thoracodorsal nerve (C6-8).
- Axillary nerve (C5,C6).
- Radial nerve (C5-8, T1).

b. **Distribution of branches of brachial plexus.**

Nerve	*Structures supplied/Distribution*
Dorsal scapular	Rhomboids and levator scapulae muscles
Long thoracic	Serratus anterior muscle
Nerve to subclavius	Subclavius muscle
Suprascapular	Supraspinatus, infraspinatus, muscle and glenohumeral joint
Lateral pectoral	Pectoralis major and pectoralis minor
Musculocutaneous	a. **Muscles of anterior/flexor compartment of arm:** Coracobrachialis biceps brachii and brachialis b. **Continues as lateral cutaneous nerve of forearm**

Contd.

Contd.

Median	6½ flexor muscles in forearm (except flexor carpi ulnaris, ulnar half of flexor digitorum profundus), and five hand muscles and skin of lateral 1/3rd of palm and lateral 1½ digits
Medial pectoral	Pectoralis minor and pectoralis major
Median cutaneous nerve of arm	Supplies skin on medial side of arm
Median cutaneous nerve of forearm	Supplies skin over medial side of forearm
Ulnar	1½ flexor muscles in forearm, most small muscles in the hand, and skin of medial 2/3rd of palm and medial 1½ digits
Upper subscapular	Upper part of subscapularis
Thoracodorsal	Latissimus dorsi
Lower subscapular	Inferior part of subscapularis and teres major
Axillary	Deltoid and teres minor, glenohumeral joint and skin over inferior part of deltoid
Radial	**All the muscles of extensor compartment of arm and forearm:** Triceps brachii, anconeus, brachioradialis and extensor muscles of forearm; supplies skin on posterior aspect of arm and forearm via posterior cutaneous nerves of arm and forearm

7. **Describe briefly:**
   a. **Erb's point and Erb's paralysis**
   b. **Klumpke's paralysis**

Ans.

a. **Erb's point (Fig. 10.3a):** Is the region on upper trunk of brachial plexus of:
- It is formed by union two roots–Ventral rami of C5 and C6.
- It divides into two divisions–Anterior and posterior divisions.
- It provides origin to two nerves–Suprascapular and nerve to subclavius.

Erb's paralysis (Erb-Duchenne Palsy): (Fig. 10.3b)
- *Site of lesion:* Erb's point, i.e., upper trunk of brachial plexus (C5,C6).
- *Cause:* Undue separation of head from the shoulder which may occur in the following conditions:

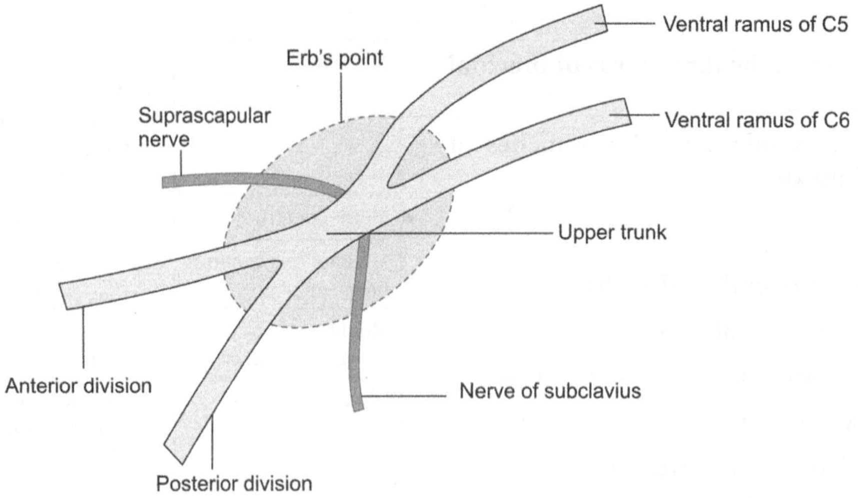

Fig. 10.3a: Erb's point

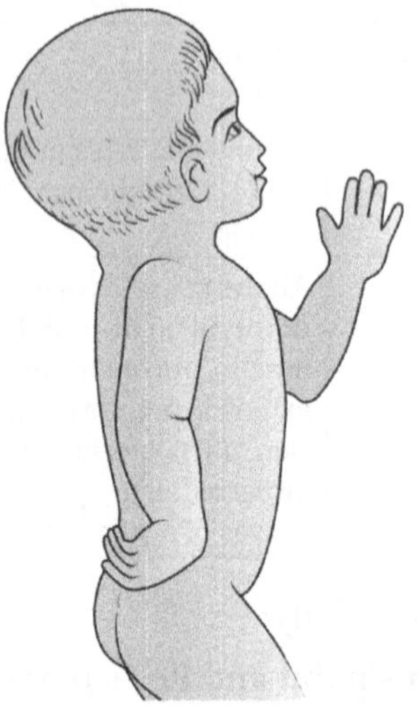

Fig. 10.3b: Erb's paralysis (waiter's tip/policeman's tip position of hand)

- Dystocia an abnormal or difficult childbirth.
- When a person falls on shoulder.

- *Position of the upper limb:* Appears like a policeman or waiter taking tip.
- *Motor loss:* Muscles paralysed are biceps brachii, brachialis, supraspinatus, infraspinatus, deltoid, brachioradialis and supinator (loss of abduction and lateral rotation of shoulder joint and flexion and supination at elbow joint).
- *Sensory loss:* Loss of sensations from the skin over the lower part of the deltoid.

b. Klumpke's paralysis: (Fig. 10.4)

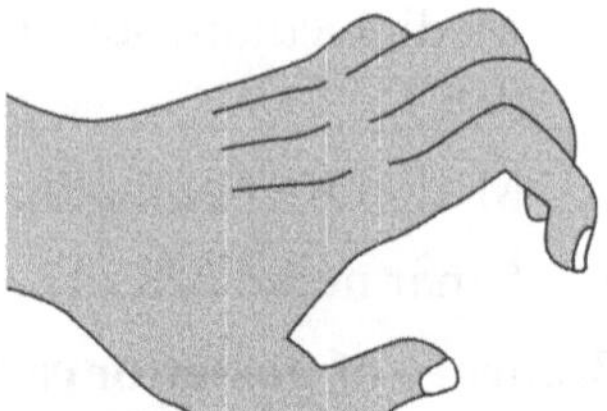

Fig. 10.4: Klumpke's paralysis (claw hand)

- *Site of lesion:* Lower trunk of brachial plexus (C8,T1).
- *Cause:* Undue separation of arm from the trunk (abduction injury) which may occur in the following conditions:
  - Birth injury.
  - Clutching something while falling from the height.
- *Position of the hand:* Complete claw hand:
  - Hyperextension at metacarpophalangeal joints.
  - Flexion at interphalangeal joints.
- *Motor loss:* Intrinsic muscles of the hand are paralysed.
- *Sensory loss:* Loss of sensations from a narrow zone along the medial side of hand and forearm.
- *Horner's syndrome:* Due to involvement of sympathetic fibers of T1 spinal nerve.

Characteristic features of Horner's syndrome are:

- Partial ptosis (drooping of upper eyelid).
- Miosis (constriction of pupil).
- Anhydrosis (absence of sweat).
- Enophthalamus.

8. **Enumerate the branches of axillary artery.**

Ans. Axillary artery extends from outer border of 1st rib to the lower border of teres major. It is divided into three parts by pectoralis minor muscle. Branches of the three parts are as follows: (Fig.10.5)

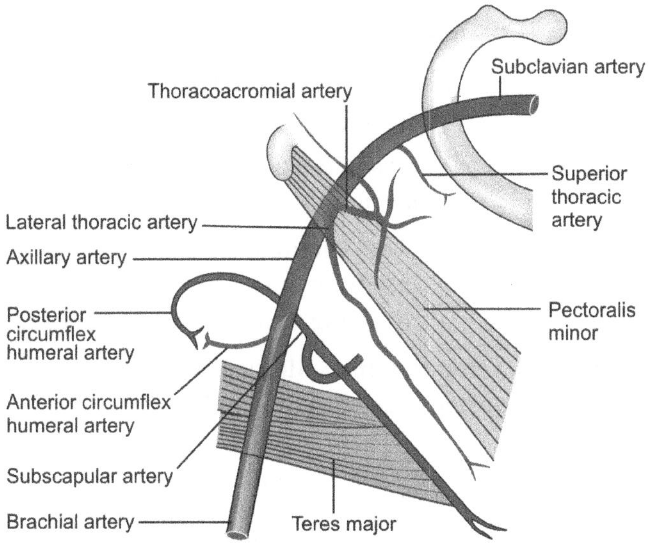

Fig. 10.5: Axillary artery–Parts and branches

a. **First part (proximal to pectoralis minor):**
   - Superior thoracic artery.

b. **Second part (deep to pectoralis minor):**
   - Thoracoacromial artery.
   - Lateral thoracic artery.

c. **Third part (distal to pectoralis minor):**
   - Anterior circumflex humeral artery.
   - Posterior circumflex humeral artery.
   - Circumflex scapular artery.

9. **Draw a schematic diagram to show the various groups of axillary lymph nodes and the areas drained by them.**

Ans. Axillary lymph nodes and areas drained by them: (Fig. 10.6a and Fig. 10.6b)

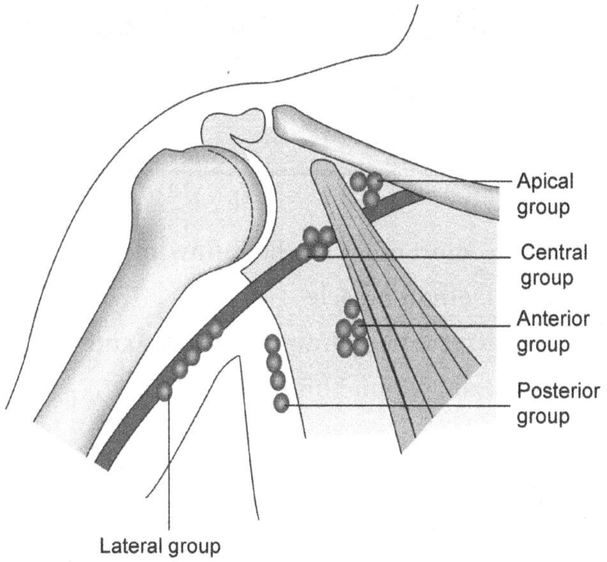

Fig. 10.6a: Axillary lymph nodes

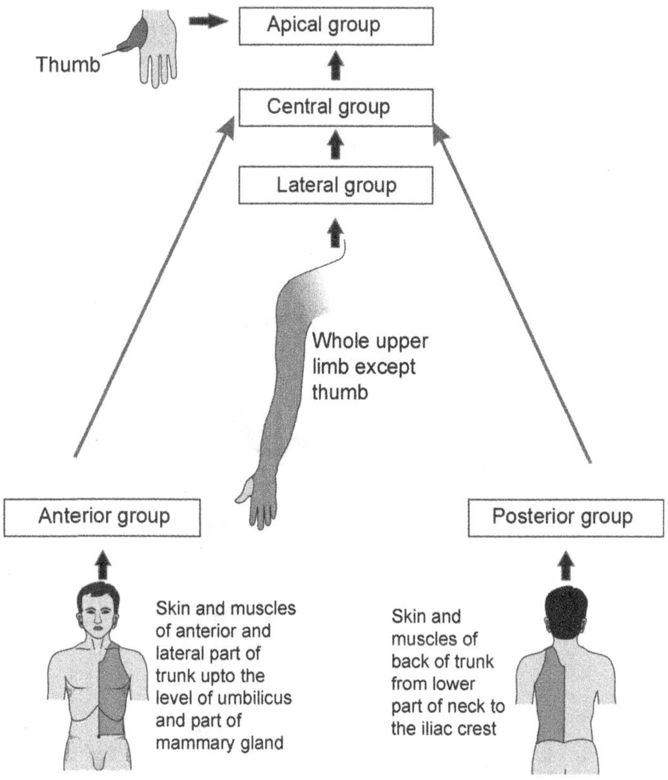

Fig. 10.6b: Areas drained by axillary lymph nodes

CHAPTER 11

SCAPULAR REGION

1. **Write short notes on the following:**
   a. **Deltoid muscle**
   b. **Musculotendinous or rotator cuff**
   c. **Subacromial bursa**

Ans.

a. **Deltoid muscle (Fig. 11.1):** It is a triangular (inverted delta) shaped muscle that forms the rounded contour of the shoulder. It is divided into three parts anterior, middle and posterior.

Origin:

- *Anterior part:* Anterior border of lateral 1/3rd of clavicle.
- *Middle (acromial) part:* Lateral border of the acromion process of scapular.
- *Posterior part:* Lower lip of the crest of spine of scapula.

Insertion: Deltoid tuberosity of humerus.

Action:

- *Anterior fibers:* Flexion and medial rotation of arm.
- *Middle fibers:* Abduction of arm from 15° to 90°.
- *Posterior fibers:* Extension and lateral rotation of the arm.

  * The deltoid also acts as a stabilizer in horizontal movements, e.g., drawing a line across a blackboard.

Nerve supply: Axillary nerve (C5,C6) from posterior cord of brachial plexus.

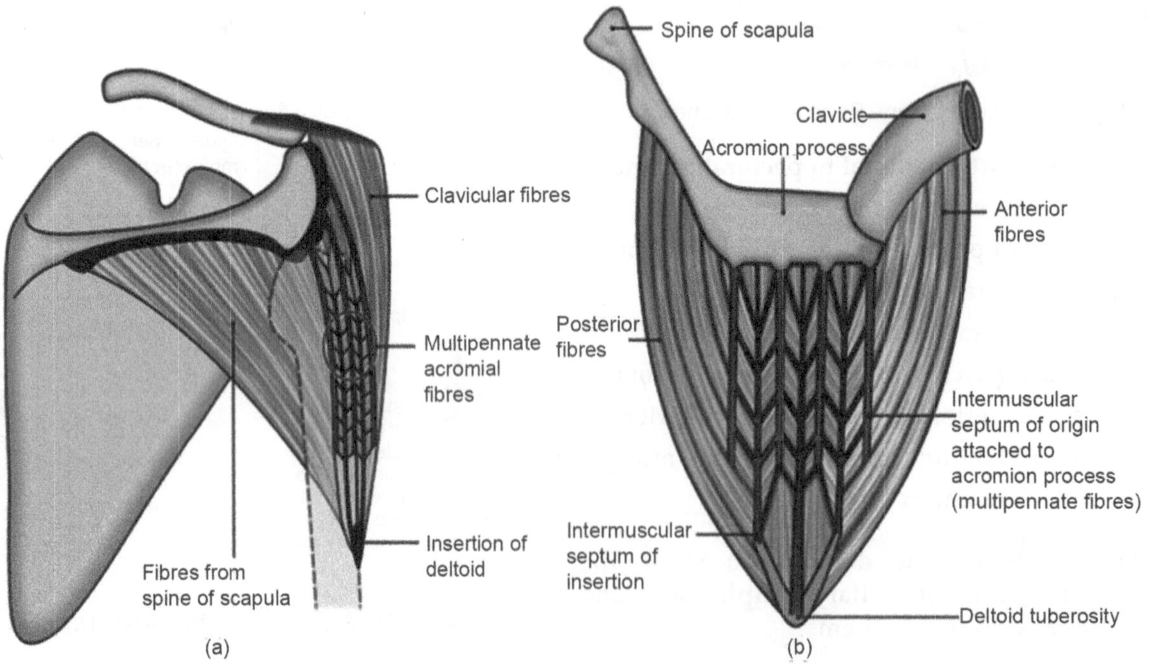

Fig. 11.1: Deltoid muscle

Applied:

- Deltoid muscle is often used to administer intramuscular injection. It should be given in the middle of the muscle to avoid injury to the axillary nerve.
- If deltoid is paralysed, rounded contour of the shoulder is lost and there is loss of power of abduction of arm up to 90°. Loss of sensation on the lateral side of the upper part of arm.

b. **Musculotendinous or rotator cuff (Fig. 11.2):** Rotator cuff is formed by a group of four muscles that surround the shoulder joint. As a group, they are responsible for stabilising the shoulder joint. Individually, they rotate the shoulder joint. The muscles that form rotator cuff are:

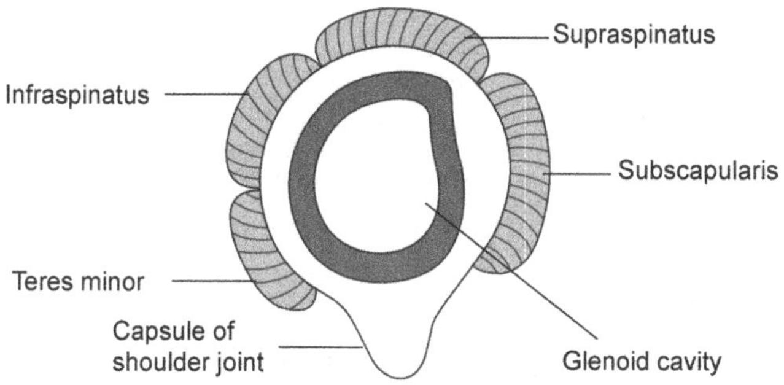

Fig. 11.2: Rotator cuff muscles

- Supraspinatus.
- Infraspinatus.
- Teres minor.
- Subscapularis.
  - The muscles take origin from scapula and are inserted on lesser and greater tubercles of humerus.
  - Their flattened tendons while crossing the shoulder joint blend with each other and with the capsule of the joint.
  - Musculotendinous cuff provides support to the capsule of the shoulder joint all around except inferiorly. The joint is supported anteriorly by subscapularis, superiorly by supraspinatus and posteriorly by infraspinatus and teres minor. As the joint is not protected inferiorly, the head of the humerus is usually dislocated inferiorly. The axillary nerve related to the surgical neck of humerus may get injured.
  - Details of the muscles forming 'Rotator cuff' are as follows:

Muscle	*Action*	*Nerve supply*
i. Supraspinatus	Abduction of arm – Initial 15	Suprascapular nerve
ii. Infraspinatus	Lateral rotation of arm	-do-
iii. Teres minor	-do-	Axillary nerve
iv. Subscapularis	Medial rotation of arm	Upper and lower subscapular nerves

* The rotator cuff muscles can be easily remembered using the acronym SITS.

c. **Subacromial bursa:**

- Is the largest bursa in the body. It is located inferior to the acromion arch and above the tendon of supraspinatus and greater tubercle of humerus.
- It is continuous with the subdeltoid bursa present beneath the deltoid muscle.
- It protects the supraspinatus tendon from friction against acromion during abduction of arm.
- ***Subacromial bursitis*** is a condition caused by inflammation of the bursa.

2. **Name the intermuscular spaces in the scapular region, write their boundaries and contents.**

Ans. Three intermuscular spaces are present in the scapular region (Fig. 11.3).

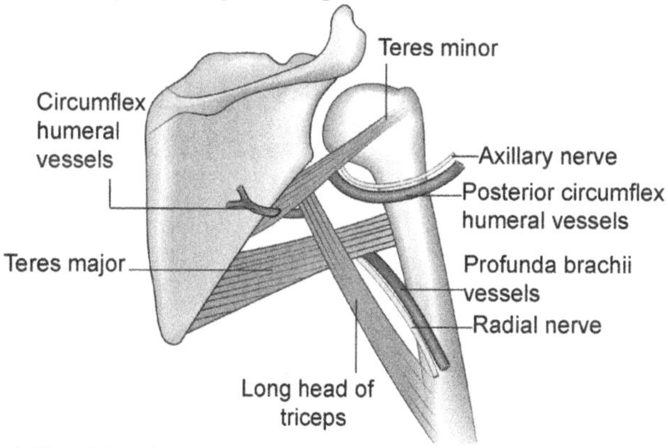

Fig. 11.3: Intermuscular spaces in the scapular region

a. **Quadrangular space:**

Boundaries

- *Superiorly*–Subscapularis, capsule of shoulder joint, teres minor (from front to back).
- *Inferiorly*–Teres major.
- *Laterally*–Surgical neck of humerus.
- *Medially*–Long head of triceps.

Contents

- Axillary nerve.
- Posterior circumflex humeral vessels.

b. **Upper triangular space:**

Boundaries

- *Laterally*–Long head of triceps.
- *Medially*–Teres minor.
- *Inferiorly*–Teres major.

Contents

- Circumflex scapular artery.

c. **Lower triangular space:**

Boundaries

- *Superiorly*–Teres major.
- *Laterally*–Shaft of humerus.
- *Medially*–Long head of triceps.

Contents

- Radial nerve and profunda brachii vessels.

3. **Draw a labeled diagram to show the anastomosis around scapula.**

Ans. Anastomosis around scapula is between the branches of first part of subclavian artery and third part of axillary artery (Fig. 11.4).

4. **Enumerate the movements possible at scapulothoracic joint and the muscles responsible for them.**

Ans. Movements possible of scapulothoracic joint

Movement	*Muscles responsible*
Elevation	Levator scapulae Trapezius (upper fibers)
Depression	Trapezius (lower fibers) Pectoralis major and minor, Latissimus dorsi Gravity
Protraction	Serratus anterior Pectoralis minor
Retraction	Rhomboids Trapezius (middle part)
Upward rotation *glenoid cavity faces upwards*	Serratus anterior (lower part) Trapezius (upper and lower part)
Downward rotation *glenoid cavity faces downwards*	Pectoralis major Latissimus dorsi Rhomboids gravity

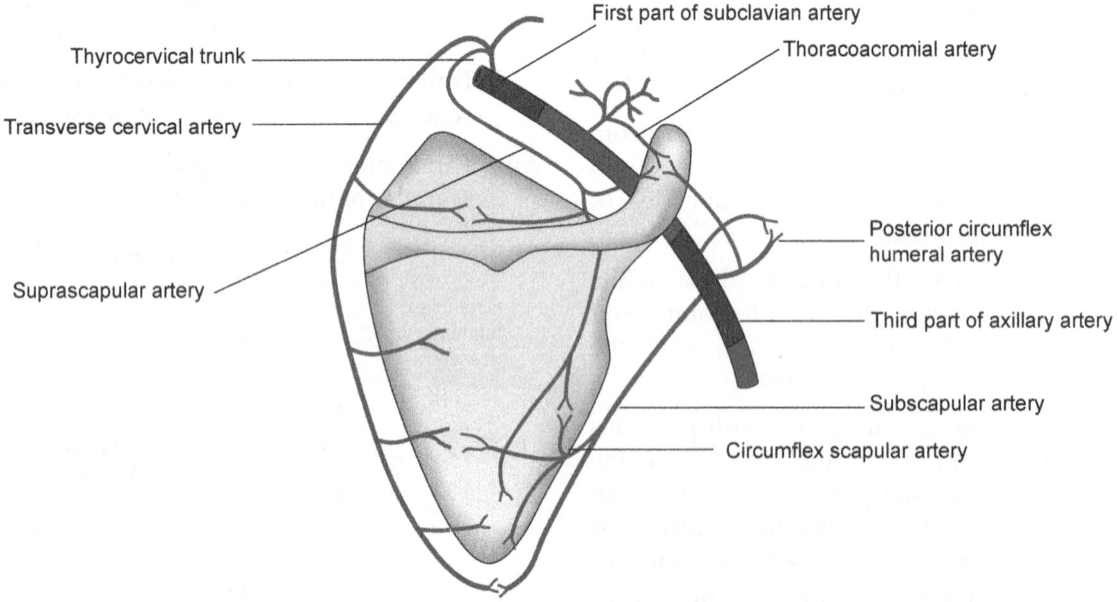

Fig. 11.4: Anastomosis around scapula

12 CHAPTER ARM AND CUBITAL FOSSA

1. **Enumerate:**

   a. **Muscles of anterior compartment of arm, their action and nerve supply**

   b. **Branches of brachial artery**

   c. **Branches of profunda brachii artery**

   d. **Nerves closely related to humerus**

Ans.

a. **Muscles of anterior (flexor) compartment of arm, their action and nerve supply:**

Muscle	*Action*	*Nerve Supply*
Biceps brachii	Flexor of forearm Supinator when the forearm is flexed **Short head**–Flexor of arm **Long head**–Prevents upward displacement of the head of humerus	Musculocutaneous
Coracobrachialis	Flexor of arm	Musculocutaneous
Brachialis	Flexor of forearm	Musculocutaneous Radial (proprioceptive)

b. **Branches of brachial artery:**

Brachial artery extends from lower border of the teres major muscle above to neck of radius below. Its branches are:

- Profunda brachii.
- Superior ulnar collateral.
- Inferior ulnar collateral.
- Muscular branches.
- Nutrient artery to humerus.
- Terminal branches–Radial and ulnar arteries.

Volkman's ischaemic contracture:

Causes of ischemia is injury/compression of brachial artery:

- Supracondylar fracture of humerus.
- Improper use of tourniquet.
- Tight plaster cast.
  - It is characterised by:

    Fibrosis and contracture of the muscles of forearm (especially FDP and FPL).
  - Deformity of hand presents:

    Flexion at wrist and at inter-phalangeal joints.

c. **Branches of profunda brachii artery:**

- Anterior descending (radial collateral).
- Posterior descending (middle collateral).
- Deltoid (ascending).
- Nutrient artery to the humerus.

d. **Nerves closely related to humerus are:**

- Axillary nerve to surgical neck of humerus.
- Radial nerve–radial groove.
- Ulnar nerve–posterior aspect of medial epicondyle.

2. **Describe cubital fossa under the following headings:**

   a. **Location**

   b. **Boundaries**

   c. **Structures forming roof**

   d. **Muscles forming floor**

   e. **Contents (from medial to lateral)**

   f. **Applied anatomy**

Ans.

a. **Location:** Triangular region in front of the elbow.

b. **Boundaries:**
- *Base:* Is formed by imaginary line joining the medial and lateral epicondyles.
- *Apex:* Is formed by the point where pronator teres meets brachioradialis.
- *Medial boundary:* Is formed by lateral border of pronator teres.
- *Lateral border:* Is formed by medial border of brachioradialis.

c. **Structures forming roof (Fig. 12.1a):**
- Skin.
- Superficial fascia containing:
  - Lateral cutaneous nerve of forearm.
  - Medial cutaneous nerve of forearm.
  - Median cubital vein.
- Deep fascia.
- Bicipital aponeurosis.

d. **Muscles forming floor:**
- Brachialis.
- Supinator.

e. **Contents (from medial to lateral) (Fig. 12.1b):**
- Median nerve.
- Brachial artery and its terminal branches – radial and ulnar arteries.
- Tendon of biceps brachii.
- Superficial branch of radial nerve.

f. **Applied anatomy:**
- The median cubital vein present in the roof of cubital fossa is the vein of choice for venipuncture.
- Blood pressure is recorded by auscultating brachial artery in the cubital fossa.

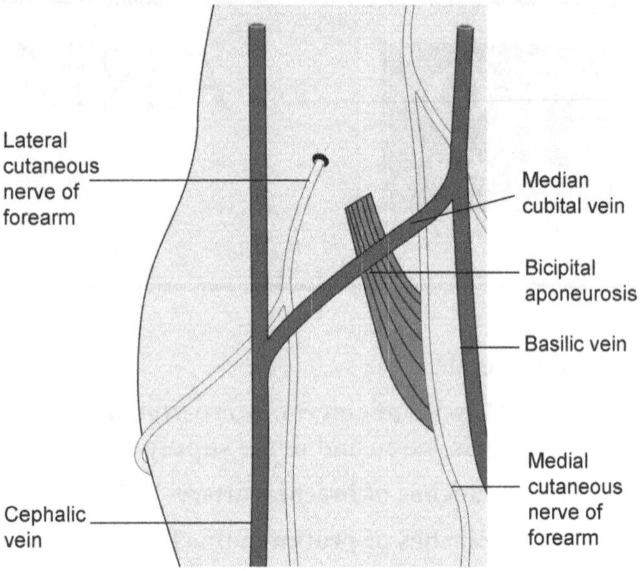

Fig. 12.1a: Structures forming roof of cubital fossa

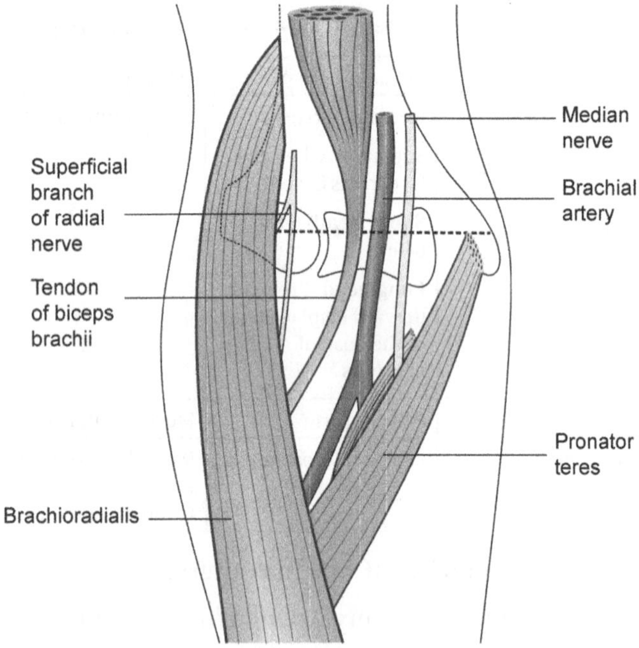

Fig. 12.1b: Boundaries and contents of cubital fossa

3. **Enumerate the:**

a. **Muscle/s of the extensor compartment of arm and its nerve supply**

b. **Structures in the spiral/radial groove**

c. **The muscular and cutaneous branches of radial nerve given in the arm**

Ans.

a. **Muscle/s of the extensor compartment of arm and its nerve supply:**
- Triceps – radial nerve.

b. **Structures in the spiral/radial groove:**
- Radial nerve.
- Profunda brachii vessels.

c. **Muscular branches of radial nerve supply in the arm are given to the following muscles:**
- Triceps.
- Brachioradialis.
- Extensor carpi radialis longus.
- Brachialis (proprioceptive fibers).

Cutaneous branches in the arm:
- Posterior cutaneous nerve of the arm.
- Lower lateral cutaneous nerve of the arm.
- Posterior cutaneous nerve of the forearm.

4. **Draw labeled diagram to show anastomosis around elbow.**

Ans. See Figure 12.2.

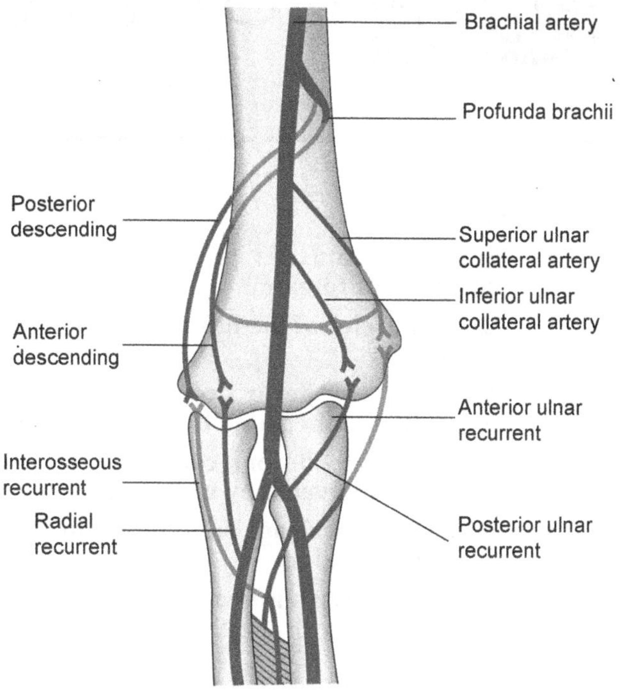

Fig.12.2: Anastomosis around elbow

13 CHAPTER

FOREARM AND HAND

1. **Enumerate the:**
   a. **Superficial muscles of the flexor compartment of forearm**
   b. **Deep muscles of the flexor compartment of forearm**
   c. **Muscles of flexor compartment of forearm are innervated by median nerve**
   d. **Muscles of flexor compartment of forearm innervated by ulnar nerve**
   e. **Structures passing superficial to the flexor retinaculum**
   f. **Structures passing deep to the extensor retinaculum**

Ans. a. **Superficial muscles of flexor compartment of forearm:**
- Pronator teres.
- Flexor carpi radialis.
- Palmaris longus.
- Flexor digitorum superficialis.
- Flexor carpi ulnaris.

b. **Deep muscles of flexor compartment of forearm:**
- Flexor pollicis longus.
- Flexor digitorum profundus.
- Pronator quadratus.

c. **6½ muscles of flexor compartment of forearm are innervated by median nerve:**
- Pronator teres.
- Flexor carpi radialis.
- Palmaris longus.
- Flexor digitorum superficialis.
- Flexor pollicis longus.
- Flexor digitorum profundus (lateral ½).
- Pronator quadratus.

d. **1½ muscles of flexor compartment of forearm innervated by ulnar nerve:**
- Flexor carpi ulnaris.
- Flexor digitorum profundus (medial ½).

e. **Structures passing superficial to the flexor retinaculum:**

From lateral to medial side:
- Palmar cutaneous branch of median nerve.
- Tendon of palmaris longus.
- Palmar cutaneous branch of ulnar nerve.
- Ulnar artery.
- Ulnar nerve.

f. **Structures passing deep to the extensor retinaculum:**

Structures passing deep to extensor rinaculum is divided into six parts. These six parts from lateral to medial are:
- Abductor pollicis longus and extensor pollicis brevis.
- Extensor carpi radialis longus and brevis.
- Extensor pollicis longus and brevis.
- Extensor digitorum, extensor indicis, posterior interosseous nerve and anterior interosseous artery.
- Extensor digiti minimi.
- Extensor carpi ulnaris.

2. **Describe briefly:**
   a. **Carpal tunnel and carpal tunnel syndrome**
   b. **Pronation and supination**

Ans. a. **Carpal tunnel: (Fig. 13.1)**

It is an osseofibrous tunnel formed posteriorly by the concave palmar surface of the carpals and bounded anteriorly by the flexor retinaculum (flexor retinaculum is attached laterally to scaphoid and crest of trapezium and medially to pisiform and hook of hamate).

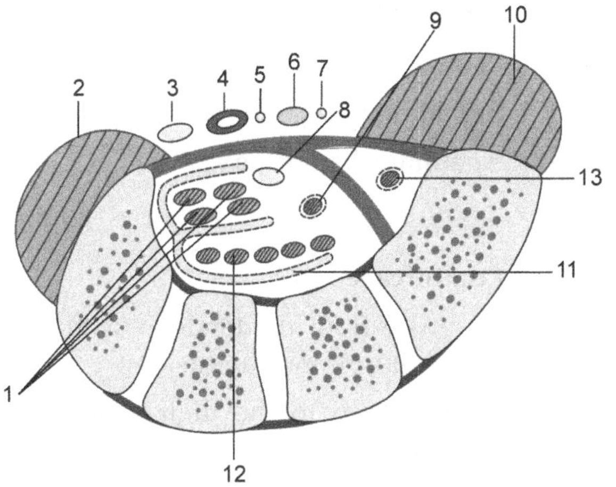

1. Tendons of flexor digitorum superficialis
2. Hypothenar eminence
3. Ulnar nerve
4. Ulnar artery
5. Palmar cutaneous branch of ulnar nerve
6. Tendon of palmaris longus
7. Palmar cutaneous branch of median nerve
8. Median nerve
9. Palmaris longus with radial bursa
10. Thenar eminence
11. Ulnar bursa
12. Tendons of flexor digitorum profundus
13. Tendon of flexor carpi radialis

Fig. 13.1: Carpal tunnel

Structures passing through the carpal tunnel are:

- Flexor digitorum superficialis tendons.
- Flexor digitorum profundus tendons.

  (Long flexor tendons share the same synovial sheath, referred to as the ulnar bursa).
- Flexor pollicis longus tendon which has its own synovial sheath, named radial bursa.
- Median nerve.

Carpal Tunnel Syndrome

- Is caused by compression of the median nerve in the carpal tunnel.
- *Cause:*
  - Osteoarthritis involving carpal bones.
  - Dislocation of carpal bones.
  - Tenosynovitis–inflammation of synovial sheaths of long flexor tendons.
- *Manifests as:*
  - Weakness and wasting of thenar muscles and loss of opposition of the thumb (Ape thumb deformity).
  - Anesthesia over palmar surface of lateral 3½ digits of the hand.
- May be treated by cutting the flexor retinaculum to relieve symptoms.

> The skin over the thenar area is not involved because it is supplied by the palmar cutaneous branch of the median nerve which enters the palm superficial to the flexor retinaculum.

b. **Pronation and supination:**

- These are rotatory movements of forearm (with hand) around a vertical axis.
- They are produced by the movement of radius around the stationary ulna.
- The movements occur at the radio-ulnar joints.
- The axis of the movement passes through the centre of the head of the radius (above) to the ulnar attachment of the articular disc (below).
- Supination is more powerful than pronation (therefore this movement is used for tightening the screws, nuts and bolts).
- In a semiflexed elbow the palm faces upwards in supination and downwards in pronation.
- ***Muscles responsible for supination:***
  - Supinator.
  - Biceps brachii (with elbow flexed).
- ***Muscles responsible for pronation:***
  - Pronator teres.
  - Pronator quadratus.

> Pronation is essentially a function of the median nerve (supplies both pronator quadratus and pronator teres, while supination depends on the musculocutaneous (biceps) and radial nerve (supplies supinator).

PALM

1. **Name the intrinsic muscles of the hand and write their nerve supply.**

Ans. Intrinsic muscles of the hand (total – 20 muscles) are grouped into five groups:

a. **Thenar muscles:**
- Abductor pollicis brevis.
- Flexor pollicis brevis.
- Opponens pollicis brevis.
- Adductor pollicis (does not form thenar eminence).

b. **Hypothenar muscles:**
- Abductor digiti minimi.
- Flexor digiti minimi.
- Opponens digiti minimi.
- Palmaris brevis.

c. **Four lumbricals** (one for each digit except thumb).

d. **Four palmar interossei** (third digit / middle finger does not have palmar interossei).

e. **Four dorsal interossei** (thumb and the fifth digit/little finger do not have dorsal interossei, whereas middle finger has two dorsal interossei).

Nerve supply: The intrinsic muscles of the hand are on the palmar aspect and are innervated by branches of the *ulnar and median nerves.*

- ***Five muscles are supplied by the median nerve:***
  - Muscles forming thenar eminence:
    - Abductor pollicis brevis.
    - Flexor pollicis brevis.
    - Opponens pollicis brevis.
  - 1st and 2nd lumbricals.
- ***Fifteen muscles are supplied by ulnar nerve:***
  - Four hypothenar muscles.
  - 3rd and 4th lumbricals.
  - Four palmar interossei.
  - Four dorsal interossei.
  - *Adductor pollicis.*

2. **Write short notes on:**

a. **Lumbricals**

b. **Interossei muscles of hand**

c. **Palmar spaces of the hand**

d. **Brachioradialis muscle**

e. **Anatomical snuff box**

Ans.

a. **Lumbricals:**
- Arise from the tendons of the flexor digitorum profundus.
- Lie deep to the digital vessels and nerves.
- Lie on the radial side of the fingers.
- Insert into the dorsal extensor expansions.
- Medial 2 lumbricals are innervated by the ulnar nerve and lateral 2 lumbricals by the median nerve.
- Flex the metacarpophalangeal joints and extend the interphalangeal joints.

b. **Interossei muscles of hand:**
- *Four dorsal interossei:*
  - Are bipennate and arise by double heads from the adjacent sides of the bodies of the metacarpals.
  - Are the abductors of digits (Dorsal **AB**duct = **DAB**).
- *Three palmar interossei:*
  - Are unipennate and arise by single head from the anterior aspect of metacarpals 2, 4 and 5.
  - Are the adductors of digits (Palmar **AD**duct = **PAD**).
- The interossei insert into the bases of proximal phalanges and into extensor expansions.
- All are innervated by the deep branch of ulnar nerve.

c. **Palmar spaces of the hand (Fig. 13.2):** The disposition of fascia and fascial septa in the hand results in the formation of potential spaces. These spaces are surgically important as they may get infected and distended with pus.

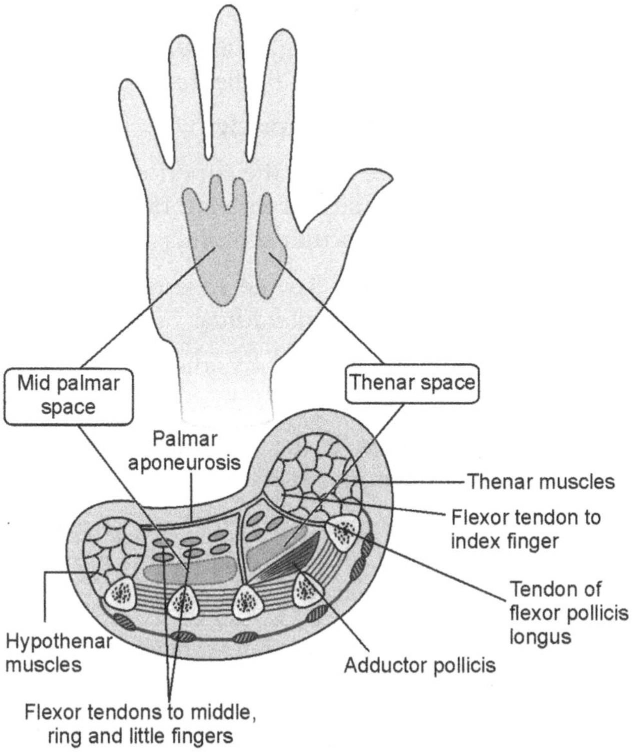

Fig. 13.2: Palmar spaces

Following are the important spaces on the palmar aspect:

- Midpalmar space.
- Thenar space.
- Pulp spaces of the fingers.
- ***Midpalmar space:***
  - *Shape:* Triangular.
  - *Location:* In the medial half of the hollow of the palm.
  - *Extent:*
    - Proximally till the distal margin of flexor retinaculum.
    - Distally till the distal palmar crease.
  - *Boundaries:*
    - Anterior: Palmar aponeurosis and flexor tendons of middle three digits (enclosed in ulnar bursa).
    - Posterior: Fascia covering interossei and middle three metacarpals.
    - Lateral: Intermediate palmar septum (extending from the palmar aponeurosis to the 3rd metacarpal).
    - Medial: Medial palmar septum (extending from the palmar aponeurosis to the 5th metacarpal).
  - *Communications:*
    - Proximally may communicate with the forearm *space of parona* through carpal tunnel.
    - Distally with the medial three web spaces (subcutaneous spaces in the interdigital cleft) through the ulnar three lumbrical canals (fascial sheaths of lumbricals).
  - *Drainage in case of infection:* Pus from this space can be drained by incision in the 3rd and 4th web spaces.
- ***Thenar space:***
  - *Shape:* Triangular.
  - *Location:* In the outer half of the hollow of the palm.
  - *Extent:*
    - Proximally till the distal margin of flexor retinaculum.
    - Distally till the proximal transverse palmar crease.
  - *Boundaries:*
    - Anterior: Palmar aponeurosis and flexor tendons of index finger and tendon of flexor pollicis longus (enclosed in radial bursa).
    - Posterior: Fascia covering adductor pollicis.
    - Lateral: Lateral palmar septum (extending from the palmar aponeurosis to the 1st metacarpal).
    - Medial: Intermediate palmar septum (extending from the palmar aponeurosis to the 3rd metacarpal).
  - *Communications:*
    - Distally with the 1st web space (subcutaneous space in the

interdigital cleft) through the 1st lumbrical canal.

- *Drainage in case of infection*: Pus from this space can be drained by incision in the 1st web space.

- ***Pulp spaces of the fingers: (Fig. 13.3)***
    - Are the subcutaneous spaces on the palmar aspect of the tips of the fingers and the thumb.
    - They are filled with subcutaneous fatty tissue that is divided into compartments by the numerous fibrous septa which extend from the distal phalanx to the skin.
    - *Boundaries:*
        - Anterior: Skin and superficial fascia.
        - Posterior: Distal 2/3rd of the distal phalanx.

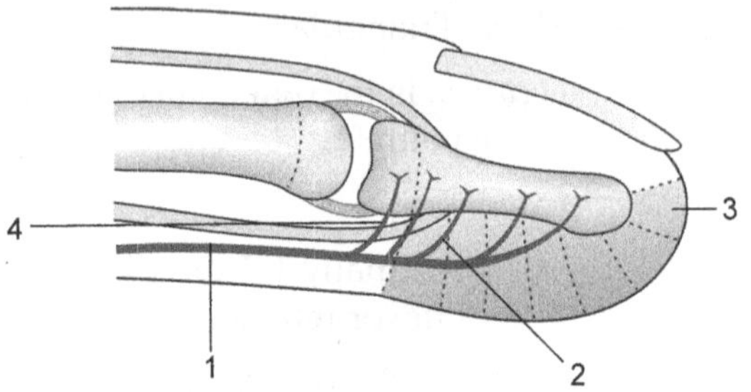

1. Digital artery
2. Branches to shaft of distal phalanx traversing the pulp space
3. Distal pulp space
4. Branch to base of distal phalanx

Fig. 13.3: Pulp spaces

Whitlow:

- Infection of the pulp spaces is known as *whitlow.*
- Pus from the pulp space is drained by lateral incision which opens all the compartments.

If neglected, the whitlow may lead to the necrosis of distal 4/5th of the distal phalanx.

This is due to the fact that the diaphysis of the distal phalanx (distal 4/5th) is supplied by the branches of the digital artery that traverse through the pulp space. The rising tension due to accumulation of pus may occlude these branches of the digital artery resulting in avascular necrosis of the distal 4/5th of the terminal phalanx. As the proximal 1/5th (epiphysis) of the distal phalanx receives blood supply proximal to the pulp space, it is not affected.

- Terminal branches of the digital artery course through the spaces to supply the diaphysis of the distal phalanx.

d. Brachioradialis muscle:

- ***Origin:*** From the superior part of the lateral supracondylar ridge and the intermuscular septum.
- ***Insertion:*** To the base of the styloid process of the radius.
- Is innervated by the radial nerve (C5, 6).
- Acts as a flexor of the forearm in midprone position.
- The radial artery and superficial radial nerve lie deep to this muscle in the forearm.

Is a flexor of forearm although it is innervated by an 'extensor' nerve (The radial nerve).

e. Anatomical snuff box:

- Is a triangular depression on the lateral aspect of dorsum of hand which becomes prominent on hyperextension of thumb.
- ***Boundaries:***
    - Anterolaterally is formed by the tendons of the abductor pollicis longus and extensor pollicis brevis.
    - Posteromedially by the tendon of extensor pollicis longus.
    - Floor is formed by scaphoid and trapezium.
    - Roof is formed by skin and superficial fascia.
- Contains radial artery.
- The cephalic vein and superficial radial nerve cross superficial to the anatomical snuff box.
- ***Applied:***
    - Tenderness in the anatomical snuff box indicates fracture of scaphoid.
    - Radial artery pulsations can be felt and the cephalic vein can be used for giving intravenous fluids at this site.

3. **Draw a labeled diagram of the following:**
   a. **Cutaneous innervation of hand**
   b. **Superficial and deep palmar arch**
   c. **Extensor expansion of finger**

Ans.

a. **Cutaneous innervations of hand: (Fig. 13.4a and Fig. 13.4b)**

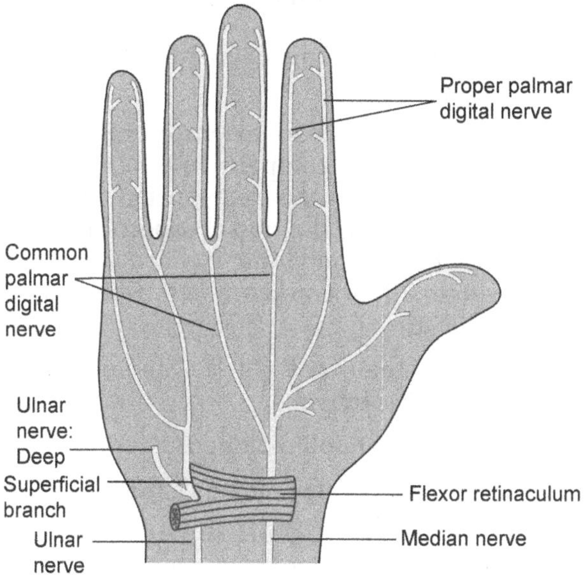

Fig. 13.4a: Cutaneous nerves on palmar surface of hand

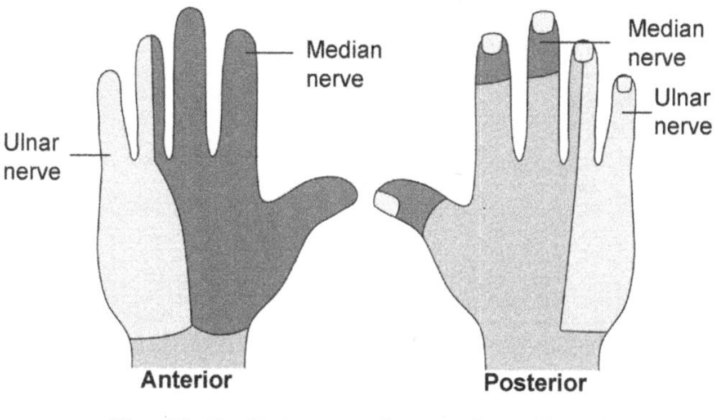

Fig. 13.4b: Cutaneous innervation of hand

b. **Superficial palmar arch:**
- Lies deep to the palmar aponeurosis.
- Is formed by the continuation of the ulnar artery and completed by a branch of radial artery.
- It gives off 4 palmar digital arteries (lateral 3 digital branches are joined by palmar metacarpal arteries from the deep palmar arch).
- Supplies the medial 3½ digits.

The deep palmar arch:
- Is formed by the radial artery that reaches the palm through the 1st metacarpal space by passing through the 1st dorsal interosseous muscle.
- Is completed medially by the deep branch of the ulnar artery.
- Gives 2 palmar digital branches (the princeps pollicis and the radialis indicis) to the lateral 1½ digits.
- Gives 3 palmar metacarpal arteries that anastomose with the palmar digital branches from the superficial palmar arch (Fig. 13.5).

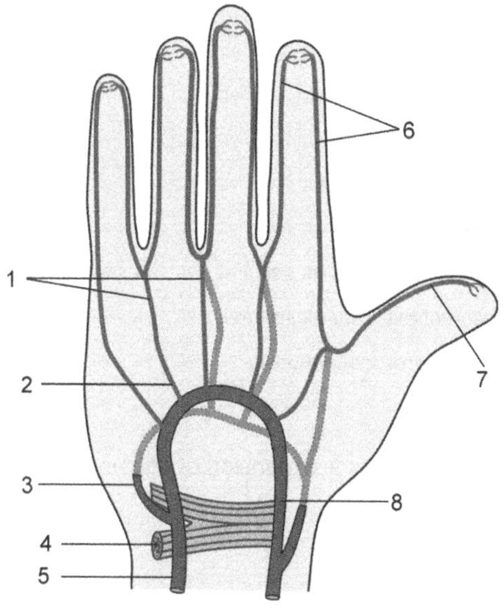

1. Common digital arteries
2. Superficial palmar arch
3. Deep branch of ulnar artery
4. Flexor retinaculum
5. Ulnar artery
6. Proper palmar digital arteries
7. Princeps pollicis artery
8. Superficial branch of the radial artery

Fig. 13.5: Superficial and deep palmar arch

c. **Extensor expansion of finger: (Fig. 13.6)**
- The tendon of extensor digitorum expands over the dorsum and sides of metacarpal head and proximal phalanx to form the extensor expansion.
- On the dorsum of the proximal phalanx, the expansion divides into

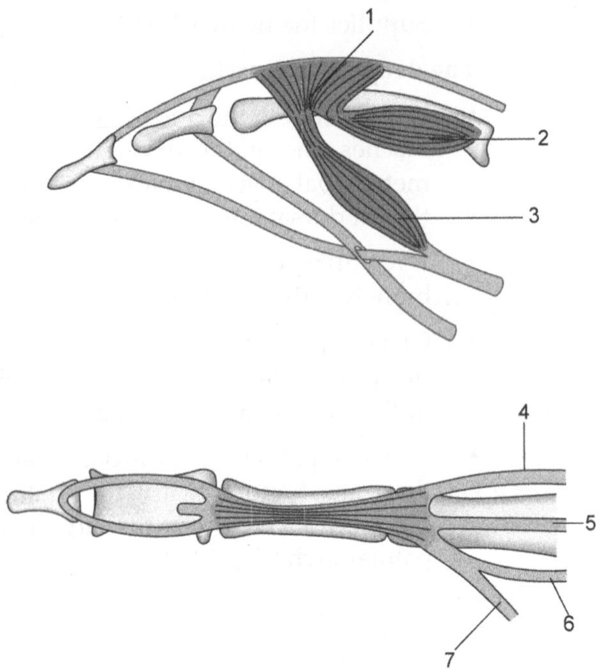

1. Extensor expansion
2. Interosseous muscle
3. Lumbrical muscle
4. Palmar interosseus muscle
5. Tendon of extensor digitorum
6. Dorsal interosseous muscle
7. Lumbrical

Fig. 13.6: Extensor expansion of right index finger

a median band (attached to the base of middle phalanx) and into 2 side bands (attached to the base of the distal phalanx).

- The tendons of lumbricals and interossei are inserted into the expansion.

4. Enumerate the structures passing deep to the extensor retinaculum.

Ans. Structures passing deep to extensor retinaculum:

The space deep to extensor retinaculum is divided into six compartments by fibrous septa extending from the deep surface of extensor retinaculum to the dorsal aspect of the lower ends of radius and ulna. The structures passing through these compartments from lateral to medial are:

- Abductor pollicis longus and extensor pollicis brevis.
- Extensor pollicis longus.
- Extensor carpi radialis longus and brevis.
- Extensor digitorum, extensor indicis, posterior interosseous nerve and anterior interosseous artery.
- Extensor digiti minimi.
- Extensor carpi ulnaris.

14 CHAPTER JOINTS OF UPPER LIMB

1. Classify the joints of upper limb and enumerate the movements possible at these joints.

Ans. Joints of upper limb: All the joints are synovial joints except intermediate radioulnar joint which is a fibrous joint.

Name of the joint	*Type of joint*
Sternoclavicular	Saddle type of synovial joint
Acromioclavicular	Plane type of synovial joint
Shoulder (glenohumeral)	Ball and socket type of synovial joint
Elbow	Hinge type of synovial joint
Superior and inferior radioulnar	Pivot type of synovial joint
Middle radioulnar	Syndesmosis type of fibrous joint
Wrist (radiocarpal)	Ellipsoid type of synovial joint
Intercarpal and carpometacarpal	Plane type of synovial joint
1st carpometacarpal	Saddle type of synovial joint
Metacarpophalangeal	Ellipsoid type of synovial joint
Interphalangeal	Hinge type of synovial joint

2. Describe shoulder joint under the following headings:

- **a. Type**
- **b. Articular surfaces**
- **c. Capsule and ligaments**
- **d. Factors providing stability**
- **e. Movements**
- **f. Applied**

Ans. Shoulder joint (Fig. 14.1a) is the most movable joint and is also more prone to dislocation than any other joint.

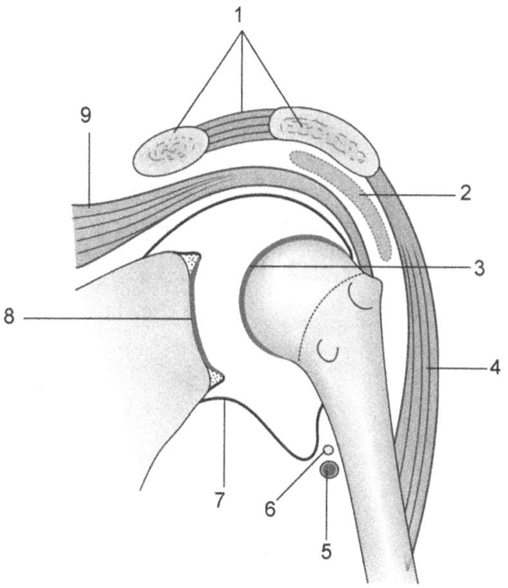

1. Coracoacromial arch
2. Subacromial bursa
3. Head of humerus
4. Deltoid
5. Posterior circumflex humeral artery
6. Axillary nerve
7. Articular capsule
8. Glenoid cavity
9. Supraspinatus

Fig. 14.1a: Shoulder joint

a. Type: Ball and socket type of synovial joint.

b. Articular surfaces:

- Large round head of the humerus.
- Small and shallow glenoid cavity.
- The fibrocartilagenous ring called glenoid labrum deepens the glenoid cavity.

c. **Capsule (Fig. 14.1b):** The capsule is thick and strong but lax.

- The fibrous capsule surrounds the joint.
- It is attached medially to the margins of the glenoid cavity beyond the glenoid labrum.
- Laterally it attached to the anatomical neck of the humerus except:
  - Inferiorly where it is attached to the surgical neck of the humerus a finger's breadth below the articular margin.
  - Superiorly at the upper end of the intertubercular groove it is deficient to allow the passage of the tendon of long head of biceps brachii.

Ligaments: (Fig. 14.1c)

- ***Glenohumeral ligaments:*** Superior, middle and inferior glenohumeral ligaments in the anterior part of the capsule.
- ***Coracohumeral ligament:*** Extends from the base of the coracoid process to the greater tubercle of the humerus.
- ***Transverse humeral ligament:*** Bridges the upper end of the intertubercular sulcus.

d. **Factors providing the stability:**

- ***Musculotendinous cuff/rotator cuff:*** Is formed by the flattened tendons of the:
  - Subscapularis anteriorly.
  - Supraspinatus superiorly.
  - Infraspinatus and teres minor posteriorly (it does not support the joint inferiorly).

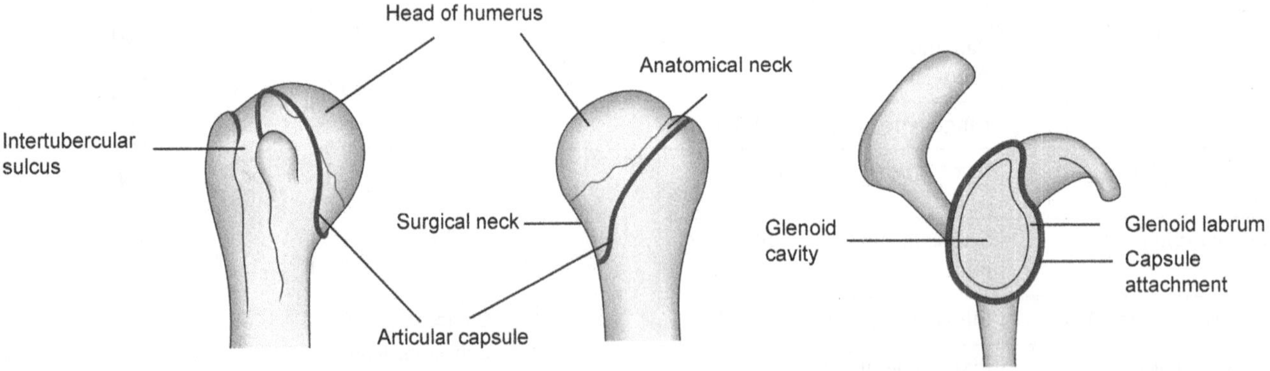

Fig. 14.1b: Capsular attachment of shoulder joint

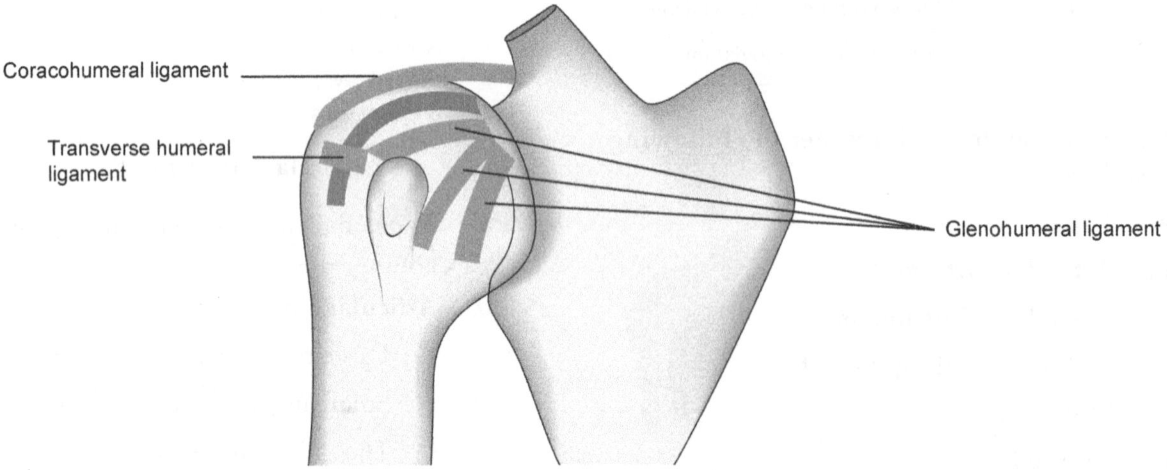

Fig. 14.1c: Ligaments of shoulder joint

- *Coracoacromial arch:* Prevents the upward dislocation of the head of the humerus.
- *Glenoid labrum:* Deepens the glenoid cavity.
- *Long head of biceps brachii:* Prevents the upward dislocation of the head of the humerus.

e. **Movements:**

Movement	*Muscles responsible for the movement*
Flexion	Pectoralis major Deltoid (anterior fibers) Coracobrachialis Biceps brachii (short head)
Extension	Deltoid (posterior fibers) Latissimus dorsi Teres major Long head of triceps
Abduction	0–15° – Spraspinatus 15–90° – Deltoid (middle fibers) **Overhead abduction:** Serratus anterior Trapezius
Adduction	Pectoralis major Latissimus dorsi Teres major
Medial rotation	Subscapularis Deltoid (anterior fibers) Pectoralis major Teres major Latissimus dorsi
Lateral rotation	Infraspinatus Teres minor Deltoid (posterior fibers)

f. **Applied:**

- ***Inferior dislocation*** of shoulder joint is common because:
  - The capsule descends downwards on the surgical neck inferiorly.
  - The capsule is not supported by the musculotendinous cuff inferiorly.
- ***Axillary nerve*** is likely to be injured in the inferior dislocation as it is related to the surgical neck of humerus.
- ***Frozen shoulder:*** Referred to as adhesive capsulitis, is a disorder in which the capsule and the connective tissue surrounding the *glenohumeral joint* becomes inflamed and stiff, greatly restricting motion and causing *chronic pain.*
- ***Painful arc syndrome:*** Thickening or calcium deposits in the supraspinatus tendon or subacromial bursitis results in pain during abduction of shoulder joint from 60° to 120°.

3. **Name the movements possible at the following joints and write the muscles responsible for producing them:**
   a. **Elbow joint**
   b. **Wrist (radiocarpal) joint**
   c. **1st carpometacarpal joint**

Ans. a. Elbow joint (Fig. 14.2a, b and c): It is a hinge variety of synovial joint. It has two parts:

- ***Humeroulnar:*** Between trochlea of humerus and trochlear notch of ulna.
- ***Humeroradial:*** Between the capitulum of humerus and superior surface of head of radius.

Movement	*Muscles responsible for the movement*
Flexion	Brachialis Biceps brachii Brachioradialis (in midprone position) Superficial flexors of forearm
Extension	Triceps Anconeus

b. **Wrist (radiocarpal joint):**

- It is ellipsoid variety of synovial joint.
- The articular surfaces are formed:
  - *Superiorly:* The inferior surface of the lower end of the radius and the triangular articular disc (ulna does not participate in the formation of wrist joint).
  - *Inferiorly:* The proximal surfaces of the scaphoid, lunate and triquetral.

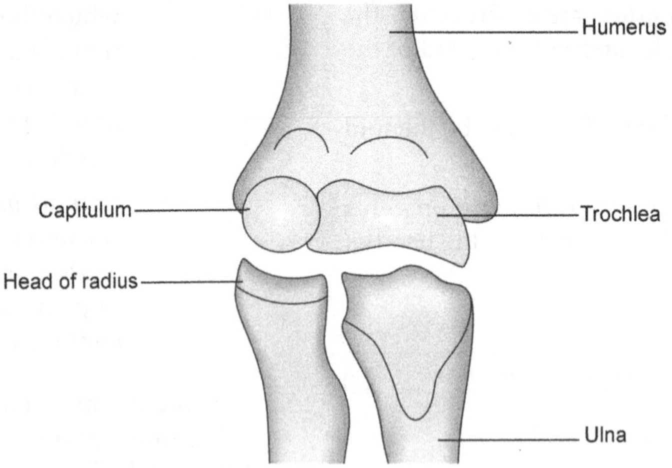

Fig. 14.2a: Elbow joint (articular surfaces)

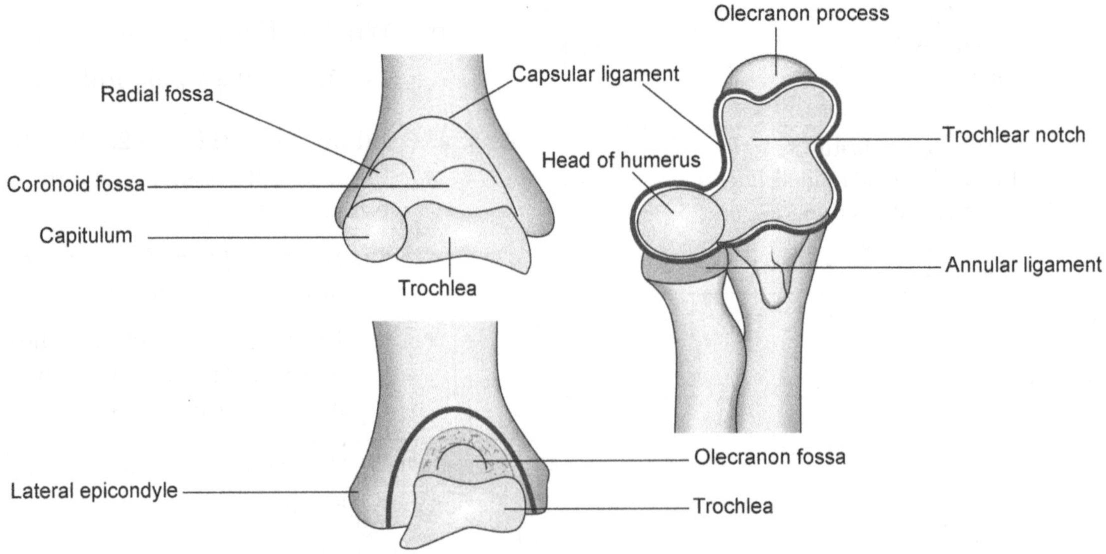

Fig. 14.2b: Capsular attachment of elbow joint

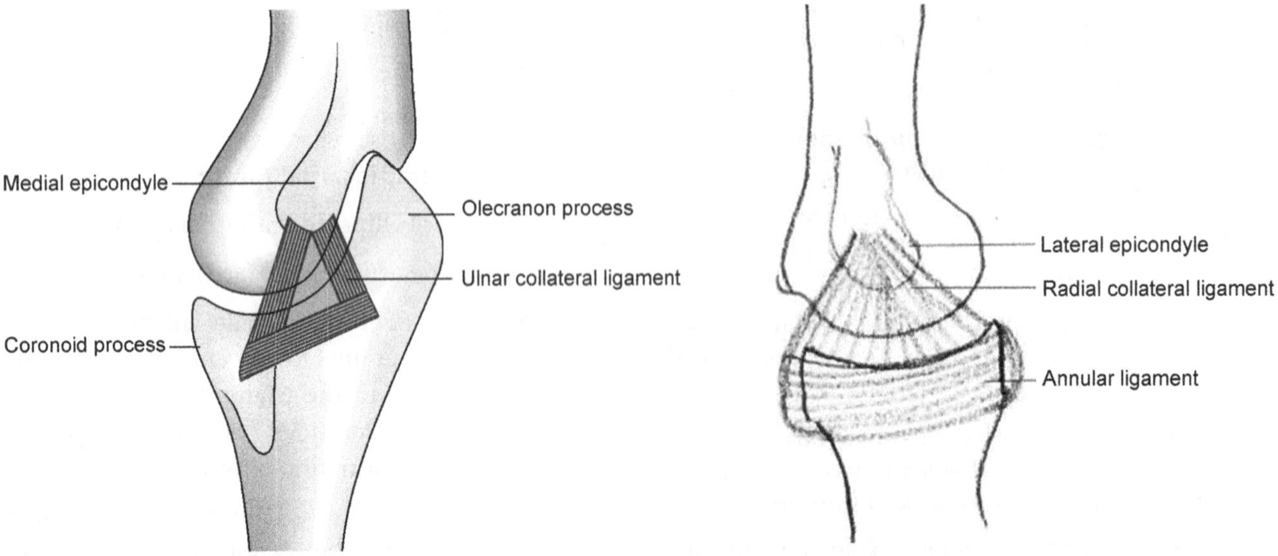

Fig. 14.2c: Ligaments of elbow joint

Movement	*Muscles responsible for the movement*
Flexion	Flexor carpi ulnaris Flexor carpi radialis Flexor digitorum superficialis Flexor digitorum profundus
Extension	Extensor carpi radialis longus and brevis Extensor carpi ulnaris Extensors of digits
Adduction	Flexor carpi ulnaris Extensor carpi ulnaris
Abduction	Flexor carpi radialis Extensor carpi radialis

c. **1st carpometacarpal joint:** It is saddle variety of synovial joint.

Movement	*Muscles responsible for the movement*
Flexion	Flexor pollicis brevis Flexor pollicis longus Opponens pollicis
Extension	Extensor pollicis longus Extensor pollicis brevis
Adduction	Adductor pollicis
Abduction	Abductor pollicis longus Abductor pollicis brevis
Opposition	Opponens pollicis Abductor pollicis longus and brevis Flexor pollicis brevis

Which squant joint movement tests the following spinal nerve?

- C5 Abduction of arm
- C6 Flexion of forearm at elbow joint
- C7 Extension of arm at elbow joint
- C8 Flexion of fingers
- T1 Abduction and adduction of the index, middle and ring fingers

15 CHAPTER NERVES AND NERVE LESIONS OF UPPER LIMB

1. Describe in brief the course, branches, distribution and applied anatomy of the following nerves:

a. Axillary nerve

b. Radial nerve

c. Median nerve

d. Ulnar nerve

Ans. a. **Axillary nerve (C_5 and C_6):**

It is a branch of the posterior cord of brachial plexus.

Course:

- It arises in the axilla and then it runs backwards through the quadrangular space and here it is closely related to the surgical neck of the humerus.
- It turns laterally deep to deltoid and divides into anterior and posterior divisions.

Branches and Distribution:

- Anterior branch supplies:
  - Teres minor muscle.
  - It continues as upper lateral cutaneous nerve of the arm which supplies the skin over the lower half of deltoid.
- Posterior branch supplies:
  - Deltoid muscle.

Applied Anatomy:

- The axillary nerve may get injured due to:
  - Inferior dislocation of head of humerus.
  - Fracture of surgical neck of humerus.
- The injury to axillary nerve results in:
  - Impaired abduction of shoulder joint due to paralysis of deltoid muscle.
  - Loss of sensation over the lower half of the deltoid.
  - Loss of rounded contour of shoulder.

b. **Radial nerve ($C_5 - T_1$):**

Is the largest nerve of the brachial plexus.

Course:

- It arises from the posterior cord of brachial plexus in the axilla.
- It enters the posterior compartment of arm at lower border of the teres major.
- It lies in the spiral groove of humerus along with the profunda brachii vessels between the long and medial heads of triceps.
- At the lower end of the spiral groove, it pierces the lateral intermuscular septum to enter the anterior compartment of arm.
- It then enters the cubital fossa and at the level of lateral epicondyle, it terminates by dividing into superficial and deep (posterior interosseous) branches.
- The superficial branch enters the forearm and runs deep to brachioradialis.
- In the lower 1/3rd of the forearm, it winds around the lateral aspect of radius to reach the anatomical snuff box on the dorsum of hand.

- It terminates by dividing into digital branches.
- The deep (posterior interosseous nerve) branch leaves the cubital fossa by passing through the supinator to enter the posterior compartment of forearm.

Branches and Distribution:

- *In the axilla:*

  Sensory:

  - Posterior cutaneous nerve of arm (skin on the back of arm).

  Motor:

  - Nerve to long head of triceps.
  - Nerve to medial head of triceps.
- *In the spiral groove:*

  Sensory:

  - Lower lateral cutaneous nerve of the arm (skin on the lateral surface of arm).
  - Posterior cutaneous nerve of the forearm (skin of the middle of the back of forearm).

  Motor:

  - Nerve to lateral head of triceps.
  - Nerve to medial head of triceps.
  - Nerve to anconeus.
- *In the anterior compartment of arm:* Motor:
  - Nerve to brachialis (proprioceptive).
  - Nerve to brachioradialis.
  - Nerve to extensor carpi radialis longus.
- *In the cubital fossa:*
  - Terminal branches:
    - Superficial branch (sensory):
      - Innervates the skin over the lateral part of the dorsum of hand and dorsal surface of lateral 3½ digits up to the distal phalanx.
  - Deep (posterior interosseous) branch (motor):
    - In the cubital fossa:
      - Extensor carpi radialis.
      - Supinator.
    - In the posterior compartment of forearm:
      - All the extensor muscles of forearm.
  - Applied anatomy: *Wrist drop* (loss of extension of wrist due to paralysis of extensors of wrist).
  - The radial nerve may get injured at the following two sites:
    - In the axilla:
      - Due to pressure of upper end of crutches (crutch palsy).
      - Drunkard falling asleep with the arm pressing over the back of chair (Saturday night palsy).
    - Injury of radial nerve in the axilla results in:
      - Loss of extension at elbow joint.
      - *Wrist drop* (loss of extension of wrist due to paralysis of extensors of wrist).
      - Loss of extension of digits.
      - Sensory loss on the skin over the posterior surface of lower part of arm, middle of the posterior part of forearm, lateral part of dorsum of hand and dorsal surface of lateral 3½ digits.
    - In the spiral groove:
      - Midshaft fracture of humerus.
    - Injury to radial nerve at this site results in:
      - *Wrist drop.*

- o Loss of extension of digits.
- o Sensory loss on the skin over the lateral part of dorsum of hand and dorsal surface of lateral 3½ digits.

> Extension of elbow joint is possible because nerves to long and medial heads of triceps arise in the axilla proximal to the site of lesion.

c. **Median nerve ($C_5 - T_1$): (Fig. 15.1a)**

Arises in the axilla by two roots (lateral and medial) from the lateral and medial cords of brachial plexus.

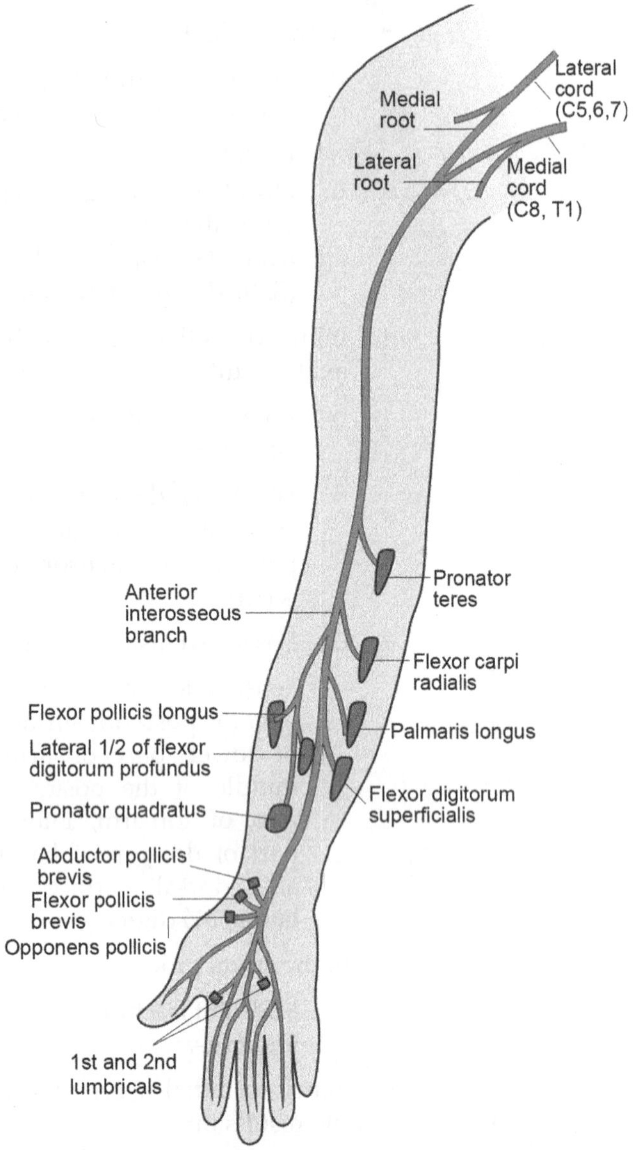

Fig.15.1a: Median nerve course and distribution

Course:

- Enters the anterior compartment of arm at the lower border of teres major.
- In the arm, initially it lies lateral to the brachial artery, then crosses in front of the artery to reach its medial side.
- Enters the cubital fossa where it lies medial to the brachial artery.
- It leaves the cubital fossa by passing between the two heads of the pronator teres and gives off anterior interosseous nerve.
- In the forearm, it passes behind the tendinous arch of flexor digitorum superficialis and runs downwards deep to the muscle.
- 5 cm proximal to flexor retinaculum it becomes superficial and lies lateral to the tendons of flexor digitorum superficialis.
- It then enters the palm through the carpal tunnel and divides into lateral and medial terminal branches.

Branches and Distribution:

- *In the axilla and arm:* No branches.
- *In the cubital fossa:*
  - Gives branches from its medial side to all the superficial flexors of the forearm except flexor carpi ulnaris.
- *In the forearm:*
  - Anterior interosseous branch supplies 2½ muscles:
    - Flexor pollicis longus.
    - Pronator quadratus.
    - Lateral half of the flexor digitorum profundus.
  - Before entering carpal tunnel it gives off palmar cutaneous branch (passes superficial to flexor retinaculum) which supplies skin over thenar eminence and lateral part of palm.
- *In the palm:*
  - Lateral branch gives:

- Motor: A recurrent branch that supplies thenar muscles except adductor pollicis.
- Sensory: Three palmar digital branches.

– Medial branch gives:
- Sensory: Two palmar digital branches.

– The five palmar digital branches supply the skin of the palmar surface of lateral 3½ digits including the nail beds and the skin on the dorsum of the distal phalanx.

Applied Anatomy:

– Median nerve may get injured at the following sites:
- At the elbow:
  - o Due to supracondylar fracture of humerus.
  - o Entrapment of nerve between the two heads of pronator teres (pronator syndrome).
- Injury to median nerve at this site results in:
  - o Loss of pronation.
  - o Weakened flexion at wrist.
  - o Ape thumb deformity: Thumb is laterally rotated and adducted. Opposition of thumb is not possible.
  - o Thenar eminence is flattened.
  - o Benediction attitude: When patient tries to make fist the index and the middle finger remain extended due to paralysis of the flexors of these two digits.
- Sensory loss over the lateral half of the palm and lateral 3½ digits (Fig. 15.1b).

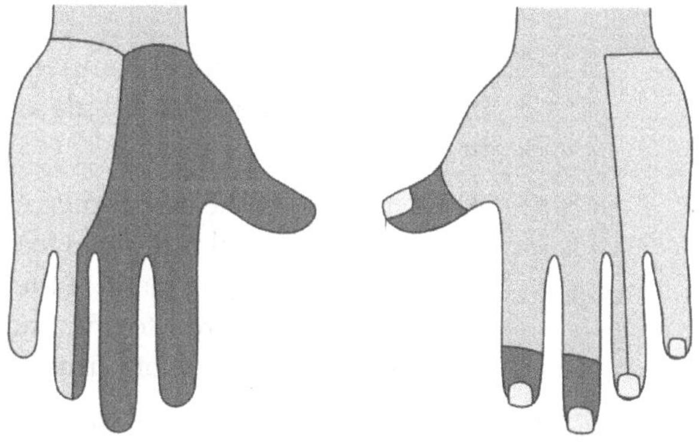

Fig. 15.1b: Area of sensory loss following injury to median nerve

– In the carpal tunnel: Refer to short note on carpal tunnel (Page No. 45).

d. Ulnar nerve (C_8 and T_1): (Fig. 15.2a)

It arises in the axilla from the medial cord of the brachial plexus.

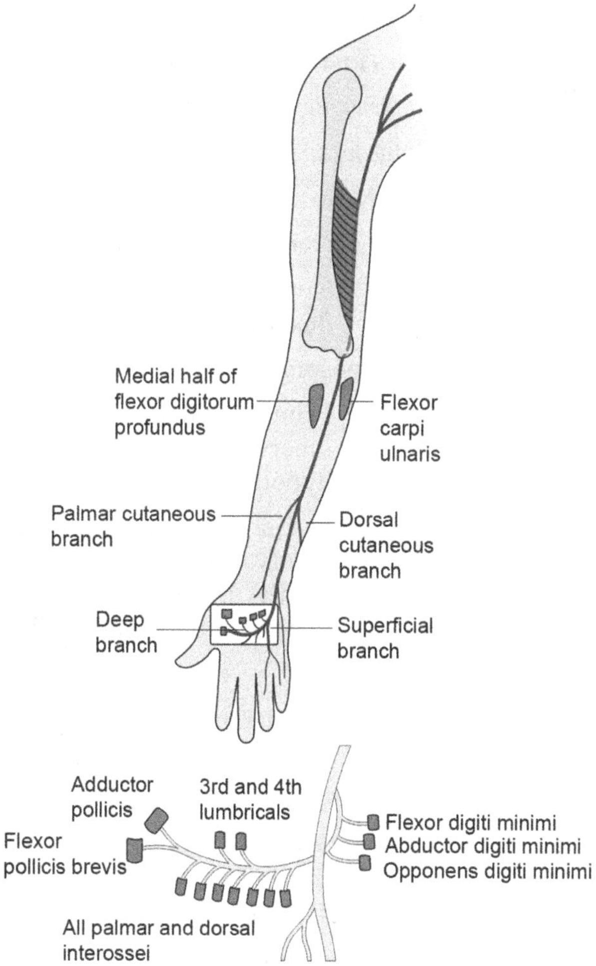

Fig. 15.2a: Ulnar nerve (Course and distribution)

Course:

- It enters the anterior compartment of arm along the medial side of the brachial artery.
- At the middle of the arm it pierces the medial intermuscular septum to enter the posterior compartment of the arm and runs downwards to the back of the medial epicondyle of humerus.
- It enters the forearm by passing between the two heads of flexor carpi ulnaris.
- In the upper 2/3rd it runs deep to flexor carpi ulnaris and then it becomes superficial and lies lateral to flexor carpi ulnaris. The nerve enters the palm by passing superficial to the flexor retinaculum and divides 3 into its terminal superficial and deep branches.

Branches and Distribution:

- *In the axilla and arm:* No branches.
- *In the forearm:*
  - Motor:
    - Nerve to flexor carpi ulnaris.
    - Nerve to medial half of the flexor digitorum profundus.
  - Sensory:
    - Palmar cutaneous branch innervates the skin over the hypothenar eminence.
    - Dorsal cutaneous branch innervates the skin over the medial 1/3rd of the dorsum of hand and medial 1½ digits.
- *In the palm:*
  - Superficial branch:
    - Motor: Nerve to palmaris brevis.
    - Sensory: Innervates skin on the palmar surface of medial 1½ digits.
  - Deep branch:
    - Purely motor: Supplies following muscles:
      - o Hypothenar muscles.
      - o Medial two lumbricals.
      - o All palmar and dorsal interossei.
      - o Adductor pollicis.

Applied Anatomy:

Ulnar nerve may get injured at the following sites: (Fig. 15.2b)

- *At elbow:* Due to fracture of medial condyle or entrapment between the two heads of flexor carpi ulnaris.

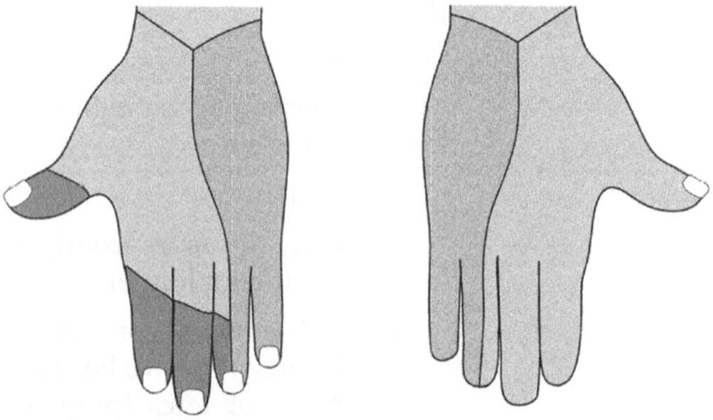

Fig. 15.2b: Area of sensory loss following injury to ulnar nerve

- *Injury at this site results in:*
  - Partial claw hand (Fig. 15.2c): Affects little and ring fingers. Hyperextension at their metacarpophalangeal joints and flexion at interphalangeal joints.

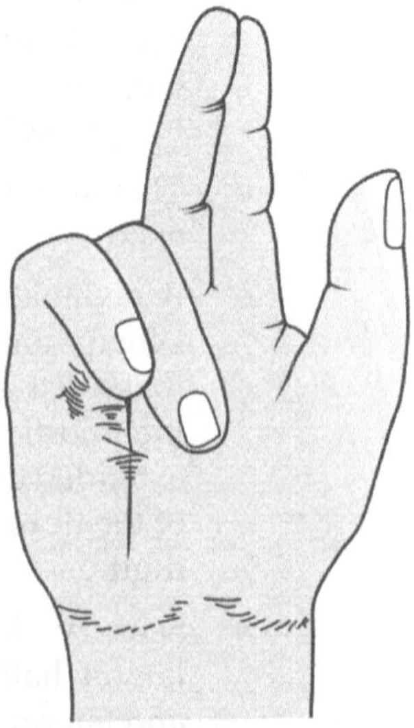

Fig.15.2c: Effect of ulnar nerve injury (Partial claw hand)

  - Flattening of hypothenar eminence.
  - Loss of abduction and adduction of fingers.
  - Loss of sensation over the palmar and dorsal surface of medial 1/3rd of hand and medial 1½ digits.
- *At wrist:* Its superficial position makes it vulnerable to cuts and wounds.
- *Injury at this site results in:*
  - Partial claw hand affecting little and ring fingers.
  - The deformity is more pronounced than the injury at elbow (ulnar paradox) because the medial half of flexor digitorum profundus is not paralysed, therefore, flexion at distal interphalangeal joint is more marked.
  - Loss of abduction and adduction of fingers.
  - Loss of sensation over the palmar surface of medial 1½ digits.
- *Complete claw hand:* Hyperextension at metacarpophalangeal joint and flexion at interphalangeal joints occurs due to paralysis of lumbricals and interossei muscles. It occurs due to:
  - Combined lesion of median and ulnar nerves.
  - Lesion of lower trunk (C_8 and T_1) of brachial plexus (Klumpke's paralysis).

VENOUS DRAINAGE OF UPPER LIMB

1. Describe briefly venous drainage of upper limb.

Ans. Venous drainage of upper limb:

- The venous drainage of the upper limb is composed of superficial and deep veins.
- The deep veins accompany the arteries.
- The deep veins are connected to the superficial veins by perforating veins.
- The superficial veins begin on the dorsum of the hand as dorsal venous arch.

a. **Cephalic vein:**
   - Begins on the radial side of the dorsal venous arch.
   - It ascends along the lateral aspect of the arm, runs in deltopectoral groove, then it pierces the deep fascia to enter the axillary vein just distal to the clavicle.

b. **Basilic vein:**
   - Begins on the medial side of the venous arch.
   - It then passes along the medial aspect of the forearm, pierces the deep fascia above the elbow and joins the venae comitantes of the brachial artery.

c. **Median cubital vein:** Links the cephalic and basilic veins in front of the elbow.
   - ***Importance of superficial veins of upper limb:***
     - *They are most commonly used for:*
       - Intravenous injections.
       - Blood transfusion.
       - Withdrawing blood for testing.

Median cubital vein is the vein of choice for venipuncture:
- Is prominent and easily accessible.
- Does not slip as it is connected to deep vein via perforator.
- Lies on bicipital aponeurosis which protects the underlying brachial artery and median nerve.

Basilic vein is preferred for inserting cardiac catheter to reach the right side of the heart.

CHAPTER 16

THE ARTERIES OF UPPER LIMB

Five primary vessels provide the upper limb's arterial feed (proximal to distal):

- Subclavian artery.
- Axillary artery.
- Brachial artery.
- Radial artery.
- Ulnar artery.

SUBCLAVIAN ARTERY

The subclavian artery is the first arterial branch which begins to supply the upper limb. The brachiocephalic trunk, on the right, gives rise to the subclavian artery. The subclavian artery directly branches off from aortic arch on the left.

In relation to the scalenes anterior muscle, it can be divided into three parts:

- **First part:** From the initiation of the subclavian artery to the medial border of the scalenes anterior muscle.
- **Second part:** Posterior to the scalenes anterior muscle.
- **Third part:** Lateral border of scalenes anterior muscle to the lateral border of the first rib.

The subclavian artery, now known as the axillary artery, as soon as it enters the axilla along the side of the first rib.

AXILLARY ARTERY (Fig. 16.1)

The axillary artery which is related to pectoralis minor lies in axillary sheath, a fibrous layer that covers the artery and the three cords of the brachial plexus.

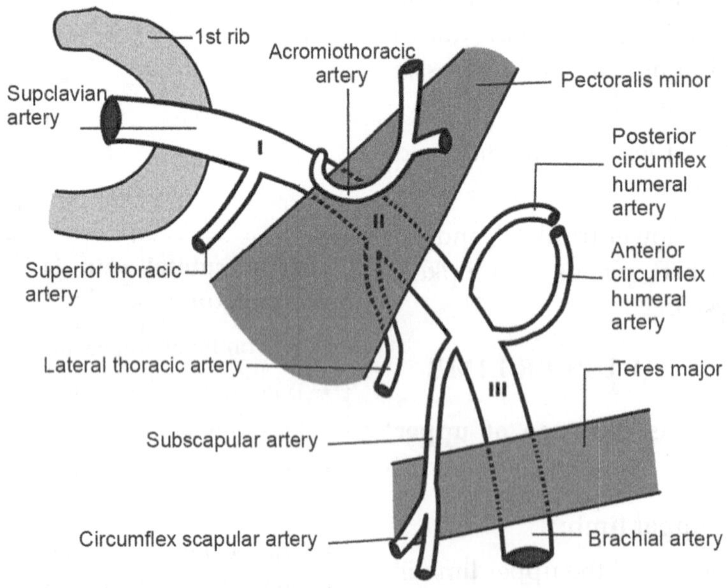

Fig. 16.1: Axillary artery

The artery, which is significant, can be divided into three parts according on where it lies in relation to the pectoralis minor muscle:

- **First part:** Proximal to pectoralis minor.
- **Second part:** Posterior to pectoralis minor.
- **Third part:** Distal to pectoralis minor.

The main branches of the axillary artery include:

First part: Superior thoracic artery.

Second part: Thoracoacromial artery and Lateral thoracic artery.

Third part: Subscapular artery, anterior and posterior circumflex humeral arteries.

The anterior and posterior circumflex humeral arteries form an anastomotic network around the surgical neck of the humerus and can be injured in cases of fracture.

At the lower border of the teres major muscle, the axillary artery continues as brachial artery.

Axillary Artery Aneurysm

A dilatation of the arterial to a size greater than double its initial value is known as an aneurysm. It is an uncommon yet significant disorder that could threaten the arteries in the upper limb. The brachial plexus may be compressed by the dilated axillary artery, resulting in neurological symptoms as paraesthesia and muscle weakness. Surgery is the only effective treatment for an axillary artery aneurysm. It entails removing the aneurysm and utilising a vascular graft to rebuild the artery wall.

BRACHIAL ARTERY (Fig. 16.2)

After the axillary artery crosses the teres major's lower border, the brachial artery continues. It is the arm's main blood vessel. The profunda brachii (deep artery), which travels with the radial nerve in the radial groove of the humerus and nourishes structures in the posterior region of the upper arm, originates from the brachial artery just distal to the teres major. By contributing to the anastomotic network surrounding the elbow joint, the profunda brachii terminates.

The actual brachial artery runs down the length of the arm. The brachial artery ends by dividing into the radial and ulnar arteries as it passes through the cubital fossa, beneath the bicipital aponeurosis.

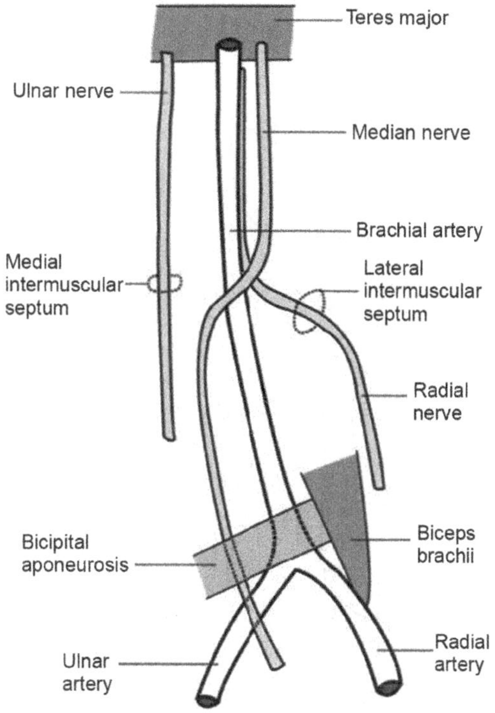

Fig. 16.2: Brachial artery

Occlusion or Laceration of the Brachial Artery

The anastomotic supply to the arm is comparatively good. This indicates that it is adequately guarded against ischaemia in situations where the brachial artery is temporarily or partially blocked. However, the ischaemia that results if the artery is totally blocked (or cut) can result in forearm muscle necrosis. Scar tissue significantly shortens and replaces muscle fibers, which might result in Volkmann's ischemic contracture, a distinctive flexion deformity.

FOREARM: RADIAL AND ULNAR ARTERIES (Figs. 16.3 and 16.4)

The brachial artery divides into two at the level of the neck of radius in the cubital fossa, forming the radial and ulnar arteries.

- The posterolateral portion of the forearm is supplied by the radial artery. It serves the anastomotic networks that encircle the wrist and carpal bones. *In the distal forearm, directly lateral to the prominent tendon of the flexor carpi radialis muscle, the radial pulse can be felt.*
- The anteromedial portion of the forearm is supplied by the ulnar artery. It also serves the anastomotic network that encircles the elbow joint. Additionally, it gives branches namely, the anterior and posterior interosseous arteries, which nourish the deeper structures of forearm.

The superficial palmar arch and the deep palmar arch are formed in the hand by the anastomosis of these two arteries.

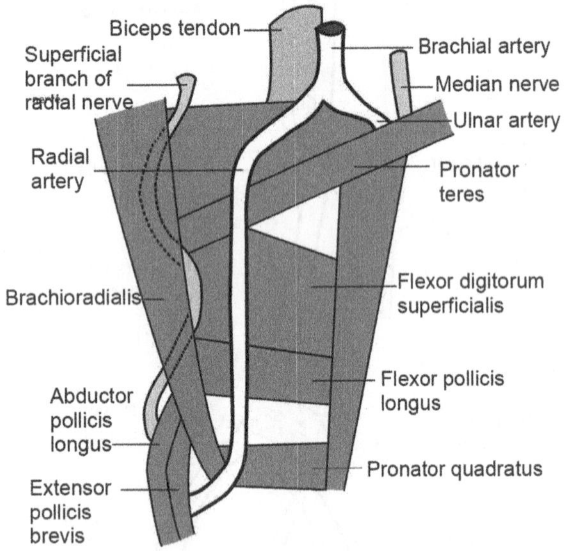

Fig. 16.3: Radial artery

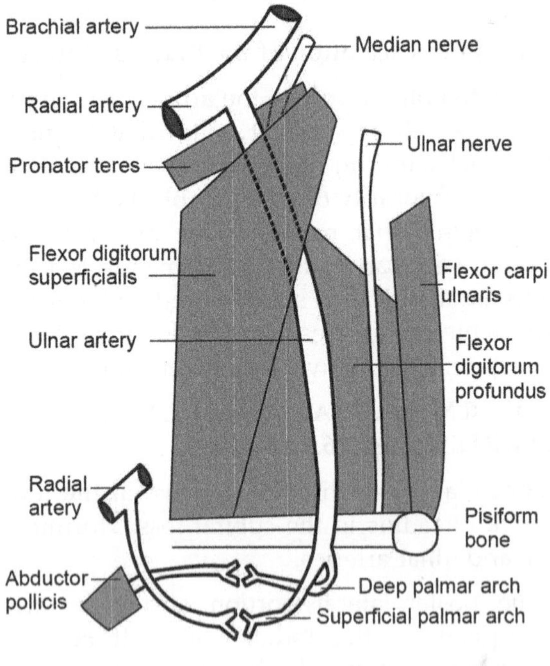

Fig. 16.4: Ulnar artery

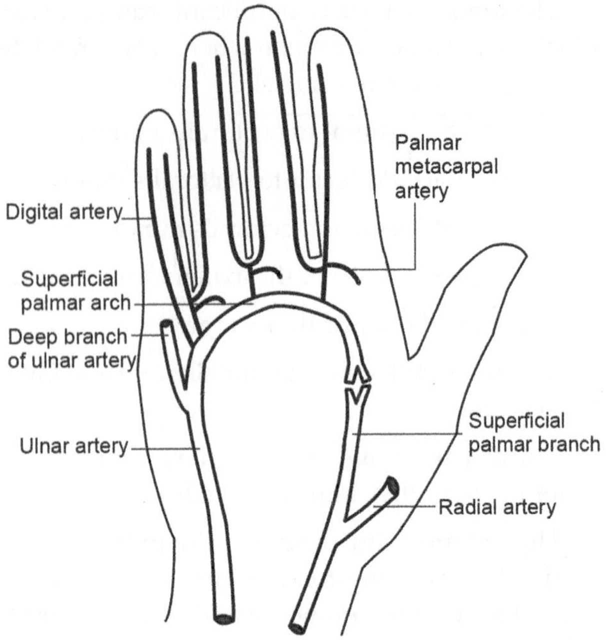

Fig. 16.5: Superficial palmar arch

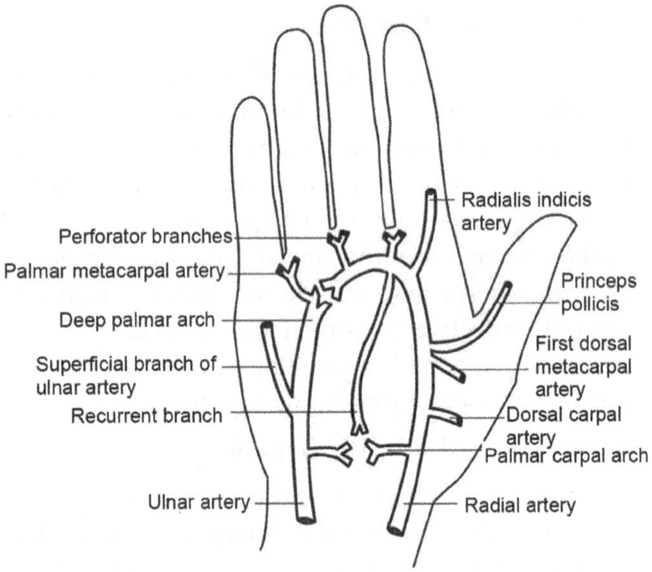

Fig. 16.6: Deep palmar arch

HAND: SUPERFICIAL AND DEEP PALMAR ARCHES (Figs. 16.5 and 16.6)

With numerous anastomoses between the vessels, the hand receives a sufficient vascular supply. This enables the hand to still be perfused despite considerable flow resistance (such as when grasping or applying pressure).

The ulnar and radial arteries are the first vessels to supply the hand's arteries with blood. The ulnar artery enters the hand lateral to the ulnar nerve and prior to the flexor retinaculum. It gives rise to the deep palmar branch and continues laterally as the superficial palmar arch across the palm.

The radial artery crosses the anatomical snuffbox's floor when it enters the hand dorsally. After that, it takes a medial turn and passes between the adductor pollicis muscle's heads. The thumb, index finger are all supplied by a branch of the radial artery and radial artery also contributes to superficial palmar arch. The radial artery subsequently continues as the deep palmar arch.

Two vascular arches are formed as a result:

- **Superficial palmar arch**, which is deep to the palmar aponeurosis and anterior to the hand's flexor tendons. The digital arteries that supply the four fingers are generated from it.
- **Deep palmar arch**, which is located deep to hand's flexor tendons. It assists in supplying blood to the wrist joint and digits.

17 CHAPTER THORACIC WALL

1. **Write vertebral level of the following:**
    a. **Jugular notch**
    b. **Sternal angle**
    c. **Xiphisternal joint**
    d. **Tip of ninth costal cartilage**
    e. **Lowest extent of costal margin**

Ans. **Vertebral levels:**
    a. *Jugular notch*–disc between T2 and T3.
    b. *Sternal angle*–disc between T4 and T5.
    c. *Xiphisternal joint*–disc between T8 and T9.
    d. *Tip of ninth costal cartilage*–L1.
    e. *Lowest extent of costal margin*–L3.

2. **Enumerate the following:**
    a. **Boundaries of superior thoracic aperture (thoracic inlet)**
    b. **Structures passing through the thoracic inlet**
    c. **Contents of atypical intercostals space**
    d. **Intrinsic muscles of the thoracic wall**
    e. **Branches of atypical intercostals nerve**
    f. **Arteries supplying thoracic wall**
    g. **Structures at the level of sternal angle**

Ans. a. **Boundaries of superior thoracic aperture (thoracic inlet):**
- Posteriorly the first thoracic vertebra.
- *Laterally:* The first pair of ribs and their costal cartilage.
- *Anteriorly:* Superior border of the manubrium.

b. **Structures that pass through the superior thoracic aperture include:**
- Trachea.
- Oesophagus.
- Thoracic duct.
- *Nerves:*
    - Phrenic nerve.
    - Vagus nerve.
    - Left recurrent laryngeal nerves.
    - Sympathetic trunks.
- ***Vessels***
    - *Arteries*
        - Left and right common carotid arteries.
        - Left and right subclavian arteries.
    - *Veins*
        - Internal jugular veins.
        - Brachiocephalic veins.
        - Subclavian veins.
- Lymph nodes and lymphatic vessels.

c. **Contents of atypical intercostals space:**
- Intercostal muscles (external, internal and innermost intercostals).
- Intercostal nerve and its branches.
- Anterior and posterior intercostals arteries.
- Anterior and posterior intercostals veins.

The neurovascular bundle in the intercostals space lies in the costal groove of rib between the internal intercost and innermost intercostals muscles. It is arranged in the following order from above downwards:
- Intercostals vein
- Intercostal artery
- Intercostal nerve

} VAN

d. **Intrinsic muscles of thoracic wall:**
   - External intercostals (outer layer).
   - Internal intercostals (intermediate layer).
   - Innermost intercostals
   - Sternocostalis
   - Subcostalis

   (Innermost intercostals, Sternocostalis, Subcostalis: Inner layer)

e. **Branches of atypical intercostals nerve (3rd – 6th intercostal nerves):**
   - ***Two communicating branches (white and gray ramus)*** which connect it to the corresponding sympathetic ganglion.
   - ***Muscular branches:***
     – Number of muscular branches that supply intercostal muscles, subcostalis and sternocostalis.
     – Collateral branch that supply parietal pleura and periosteum of rib besides supplying intercostal muscles.
   - ***Cutaneous branches:***
     – Lateral cutaneous branch (reaches skin by piecing muscles at midaxillary line and divides into anterior and posterior branches).
     – Anterior cutaneous branch (reaches skin by piecing muscles about 1 cm lateral to the sternum and divides into medial and lateral branches.

f. **Arteries supplying thoracic wall:**
   - Superior intercostal artery (a branch of costocervical trunk from the second part of subclavian trunk) gives posterior intercostal arteries first two intercostal spaces.
   - Two anterior intercostal arteries for each intercostal space (in upper six intercostal spaces they are direct branches of internal thoracic artery (ITA) and in 7th, 8th and 9th they arise from musculophrenic artery, a branch of ITA, 10th and 11th intercostal spaces don't have anterior intercostal arteries).
   - Posterior intercostal arteries (for 3rd to 11th intercostal space they arise from descending thoracic aorta).

g. **Structures at the level of sternal angle:**
   - Ascending aorta ends.
   - Arch of aorta begins and ends.
   - Descending aorta begins.
   - Trachea bifurcates into right and left principal bronchii.
   - Pulmonary trunk divides into right and left pulmonary arteries.
   - Azygous veins drains into superior vena cava.
   - Upper border of heart lies at this level.

Sternal angle (angle of Louis) which can be easily palpated is used for counting ribs. The second costal cartilage articulates with sternum at this level.

2. **Draw labeled diagram of the following:**
   a. **Structures passing through the thoracic inlet (transverse section)**
   b. **Typical intercostals space**
   c. **Typical intercostals nerve**
   d. **Azygous system of veins**

Ans. a. **Structures passing through the thoracic inlet (transverse section) (Fig. 17.1).**
   b. **Typical intercostals space (Fig. 17.2).**
   c. **Typical intercostals nerve (Fig. 17.3).**
   d. **Azygous system of veins (Fig. 17.4).**

3. **Enumerate the factors responsible for the increase in various diameters of the thoracic cavity during inspiration.**

Ans. During inspiration the volume of thoracic cavity increases to allow expansion of lungs. The following factors are responsible for increase in the diameters of thoracic cavity:
   - **Vertical** diameter is increased by contraction of diaphragm.
   - **Anteroposterior** diameter is increased by anterior movement of sternum due to elevation of vertebrosternal (1st-7th) ribs (Pump handle movement).
   - **Transverse** diameter is increased due to elevation of vertebrochondral (8th, 9th and 10th) ribs (bucket handle movement).

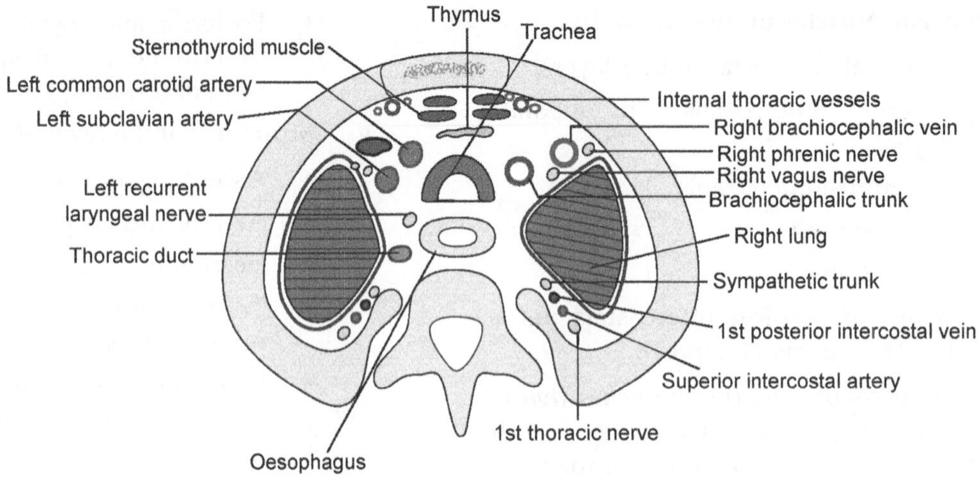

Fig. 17.1: Thoracic inlet

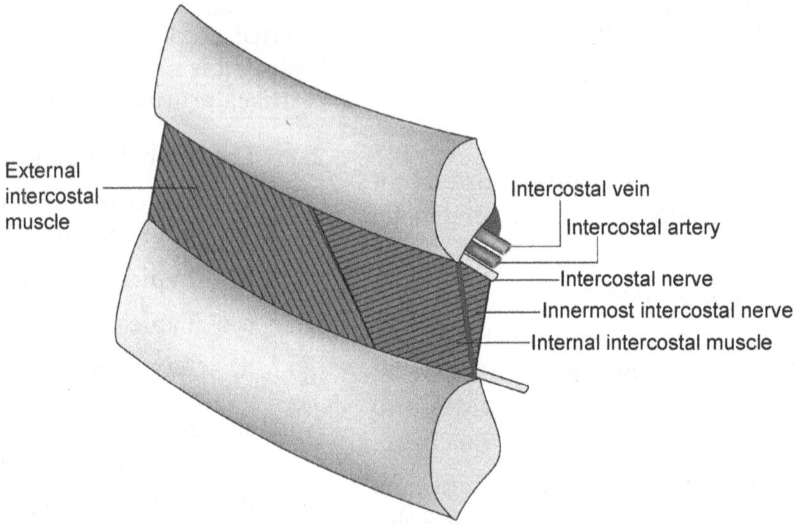

Fig. 17.2: Typical intercostals space

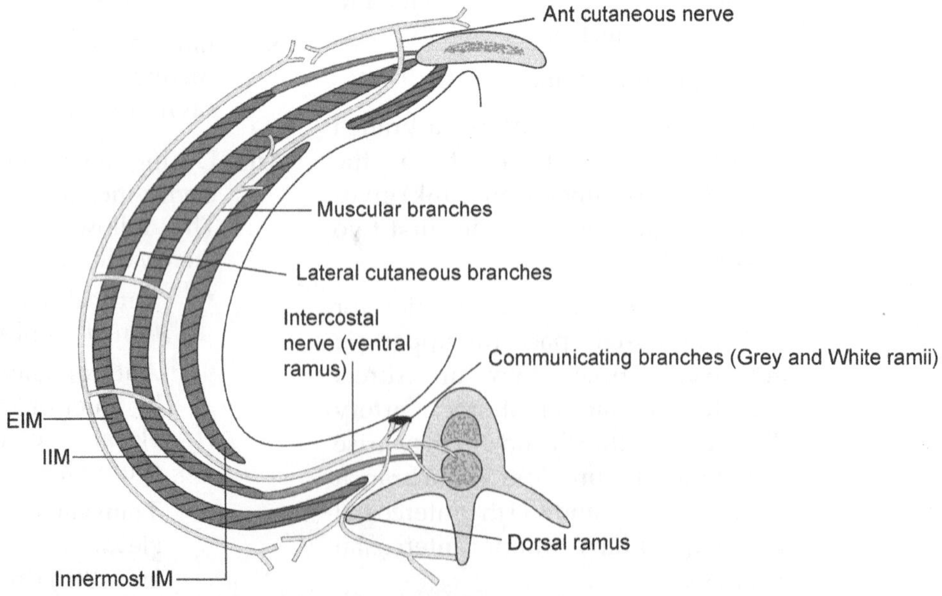

Fig. 17.3: Course and branches of typical intercostals nerve

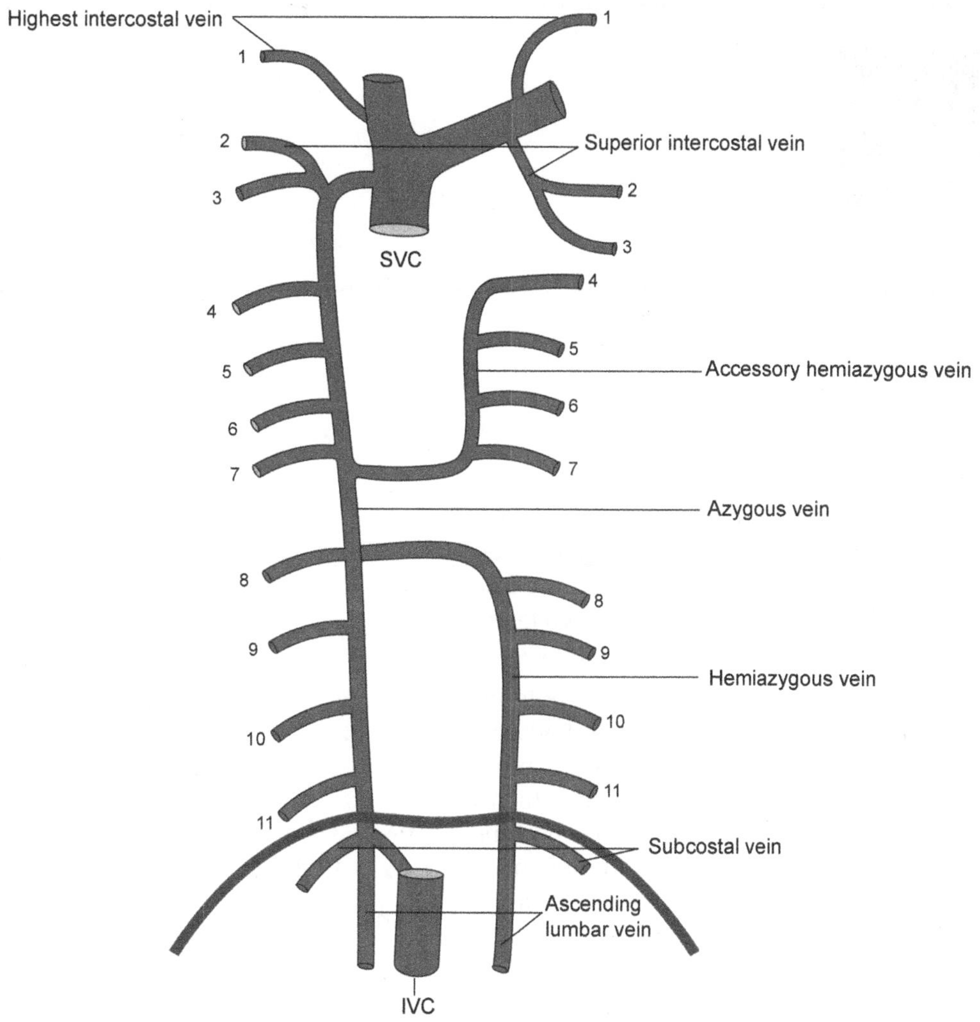

Fig. 17.4: Azygous system of veins

4. **Name the muscles that act during inspiration and expiration.**

Ans. See following Table.

	Inspiration	*Expiration*
Quite respiration	• Diaphragm • External intercostal muscles	• Passive diaphragm and intercostals relax
Forced respiration	• Diaphragm and intercostals • Sternocleidomastoid • Scalene muscles (raise 1st and 2nd ribs) • Pectoralis major (when arm is fixed) • Levator scapulae, trapezius and rhomboids major and minor (fix and elevate scapula) • Quadratus lumborum (fixes last rib)	• Anterior abdominal wall muscles • Internal intercostals • Serratus posterior muscles

18
CHAPTER

PLEURA

1. **Define:**
   a. **Pleura**
   b. **Pleural cavity**

Ans. a. **Pleura** is a serous membrane lined by mesothelium (simple squamous epithelium) that is present as a closed sac around the lungs. It comprises two layers, outer parietal and inner visceral layer.

b. **Pleural cavity** is a closed potential space between the parietal and visceral layers of pleura. It normally contains only a thin film of serous fluid which is secreted by the pleura. The space becomes apparent if there is accumulation of air (pneumothorax), blood (haemothorax) or pus (empyema).

2. **What are the characteristic features of:**
   a. **Parietal pleura**
   b. **Visceral pleura**

Ans. a. **Characteristic features of parietal pleura:**
- It is the inner layer of the two layers of pleura.
- It is tightly adherent to the outer surface of lung.
- It also lines the fissures of the lung.
- It does not cover the hilum of the lung and the area along which pulmonary ligament is attached.
- It develops from the splanchnopleuric layer of the mesoderm.
- It is innervated by the autonomic nervous system and is therefore pain insensitive.
- It is continuous with the parietal layer at the root of lung.

b. **Characteristic features of visceral pleura:**
- It is the outer layer of the two layers.
- It lines the corresponding half of the thoracic wall separated from it by endothoracic fascia (areolar tissue), covers the thoracic surface of diaphragm and the mediastinum.
- It develops from the somatopleuric layer of the mesoderm.
- It innervates by the somatic nervous system and is therefore sensitive to pain.

3. **What are the various subdivisions of parietal pleura?**

Ans. Parietal pleura is given different names that correspond to the structures with which it is associated.

a. **Cervical:** Dome shaped pleura extending into the neck (summit is 2.5 cm above).

b. **Costal:** Lines the ribs and intercostal spaces.

c. **Diaphragmatic:** Pleura covering the diaphragm.

d. **Mediastinal:** Pleura covering the mediastinum.

> Sites where the parietal pleura extends beyond the thoracic cage and is in danger of being injured.
> - Above the medial 1/3rd of the clavicle on both the sides.
> - Beyond the right xiphicostal angle.
> - Below costovertebral angle on both the sides.

4. **Draw labeled diagram to show the costomediastinal, costodiaphragmatic and costovertebral lines of reflection of parietal pleura and surface marking of pleura and lungs.**

Ans. See Figure 18.1a and Figure 18.1b.

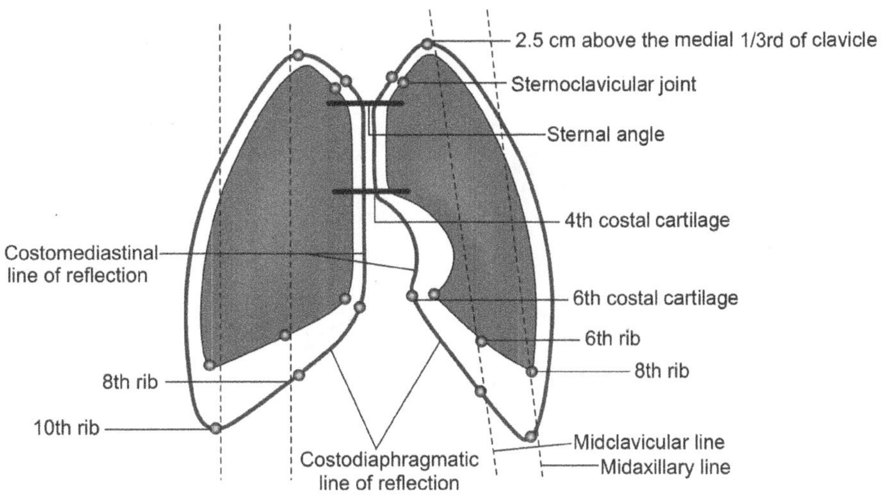

Fig. 18.1a: Costomediastinal and costodiaphragmatic lines of pleural reflection and surface marking of lungs and pleura

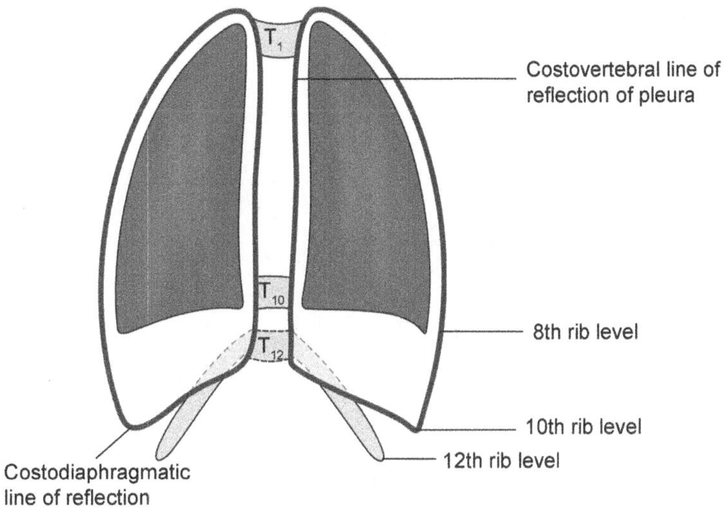

Fig. 18.1b: Costovertebral and costodiaphragmatic lines of pleural reflection and surface marking of lungs and pleura

5. **Describe briefly:**
   a. **Pulmonary ligament**
   b. **Pleural recesses**
   c. **Nerve supply of pleura**

Ans. a. **Pulmonary ligament:** The narrow fold of parietal pleura that extend below the root of lung. Functions of the pulmonary ligament are:

- Allows the descent of structures of root of lung during inspiration.
- Provides dead space into which pulmonary vein can expand during increased venous return (e.g., during exercise).

b. **Pleural recesses:** Anterior and inferior regions of pleural cavities are normally not occupied by the lungs. In these regions, the two layers of parietal pleura are opposed to each other resulting in formation of recesses. These recesses allow expansion of lungs inspiration. The recesses of the pleura are:

- Right and left costodiaphragmatic recesses (Fig. 18.2a).
- Right and left costomediastinal recesses (Fig. 18.2b).
  - *Costodiaphragmatic recess:*
    - Is the largest and clinically most important recesses.

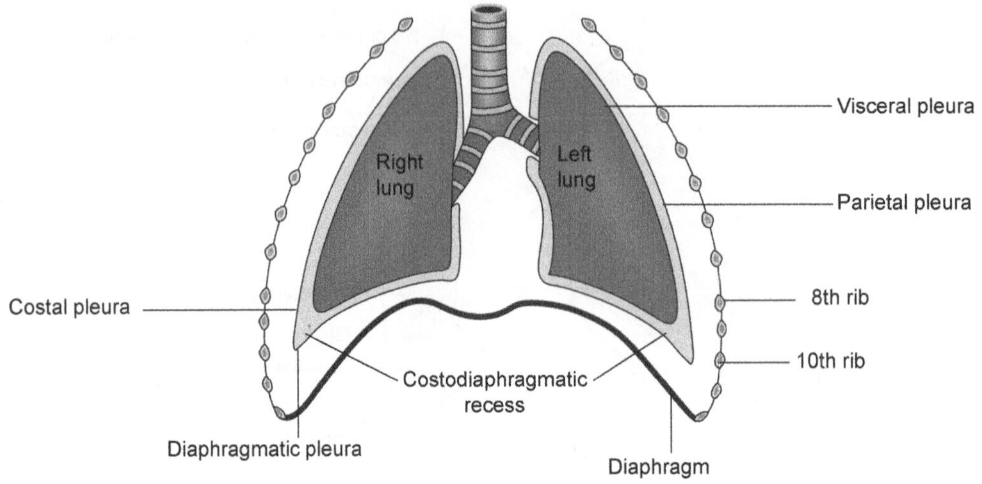

Fig. 18.2a: Costodiaphragmatic recess

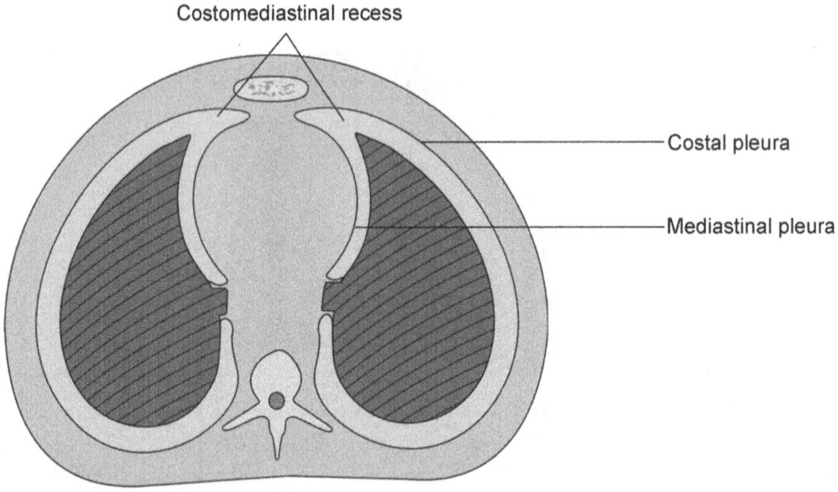

Fig. 18.2b: Costomediastinal recess

- Is present between the costal and diaphragmatic parts of parietal pleura.
- Is C-shaped and present between the inferior margins of the lungs and the inferior margin of the pleural cavities.
- The maximum vertical distance is 5 cm along the midaxillary line opposite to 8th–10th ribs.
- Is the most dependent part of the pleural cavity and therefore the fluid of pleural effusions first collect here.

– *Costomediastinal recess:*

- Is present anteriorly between the costal and mediastinal pleura.
- The left costomediastinal recess is larger due to the presence of cardiac notch along the anterior border of the left lung.

c. **Nerve supply of pleura:**

- ***Parietal pleura:*** Is pain sensitive.
  - *Costal and peripheral part of diaphragmatic pleura*–Intercostal nerves.
  - *Mediastinal and central part of diaphragmatic pleura*–Phrenic nerve.

- ***Visceral pleura:*** Is insensitive to pain.
  - *Is supplied by autonomic (sympathetic) nerves* –T_2 –T_5.

In inflammation of the mediastinal and central part of diaphragmatic pleura, the pain is referred to the root of neck and the shoulder region as their parts of pleura are supplied by phrenic nerve (C3, C4, C5) and the skin at the above mentioned sites is innervated by the same spinal segments via supraclavicular nerves (C3, C4). When lower costal or peripheral part of diaphragmatic pleura are affected, the pain may be referred to the anterolateral abdominal wall along the distribution of lower intercostal nerves which also innervate the anterior abdominal wall.

6. **Describe briefly the following:**
   a. **Pleurisy or Pleuritis**
   b. **Pleural tap**
   c. **Pneumothorax**
   d. **Pleural effusions**

Ans. a. **Pleurisy or Pleuritis:** Pleurisy is inflammation of the pleural membranes. The condition is very painful especially when a person takes deep breath. During respiratory movements, the parietal and visceral layers slide past other. Normally the pleural fluid in the pleural cavities lubricates the surfaces of these membranes. When the pleural membranes are inflamed, their surfaces become rough, the rough surfaces rub against each other and produce pain. Due to the friction between the two layers of pleura during the respiratory movements, pleural rub can be with the stethoscope.

b. **Pleural tap:** It is aspiration of pleural effusion from the pleural cavity. It is usually done in the 6th intercostal space in the midaxillary line. The needle is inserted just above the upper border of the rib in the lower part of the intercostal space to avoid injury to the intercostal nerves and vessels. The needle should not be inserted below the 9th intercostal space, lest it may injure the spleen on the left side and liver on the right side.

c. **Pneumothorax:** Presence of air in the pleural cavity is known as pneumothorax. The increased air pressure in the pleural cavity may result in the collapse of the lung. It could be caused due to the penetrating thoracic wound, spontaneous rupture of pulmonary bulla (spontaneous pneumothorax), fractures rib, anaesthetist's needle puncturing the pleura during stellate ganglion block, in making a loin incision kidney, to perfom adrenalectomy or to drain a subphrenic abscess.

Tension pneumothorax is a condition in which the ruptured tissues of thoracic wall form a valve that permits air to enter the pleural cavity upon inspiration, but does not allow air to escape during expiration and therefore greatly increases the pressure inside and pushing the mediastinal structures to the opposite side.

d. **Pleural effusions:** The excessive accumulation of fluid in the pleural cavity is called pleural effusion. It is usually due to inflammation of the pleura. The progressive accumulation of fluid may cause retraction of lung towards the hilum and may displace the mediastinum to the opposite side. The fluid may be in the form of:

- Blood – Haemothorax.
- Pus – Pyothorax/empyema.
- Lymph – Chylothorax.

19

CHAPTER

LUNGS

1. **Describe lungs under the following headings:**
   a. **Gross features**
   b. **Fissures and lobes**
   c. **Root of lung**

Ans. a. **Gross features:** Each lung has: (Fig. 19.1a and Fig. 19.1b)

- *Apex:*
  - Is blunt.
  - Extends into the neck, an inch above the medial 1/3rd of the clavicle.
  - Is covered by cervical pleura and suprapleural membrane.
  - Is related anteriorly to the subclavian artery and scalenus anterior muscle.
  - Is related posteriorly to the neck of the 1st rib.

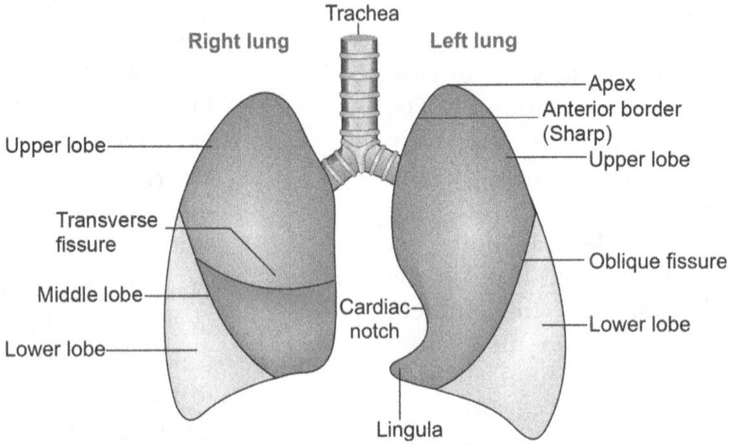

Fig. 19.1a: Gross features of right and left lungs (anterior aspect)

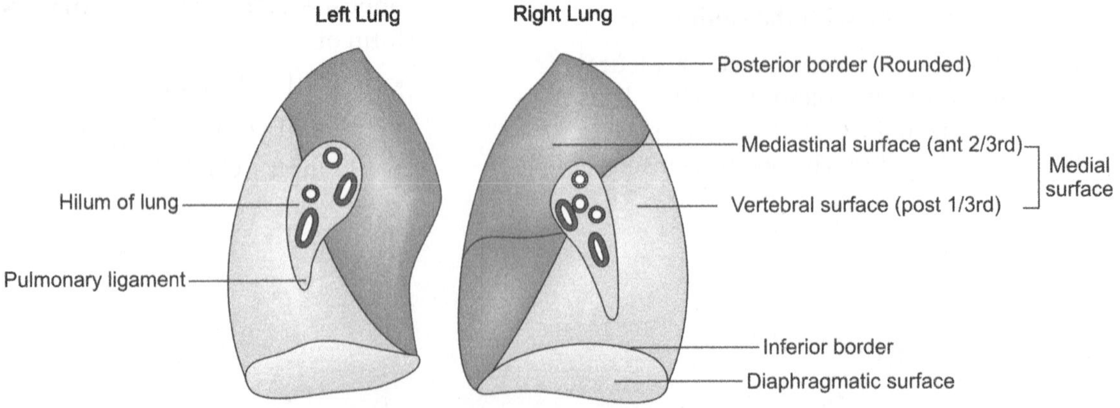

Fig. 19.1b: Gross features of right and left lungs (medial aspect)

- *Base:*
  - Is semilunar and concave.
  - Is related to the dome of the diaphragm.
  - On the right side it is separated from the liver by the right dome of the diaphragm.
  - On the left side it is separated from the fundus of the stomach and spleen by left dome of diaphragm.
- *Borders:*
  - *Anterior:* Is sharp and shorter than the posterior boder.
    * Anterior border of left side presents a concave CARDIAC NOTCH and the tongue shaped projection below the cardiac notch is LINGULA.
  - ***Posterior:*** Is thick and rounded.
  - ***Inferior:*** Is semilunar in shape.
- *Surfaces:*
  - *Costal:* Is covex and is related to ribs and intercostals.
  - *Medial:* Is divided into two parts:
    - ◆ Mediastinal: Anterior 2/3rd of medial surface. Is related to the mediastinal structures.
    - ◆ Vertebral: Posterior 1/3rd of medial surface. Is related to vertebral bodies and intervertebral discs.

b. **Fissures and lobes:**

- ***Right lung has:***
  - *Two fissures* – Oblique and transverse/horizontal.
  - *Three lobes* – Superior, middle and inferior.
- ***Left lung has:***
  - *One fissure* – Oblique.
  - *Two lobes* – Superior and inferior.

c. **Root of lung:**

- Lung root consists of the structures passing to and from the hilum of the lung to the mediastinum.
- Lung roots lie opposite to T5 – T7 vertebrae.
- The structures of the lung root are embedded in the connective tissue and surrounded by extension of mediastinal pleura. Following structures are present in the lung root:
  - Principal bronchus in the left lung and eparterial and hyparterial bronchi in the right lung.
  - Pulmonary artery.
  - Superior and inferior pulmonary veins.
  - Bronchial arteries (one on the right side and two on the left side).
  - Bronchial veins.
  - Nerves (anterior and posterior pulmonary plexus).
  - Lymphatics from the lung.

> Lung roots move downward and forward in full inspiration to allow expansion of the posterior part of the lung.

2. **Enumerate the differences between:**
   a. **Fetal and adult lung**
   b. **Right and left lung**

Ans. a. Differences between fetal and adult lung

S. No.	*Fetal lung*	*Adult lung*
1.	Solid	Porus
2.	Sinks in water	Float in water
3.	Does not crepitate on touch	Crepitates on touch
4.	Colour-pink	Colour-Grey to mottled black (due to deposition of carbon)
5.	No air in alveoli	Air in alveoli

b. Differences between right and left lung

S. No.	*Right lung*	*Left lung*
1.	Shorter	Longer
2.	Wider	Longer
3.	Heavier	Lighter
4.	Usually has two fissures–oblique and transverse	Usually has one fissure–oblique
5.	Has usually three lobes–Superior, middle and inferior	Has usually two lobes–Superior and inferior
6.	Anterior border is straight	Anterior border has a concave cardiac notch
7.	Base is more concave (higher dome of diaphragm due to liver below it).	Base is less concave

3. **Define hilum of lung and enumerate the important structures passing through the hilum of right and left lungs:**
   a. **From above downwards**
   b. **From before backwards**

Ans. a. From above downwards:

Right lung	*Left lung*
Eparterial bronchus	Pulmonary artery
Pulmonary artery	Principal bronchus
Hyparterial bronchus Inferior pulmonary vein	Inferior pulmonary vein

b. **From before backwards:** Superior pulmonary vein, Pulmonary artery, Bronchus.

4. **Draw labeled diagram of the following:**
   a. **Hilum of right and left lungs**
   b. **Mediastinal surface of right and left lung**

Ans. a. **See Figure 19.2.**
   b. **See Figure 19.3a and Figure 19.3b.**

5. **Describe bronchopulmonary segment under the following headings:**
   a. **Definition**
   b. **Characteristic features**
   c. **Nomenclature**
   d. **Clinical significance**

Ans. a. Definition: Bronchopulmonary segment is a wedge shaped self contained functionally independent respiratory unit of lung which is aerated by tertiary or segmental bronchus (Fig. 19.4).

b. **Characteristic features:**
- Is pyramidal in shape with apex directed towards the hilum and base towards the surface of the lung.
- Each segment is separated from the adjacent segments by connective tissue.
- Segmental/tertiary bronchus with bronchial vessels and a branch of

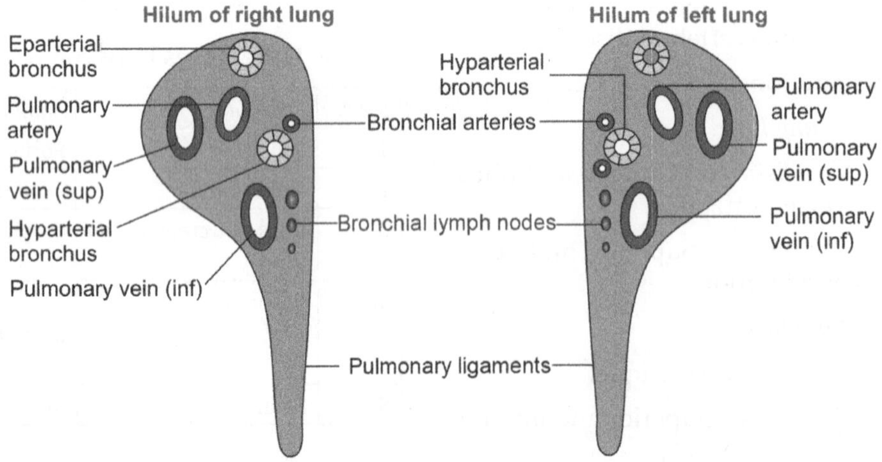

Fig. 19.2: Structures passing through the hilum of the right and left lungs

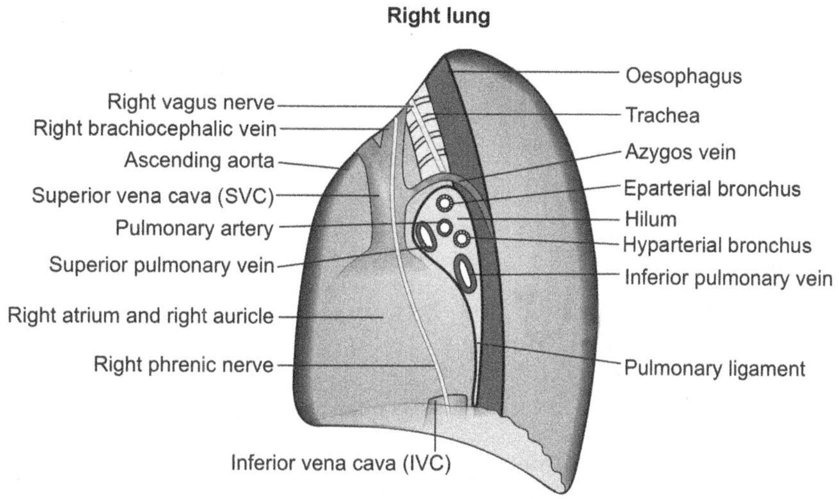

Fig. 19.3a Structures related to the mediastinal surface of right lung

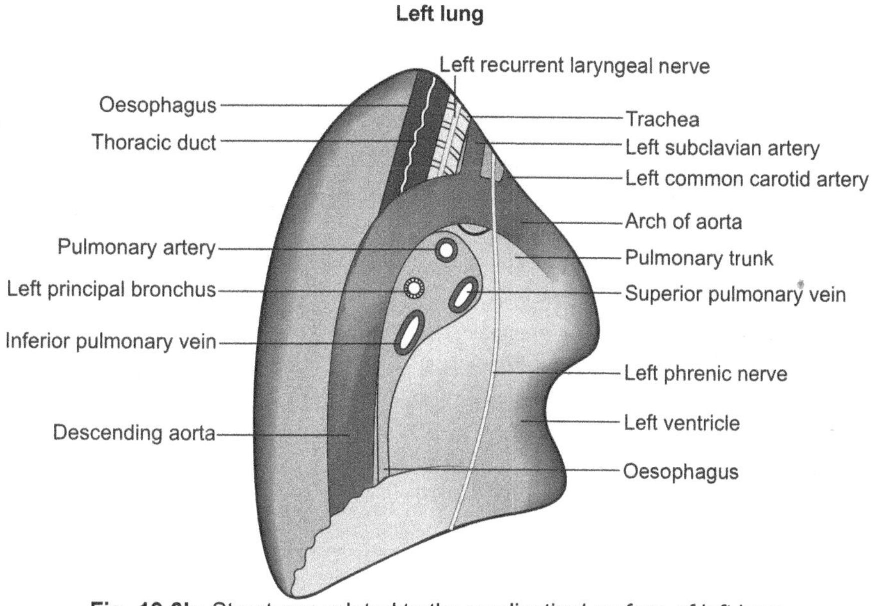

Fig. 19.3b: Structures related to the mediastinal surface of left lung

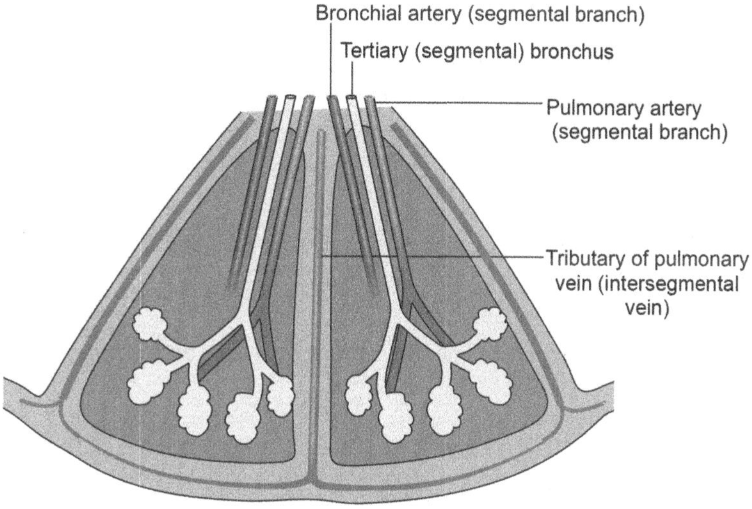

Fig. 19.4: Two adjacent bronchopulmonary segments

pulmonary artery accompanying it are central in position.

- There is little anastomosis between the arteries of adjacent segments.
- Tributaries of pulmonary vein are intersegmental running in the connective tissue septa.
- Intersegmental veins act as guide for separating the segments during surgical resection.

c. **Nomenclature:**

- There are 10 bronchopulmonary segments in each lung (Fig. 19.5).

Right lung	*Left lung*
A. Superior lobe	**A. Superior lobe**
1. Apical 2. Posterior 3. Anterior	1. Apical 2. Posterior 3. Anterior 4. Superior lingular 5. Inferior lingular
B. Middle lobe	
4. Lateral 5. Medial	
C. Inferior lobe	**B. Inferior lobe**
6. Apical 7. Medial basal 8. Anterior basal 9. Lateral basal 10. Posterior basal	6. Apical 7. Medial basal 8. Anterior basal 9. Lateral basal 10. Posterior basal

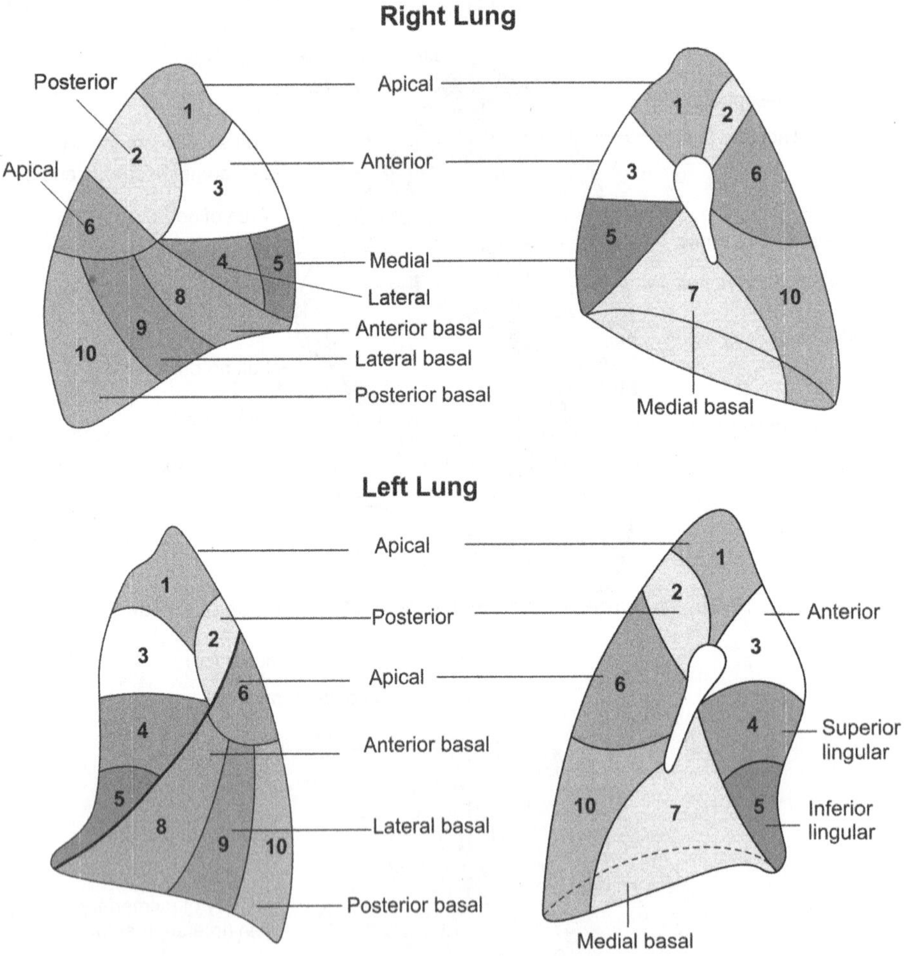

Fig.19.5: Bronchopulmonary segments of right and left lungs

d. **Clinical significance:**

- The connective tissue septa between the adjacent bronchopulmonary segments acts as a natural barrier and prevents spread of infection between the segments.

  * Carcinoma and tuberculosis break through the barrier.
- The knowledge of bronchopulmonary segments helps in:
  - Performing bronchoscopy.
  - Correct interpretation of bronchogram.
  - Understanding why abscessors are more common in some segments.
    - Posterior segment of upper lobe.
    - Apical segment of the lower lobe.
  - Natural drainage from the infected segment by adopting different postures, e.g., for drainage of apical segment of the lower lobe the patient should be asked to lay prone with head turned to one side.

6. **Describe briefly:**

   a. **Nerve supply of lungs**

   b. **Lymphatic drainage of lungs**

Ans. a. **Nerve supply of lungs:**

Lungs are supplied by autonomic nervous system. Sympathetic and parasympathetic fibers form anterior and posterior pulmonary plexuses in the roots of the lungs before supplying it.

- ***Sympathetic fibers are:***
  - Derived from T2–T5 spinal segments.
  - Bronchodilator.
  - Vasomotor.
  - Inhibitor of secretions from the glands of bronchial tree.

* Sympathomimetic drugs such as epinephrine cause bronchodilation and relieve bronchial asthma (bronchospasm).

- ***Parasympathetic fibers are:***
  - Derived from the vagus nerves.
  - Bronchoconstrictor.
  - Secretomotor.

  * Also carry afferent (sensory) fibers which are sensitive to stretch and play important role in reflex control of respiration.

b. **Lymphatic drainage of lungs:**

Lymph from the lungs is drained by two sets of lymph vessels.

- ***Superficial lymph vessels:***
  - Drain the peripheral lung tissue.
  - Form the superficial (subpleural) plexus beneath the pleura.
  - Pass around the borders and fissures of lungs to drain into the *bronchopulmonary lymph nodes* at the hilum.
- ***Deep lymph vessels:***
  - Drain the bronchial tree.
  - Begin from the submucosa of bronhii.
  - Form deep plexus around the bronchii and first drain into *pulmonary lymph nodes* located within lungs around lobar bronchii.

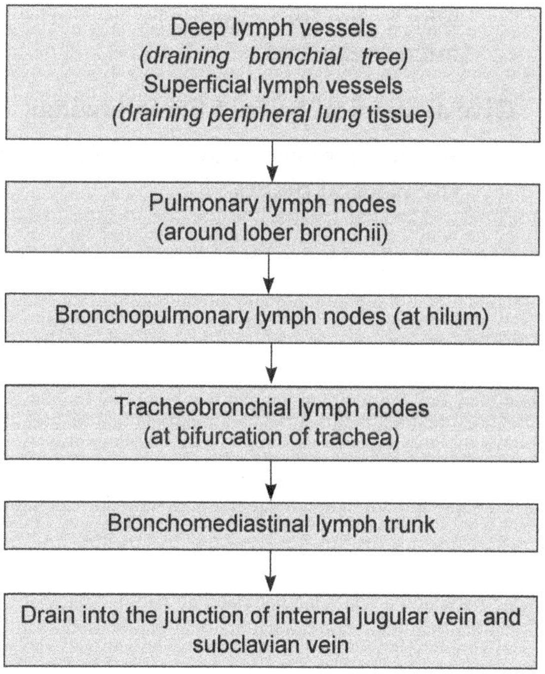

Flowchart: Showing lymphatic drainage

- Finally from pulmonary lymph nodes the lymph is drained into *bronchopulmonary lymph nodes* located at the hilum.

7. **Explain the following terms:**
   a. **Bronchitis**
   b. **Bronchiectasis**
   c. **Atelectasis**
   d. **Emphysema**
   e. **Pneumonia**

Ans. a. **Bronchitis:** Inflammation of the mucous membrane lining the bronchial tree.

b. **Bronchiectasis:** Localized or widespread dilation of bronchi which become seats of infection.

c. **Atelectasis:** A collapsed or airless state of the lung, which may involve all or part of the lung. The primary cause of atelectasis is obstruction of the bronchus serving the affected area. In fetal atelectasis, the lungs fail to expand normally at birth.

d. **Emphysema:** Chronic respiratory obstruction leads to considerable dilation of alveoli which may lead to destruction of the walls of alveoli.

e. **Pneumonia:** Pneumonia is a general term that refers to an infection of the lungs, which can be caused by a variety of microorganisms.

8. **Give anatomical basis of the following:**
   a. **Black lines seen or deposits seen deep to the visceral pleura**
   b. **Lung fields seen in X-ray chest are more dense in infants than in adults**
   c. **Common sites of formation of lung abscess**
   d. **Aspirated foreign bodies usually pass into right principal bronchus**
   e. **Tuberculosis invariably begins in the upper portion of upper lobe of lung**

Ans. a. The black lines or deposits beneath the visceral pleura forming honeycomb pattern are carbon particles deposited in the subpleural lymphatic plexus.

b. Lung fields appear more dense in infants because thinning of the alveolar septa continues during first few years of life. The thinning increases the air : soft tissue ratio and hence the ability of the X-rays to penetrate the lungs.

c. Apical segment of the lower lobe and posterior segment of the upper lobe are common sites of lung abscess because these segments are the most dependent in supine position.

d. Aspirated foreign bodies usually pass into the right principal bronchus because it is shorter, wider and more in line with the trachea.

e. Tuberculosis begins almost invariably in the upper portion of the upper lobe due to the higher oxygen tensions in the apical parts of the lung, as Mycobacterium tuberculosis is an aerobe and thrives best in tissues with high oxygen tension.

20 CHAPTER PERICARDIUM

1. **Describe pericardium under the following headings:**
   a. **Definition**
   b. **Layers**
   c. **Functions**
   d. **Contents**
   e. **Nerve and arterial supply**

Ans. a. **Definition:** It is a conical, double layered fibroserous sac that encloses the heart and the roots of the great blood vessels.

b. **Layers:** It consists of a strong outer layer composed of tough fibrous tissue called fibrous pericardium and an internal double layered sac called serous pericardium. Serous pericardium consists of two layers:
   - *Parietal layer:* Lines the inner surface of fibrous pericardium.
   - *Visceral layer:* Covers the heart and the roots of the great blood vessels.

c. **Functions:**
   - *Fibrous pericardium*
     – Keeps the heart in position.
     – Protects the heart.
   - *Serous pericardium*
     – Allows smooth contraction and dilatation of the heart within the pericardium.

d. **Contents:**
   - Heart with coronary vessels.
   - Ascending aorta.
   - Pulmonary trunk.
   - Terminal part of superior and inferior vena cava.
   - Terminal part of pulmonary veins.

e. **Nerve and arterial supply:**
   - *Nerve supply:*
     – Fibrous and parietal layer of serous pericardium – Phrenic nerve.
     – Visceral layer of serous pericardium–vagus and sympathetic nerves via coronary plexus.
   - *Arterial supply:*
     - ***Fibrous and parietal layer of serous pericardium:*** Branches of internal thoracic, musculophrenic and descending thoracic aorta.
     - ***Visceral layer of serous pericardium:*** Coronary arteries.

2. **Enumerate:**
   a. **Structures piercing fibrous pericardium**
   b. **Structures present between the mediastinal pleura and fibrous pericardium**

Ans. a. **Structures piercing fibrous pericardium:**
   - Ascending aorta.
   - Right and left pulmonary arteries.
   - Superior and inferior vena cava.
   - Four pulmonary veins.

b. **Structures present between the mediastinal pleura and fibrous pericardium:**
   - Phrenic nerve.
   - Pericardiophrenic vessels.

3. **Define pericardial cavity and describe briefly the transverse and oblique sinuses.**

Ans. Pericardial cavity is a potential space between the parietal and visceral layers of serous pericardium.

It contains a capillary layer of serous fluid (pericardial fluid) which lubricates the opposed surfaces of serous pericardium and allows the heart to contract and dilate smoothly. Pericardial cavity presents two sinuses: (Fig. 20.1)

- Transverse sinus.
- Oblique sinus.

a. **Transverse sinus:** It is a transverse gap between the tubular sheaths of visceral pericardium enclosing the arterial and venous ends of the heart. Its boundaries are:
   - *Anteriorly:* Ascending aorta and pulmonary trunk.
   - *Posteriorly:* Left atrium and superior vena cava.
   - *Superiorly:* Bifurcation of pulmonary trunk.
   - *Inferiorly:* Upper surface of left atrium.
   - On either side it communicated with the pericardial cavity.

During cardiac surgery a temporary ligature may be passed to occlude aorta and pulmonary trunk.

b. **Oblique sinus:** It is a cul-de-sac behind the left atrium of the heart. It is bounded by the visceral pericardium covering the left atrium anteriorly and parietal pericardium posteriorly. It is closed on all sides except below. It is bounded by the following structures:
   - *Anteriorly:* Left atrium.
   - *Posteriorly:* Parietal peritoneum.

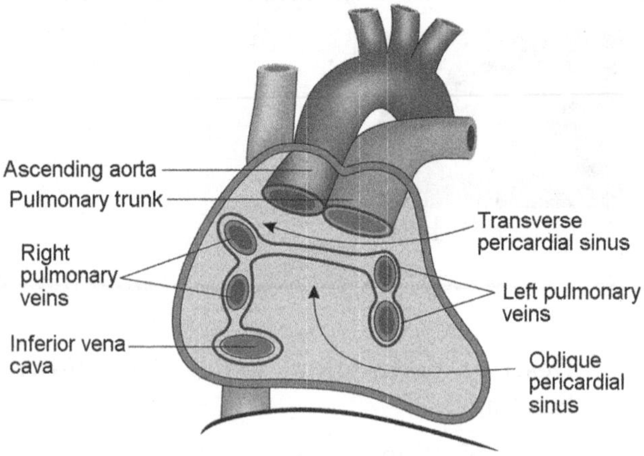

Fig. 20.1: Transverse and oblique pericardial sinuses

   - *Right:* Right pulmonary veins and inferior vena cava.
   - *Left:* Left pulmonary veins.
   - *Superiorly:* Upper margin of left atrium.
   - *Inferiorly:* Communicated with the pericardial cavity.

Oblique sinus allows the distension of left atrium.

3. **What is pericardial temponade?**

Ans. **Accumulation of fluid in the pericardial cavity:** It will compress the heart and thereby decrease the diastolic capacity. This in turn results in diminished cardiac output.

Sites used for aspiration of pericardial fluid and for giving intracardiac injections:

- ***Parasternal route:*** Through the left 4th or 5th intercostal space close to the lateral margin of sternum to avoid injury to the anterior margin of lung, pleura and internal thoracic vessels.
  - *Intrathoracic injections are preferred through this site.*
- ***Subcostal route:*** Through the left costoxiphoid angle. The needle should be directed upwards, backwards and to the left.

21 CHAPTER HEART

1. **Describe heart under the following headings:**
   a. **Location**
   b. **Dimensions and weight**
   c. **External features**

Ans. a. **Location:** Heart lies in the middle mediastinum. 1/3rd of the heart lies to the right and 2/3rd to the left of the midline. In supine position it lies opposite to T5 – T8 vertebra and in erect position descends by one vertebra (T6 – T9).

b. • **Dimensions:**
   – *Base to apex:* 12 cm.
   – *Transversely:* 8–9 cm.
   – *Anteroposteriorly:* 6 cm.

• **Weight:**
   – *Males:* 280–340 gm.
   – *Females:* 230–280 gm.

c. **External features:**

The heart has:

• *An apex:*
   – Is formed by the left ventricle.
   – Lies in the fifth intercostal space 9 cm from the median plane.

Apex beat:
- Is the lowermost and outermost thrust of the heart felt on the front of the chest.
- In *adults* it is felt in the left 5th intercostals space 9 cm from the median plane (just medial to the midclavicular line.
- In *infants* it is felt in the 2nd or 3rd intercostals space just lateral to the midclavicular line.

• *A base:*
   – Is quadrilateral in shape.
   – 2/3rd is formed by posterior surface of left atrium and 1/3rd by right atrium.
   – Lies opposite to T5-T8 vertebra in supine position.
   – Posterior relations of the base of heart are:
      ◆ Oblique sinus of pericardial cavity.
      ◆ Right pulmonary veins.
      ◆ Oesophagus.
      ◆ Descending thoracic aorta.
      ◆ Middle four thoracic vertebrae.

• ***Three surfaces: (Fig. 21.1a and 21.1b)***
   – *Sternocostal:* Is formed by right atrium, right ventricle, left auricle and left ventricle.
   – *Diaphragmatic:* 2/3rd is formed by left ventricle and 1/3rd by right ventricle.
   – *Left surface:* Is formed by left auricle and left ventricle.

• ***Four borders:***
   – *Superior:* Is formed by the two atria.
   – *Inferior:* Right atrium.
   – *Right:* Mainly by right ventricle and near the apex by left ventricle.
   – *Left:* Is formed by left auricle and left ventricle.

• ***Five sulci:***
   – *Atrioventricular sulcus:* Separates atria from ventricles.

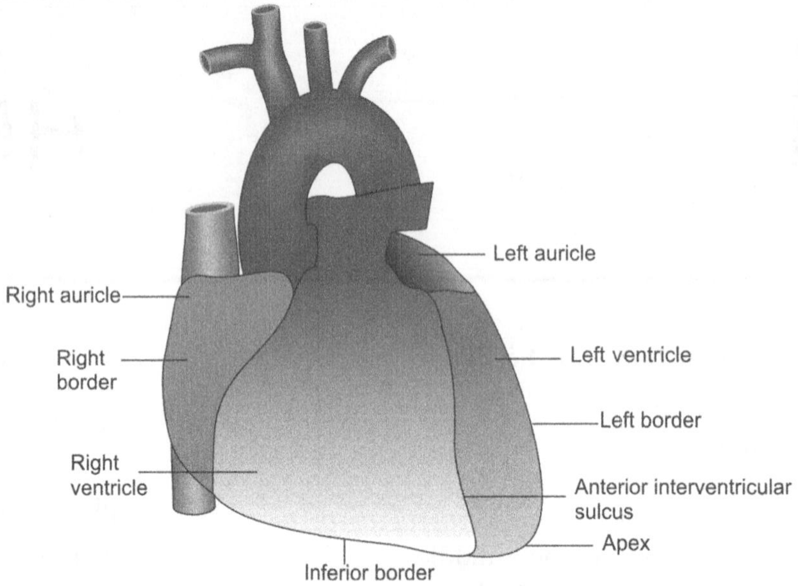

Fig. 21.1a: Sternocostal surface of heart

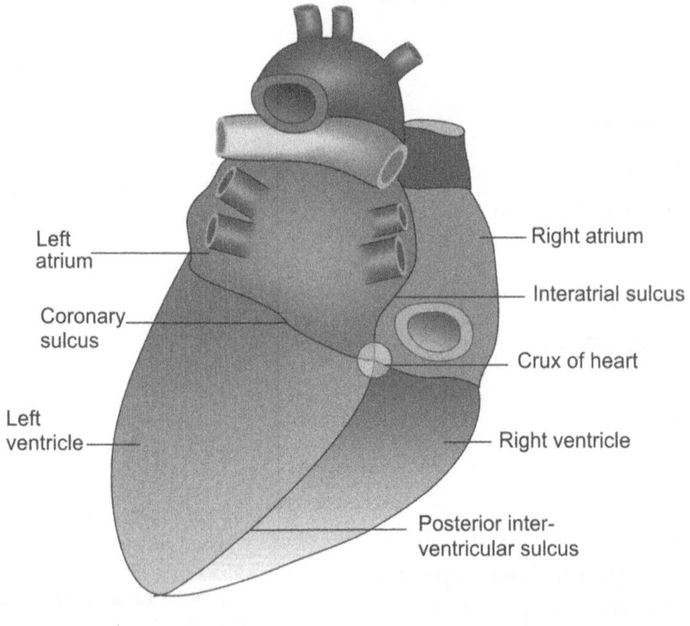

Fig. 21.1b: Posterior surface (base) and diaphragmatic surface of heart

- *Anterior interventricular sulcus:* Separates right and left ventricles on the sternocostal surface.
- *Posterior interventricular sulcus:* Separates right and left ventricles on the diaphragmatic surface.
- *Interatrial sulcus:* Separates right atrium from the left atrium.
- *Sulcus terminalis:* Extends from the opening of SVC to IVC and separates the rough part from the smooth part of the right atrium.

2. **Enumerate:**
   a. **Chambers of the heart**
   b. **Veins opening into the right atrium**

Ans. a. **Heart consists of four chambers:**

- ***Right atrium:*** Receives the impure blood from the body and the heart itself.
- ***Right ventricle:*** Receives the impure blood from the right atrium and outflows the blood into the pulmonary circulation through the pulmonary trunk.
- ***Left atrium:*** Receives oxygenated blood from the lungs via pulmonary veins.
- ***Left ventricle:*** Receives oxygenated blood from the left atrium and outflow the blood into the systemic circulation via aorta.

b. **Veins opening into the right atrium:**

- Superior vena cava.
- Inferior vena cava.
- Coronary sinus.
- Anterior cardiac veins.
- Venae cordis minimae (Thebesian veins).

3. **Draw a labeled diagram to show:**
   a. **The internal features of the right atrium**
   b. **Surface marking of valves and auscultatory areas of heart**

Ans. See Figure 21.2 and Figure 21.3.

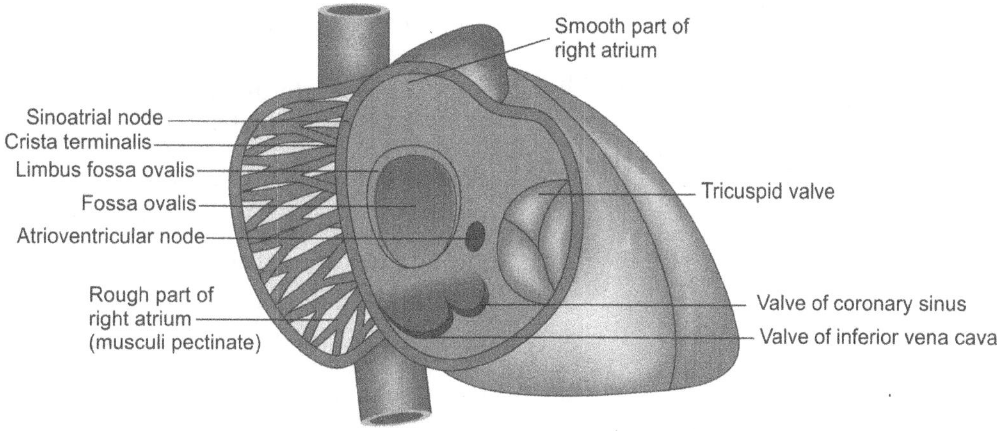

Fig. 21.2: Internal features of right atrium

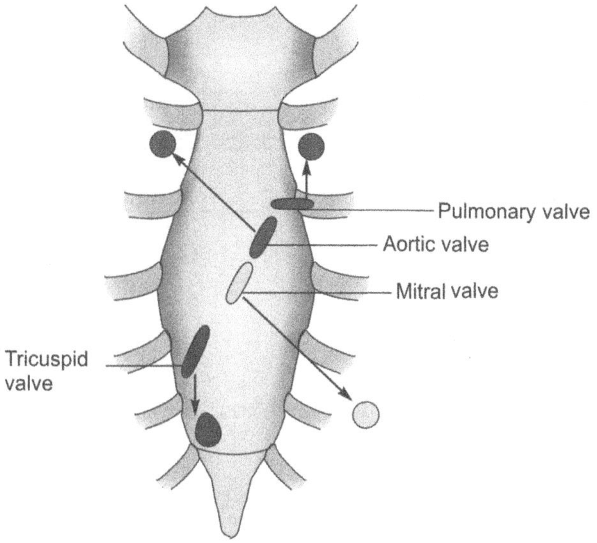

Fig. 21.3: Surface marking of valves and auscultatory areas of heart

4. **Describe briefly:**
   a. **Fossa ovalis**
   b. **Right atrioventricular orifice and tricuspid valve complex**

Ans. a. Fossa ovalis:

- It is a shallow oval depression in the lower part of the interatrial septum.
- It marks the site of the foramen ovale, an opening in the interatrial septum of the fetal heart.
- It represents septum primum.
- Limbus fossa ovalis (free edge of septum secundum) forms the margins of fossa ovalis except inferiorly.

b. • **Right atrioventricular orifice:**
   - Is the opening between right atrium and ventricle.
   - Is elliptical in shape and about 3 cm wide.
   - Is guarded by tricuspid valve.
- **Tricuspid valve complex:**
   - It guards the right atrioventricular orifice.
   - *The complex includes:*
     - Tricuspid annulus (a collagenous ring to which the bases of cusps are attached).
   - *Three cusps:*
     - *Chordae tendinae:* Endothelial covered collagenous threads that connect the apical 1/3rd of the papillary muscles to the free margins and ventricular surface of the tricuspid valve complex.
     - *Papillary muscles:* Are conical shaped muscles, their base is attached to the walls of the ventricles and apex provide attachment to chordae tendinae. Right ventricle has three papillary muscles:
       - Anterior.
       - Posterior.
       - Septal.

5. **What is moderator band or septomarginal trabecula?**

Ans. Moderator band:

- It is a specialized trabecula in the right ventricle that extends from the right side of the ventricular septum to the base of the anterior papillary muscle.
- It carries the right branch of bundle of His.
- It ensures the closure of right atrioventricular orifice before the systole so that there is no regurgitation of blood into the right atrium.
- It prevents overdistension of right ventricle.

6. **Enumerate the differences between the right and left ventricle.**

Ans. See the following Table.

	Right ventricle	*Left ventricle*
1.	The walls are thinner	The walls are 3 times thicker
2.	In TS – the cavity is crescentic shape	In TS – the cavity is oval shaped
3.	Trabeculae carneae are coarse and few	Trabeculae carneae are fine and numerous
4.	Has three papillary muscles	Has 2 papillary muscles
5.	Chordae tendinae are few and short	Chordae tendinae are more and long
6.	Atrioventricular orifice is guarded by tricuspid valve	Atrioventricular orifice is guarded by bicuspid valve
7.	Inlet and outlet lie at obtuse angles	Inlet and outlet lie at acute angle

7. **Give anatomical basis of:**
   a. **Fallot's tetralogy**
   b. **Dextrocardia**

Ans. a. Fallot's tetralogy: Is a congenital heart anomaly which involves four anatomical abnormalities. It is the most common cyanotic defect, and the most common cause of blue baby syndrome. It is characterized by the following four defects (Fig. 21.4):

- Ventricular septal defect.
- Pulmonary stenosis.
- Overriding aorta over the ventricular septal defect.
- Right ventricular hypertrophy.

b. **Dextrocardia:** It is a congenital anomaly in which the heart lies on the right side of the thoracic cavity. This may be associated with the reversal of all the abdominal organs, a clinical condition known as situs inversus.

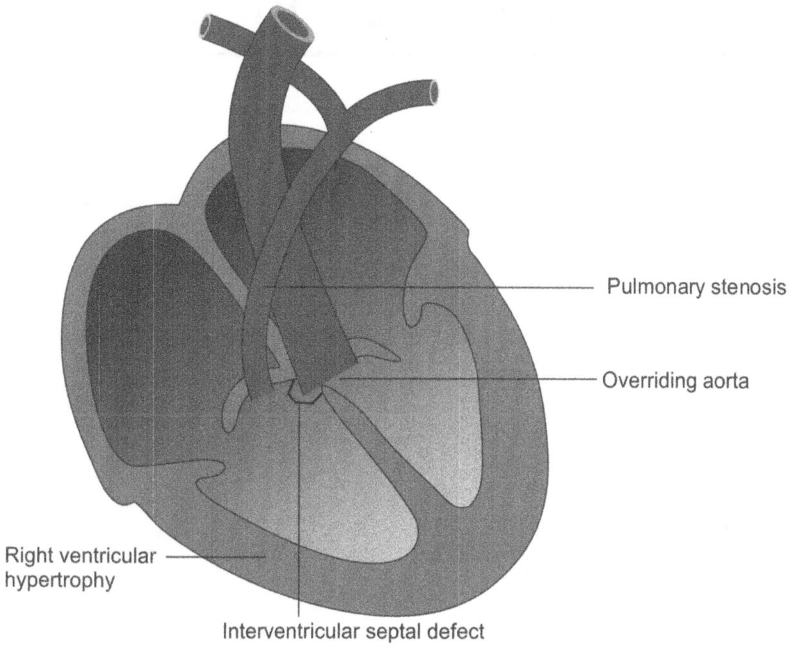

Fig. 21.4: Features of Fallot's tetralogy

22 CHAPTER

BLOOD SUPPLY AND CONDUCTING SYSTEM OF HEART

1. What are the characteristic features of coronary arteries?

Ans. Coronary arteries are:

- Highly enlarged vasa vasorum that supply the heart.
- The only arteries that get filled up during diastole of the heart.
- The first branches of aorta.
- Functional end arteries, i.e., the anastomoses between the branches of coronary arteries is inadequate to compensate for the sudden occlusion.

2. Describe the arterial supply of heart.

Ans. The heart's blood supply is derived from the right and left coronary arteries which are the branches of ascending aorta (Fig. 22.1).

a. **Right coronary artery:**
   - ***Origin:*** It arises from right (anterior) aortic sinus.
   - ***Course:*** Passes forward between the pulmonary trunk and the right auricle.
     - Descends to the right in the atrioventricular sulcus (coronary sulcus).
     - Turns posteriorly at the junction of right and inferior border.
     - Continues along the posterior part of coronary sulcus to anastomose with the branch of left coronary artery.
   - ***Branches:***
     - Right conus artery.
     - Artery to SA node (65% of cases).
     - Right marginal artery.

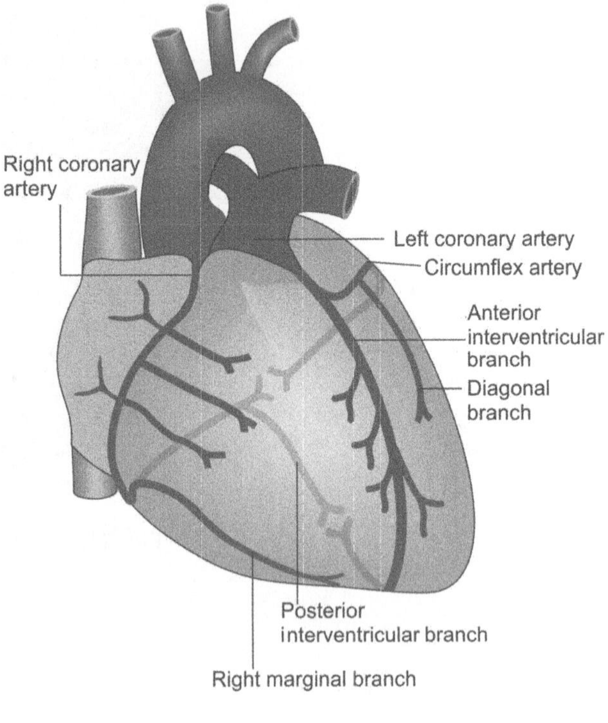

Fig. 22.1: Arterial supply of heart

     - Posterior interventricular branch–gives a branch to AV node.
     - Unnamed branches to right atrium and ventricle.
   - ***Areas supplied:***
     - Most of the right atrium.
     - Right ventricle except the area adjoining anterior interventricular groove.
     - Left ventricle adjacent to the posterior interventricular sulcus.
     - Posterior 1/3rd of the interventricular septum.

  - SA node in 65% of the cases.
  - AV node and bundle of His, except left branch of bundle of His.

b. Left coronary artery:

- *Origin:* It arises from left (left posterior) aortic sinus.
- *Course:* Passes first behind and then to the left of the pulmonary trunk to reach the left part of the atrioventricular sulcus:
  - Divides into anterior interventricular and circumflex branches.
  - The circumflex branch represents the continuation of the left coronary artery. It turns round the left border of heart and continues along the posterior part of coronary sulcus to anastomose with the branches of right coronary artery.
- *Branches:*
  - Left conus artery.
  - Anterior interventricular artery.
  - Circumflex artery.
  - Diagonal artery.
  - Unnamed branches to left atrium and ventricle.
- *Areas supplied:*
  - Left atrium.
  - Left ventricle except the area adjoining posterior interventricular groove.
  - Right ventricle adjacent to the anterior interventricular sulcus.
  - Anterior 2/3rd of the interventricular septum.
  - SA node in 35% of the cases.
  - Part of the left branch of bundle of His.
- The left coronary artery is larger than the right coronary artery.
- Right coronary artery supplies most of the conducting system of heart.
- Interatrial septa and interventricular septa are supplied by branches of both coronary arteries.

3. Describe briefly the 'cardiac dominance'.

Ans. Coronary artery dominance:

- The artery from which the posterior interventricular artery (posterior descending artery (PDA)) arises determines the coronary dominance.
- If the posterior interventricular artery is a branch of right coronary artery then the coronary circulation is said to be "right-dominant".
- If the posterior interventricular artery arises from circumflex artery, a branch of the left artery, then the coronary circulation is "left-dominant".
- If the posterior interventricular artery arises from both the right coronary artery and the circumflex artery, then the coronary circulation is "codominant/ balanced".
- Approximately 70% of the general population are right-dominant, 20% are codominant and 10% are left-dominant.
- Anterior interventricular branch of left coronary artery is the most common to be involved in coronary thrombosis leading to myocardial ischemia or infarction.
- Right coronary artery supplies most of the conducting system of the heart, therefore, its involvement causes arrhythmia.

4. Give anatomical basis of the following:

a. Angina pectoris

b. The cardiac pain due to angina pectoris or myocardial infarction is usually referred to the left precordium and medial aspect of left arm and forearm

c. Prognosis of coronary disease is better in old age than in young

Ans. a. Narrowing of coronary arteries is responsible for reduced blood flow which in turn results in decreased oxygen supply to cardiac muscle. The limited anaerobic metabolism of cardiac muscle results in built up of lactic acid which stimulates the pain receptors and as a result there is moderate to severe pain in the left precordium. The condition is called 'angina pectoris'. The pain is often referred to left shoulder, ulnar side of left arm and forearm.

b. The heart is innervated by upper four thoracic spinal segments (T1-T4). The skin over the precordium is supplied by T2-T4 spinal segments and the skin over the medial aspect of forearm and arm by T1 and T2 spinal segments respectively. The cardiac pain is therefore referred to the precordium and medial aspects of arm and forearm because of the same segmental innervations.

c. The coronary arteries are functional end arteries but not anatomical end arteries. Anatomically, the coronary arteries anastomose with each other by their trunks, branches and mostly at the precapillary level. In case of block in the coronary artery, as a result of thrombosis or atherosclerosis, these anastomoses are not effective in young people and as a result the coronary disease can be fatal in young. The coronary disease is less dangerous in old age because the anastomoses increase and collateral channels develop with the advancement of age.

5. **Describe briefly:**

 a. **Venous drainage of the heart**

 b. **Conducting system of the heart**

 c. **Nerve supply of heart**

Ans. a. **The venous blood from the heart is drained by three system of veins: (Fig. 22.2)**

- Coronary sinus.
- Anterior cardiac veins.
- Venae cordis minimae.
- *Coronary sinus:*
  - Drains most of the venous blood from the heart.
  - Is a short, wide venous channel about 2.5 cm long and lies in the posterior part of the coronary sulcus.
  - Its left end is continuous with the great cardiac vein.

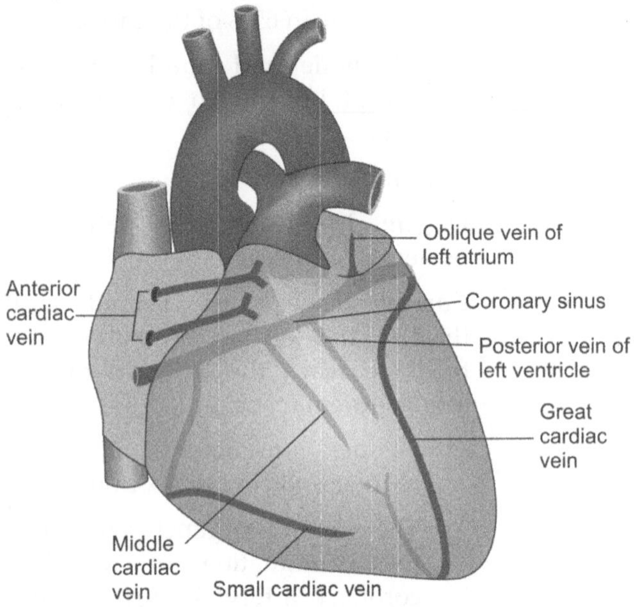

Fig. 22.2: Venous drainage of heart

  - Its right end opens in the right atrium of the heart between the openings of inferior vena cava and right atrioventricular orifice.
  - *Tributaries*
    - Great cardiac vein – lies along anterior interventricular sulcus.
    - Middle cardiac vein – lies along inferior border of the heart.
    - Small cardiac vein – lies along the posterior interventricular sulcus.
    - Oblique vein of the left atrium.
- *Anterior cardiac veins:*
  - Several small veins, that drain blood from the anterior aspect of right ventricle.
  - They open into the right atrium.
- *Venae cordis minimae:*
  - Drain venous blood from the endocardium and deep part of myocardium.
  - Open directly into the chambers of heart.

b. **Conducting system of the heart: (Fig. 22.3)**

- It is meant for initiating and maintaining cardiac rhythm and establish

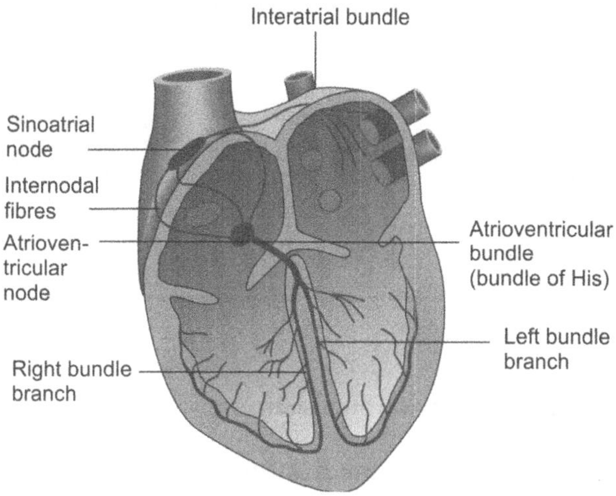

Fig. 22.3: Conducting system of heart

proper co-ordination between the atrial and ventricular contractions.

- Is made up of specialized cardiac muscle fibers having a high degree of sensitivity and auto rhythmicity.
- ***Components:***
  - *Sinoatrial node (SA node):*
    - Is also known as pacemaker.
    - Initiates the cardiac impulse.
    - Is located in the upper part of crista terminalis by the side of the opening of superior vena cava.
    - Impulse from SA node to AV node is carried by intermodal fibers.
  - *Atrioventricular node (AV node):*
    - Is situated in the right atrium, in the lower part of interatrial septum.
    - It lies in the triangle of Koch, which is bounded by:
      - Base of septal cusp of tricuspid valve.
      - Orifice of coronary sinus.
      - Tendon of Todaro.
  - *Atrioventricular bundle of HIS:*
    - From the AV node it descends in the interventricular septum and divides into:
      - Right ventricular branch.
      - Left ventricular branch.
  - The two branches descend in the interventricular septum and spread out in the walls of the respective ventricles to end in Purkinje fibers.

> Moderator band (branch of right bundle of His) passes from the interventricular septum to anterior papillary muscle in the septomarginal trabecula.

c. **Nerve supply of heart:**

The heart rate and the cardiac output are controlled by autonomic nervous system.

- Sympathetic fibers are provided by the cardiac branches of superior, middle and inferior cervical ganglia (from T2-T5 spinal segments).
- Parasympathetic fibers are provided by the cardiac branches (superior, inferior and recurrent) of the left and right vagus nerves.
- The sympathetic and parasympathetic fibers reach heart via the superficial and deep cardiac plexuses.
  - The superficial cardiac plexus is located below the arch of aorta, it is formed by:
    - Cardiac branch of superior cervical ganglion of left sympathetic chain.
    - Inferior cervical cardiac branch of left vagus.
  - The deep cardiac plexus is located behind the arch of aorta and in front of tracheal bifurcation. It is formed by:
    - Cardiac branches of middle and inferior cervical ganglion of both the sympathetic chain and from the superior cervical ganglion of right sympathetic chain.
    - Cardiac branches of T2-T5 ganglion of both the sympathetic chain.
    - Superior and recurrent branches of both the vagi and inferior cardiac branch of right vagus.

23 CHAPTER

MEDIASTINUM

1. Define mediastinum and what are its subdivisions?

Ans. Mediastinum comprises all the structures that form a median septum which separates the two halves of the thoracic cavity (Fig. 23.1).

- It extends from sternum in front to thoracic vertebrae behind.
- It is divided by an imaginary plane passing at the level of sternal angle into:
  - Superior mediastinum.
  - Inferior mediastinum which is further subdivided into:
    - Anterior mediastinum.
    - Middle mediastinum.
    - Posterior mediastinum.

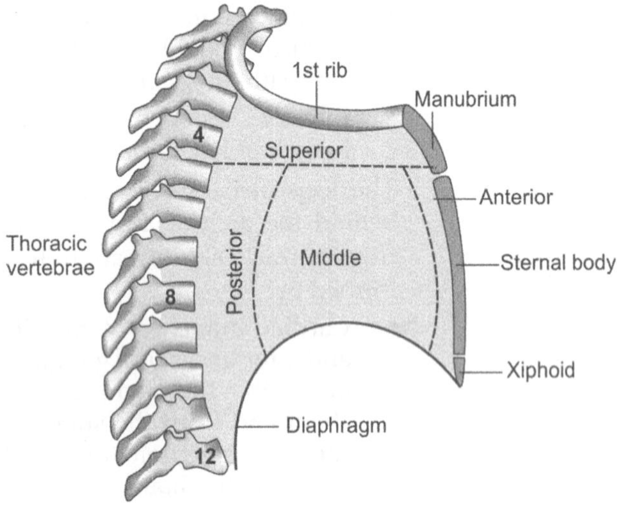

Fig. 23.1: Subdivisions of mediastinum

2. Enumerate the contents of:

a. Superior mediastinum

b. Anterior mediastinum

c. Middle mediastinum

d. Posterior mediastinum

Ans. a. Superior mediastinum:

- *Veins:* Superior vena cava and right and left brachiocephalic veins.
- *Arteries:* Arch of aorta and its three branches – brachiocephalic trunk, left common carotid artery and left subclavian artery.
- *Nerves:* Right left vagus, right and left phrenic, left recurrent laryngeal and superficial and deep cardiac plexus.
- Thoracic duct.
- Trachea.
- Oesophagus.
- Thymus.

b. Anterior mediastinum:

- Superior and inferior sternopericardial ligaments.
- Remains of thymus.
- Sternal branches of internal thoracic artery.
- Connective tissue.

c. Middle mediastinum:

- Heart and pericardium.
- *Blood vessels:*
  - Ascending aorta.
  - Pulmonary trunk.
  - Pulmonary veins.
  - Inferior half of superior vena cava.
  - Arch of azygous vein.
  - Pericardial vessels.

- *Nerves:* Right and left phrenic nerve.
- Right and left bonchii.

d. **Posterior mediastinum:**
- Oesophagus.
- Thoracic duct.
- Descending thoracic aorta.
- Azygous and hemiazygous veins.
- Greater, lesser and lowest splanchnic nerves.

3. **Write short notes on:**
   a. **Oesophagus**
   b. **Thoracic duct**
   c. **Thoracic part of sympathetic trunk**

Ans. a. **Oesophagus:**
- Is a muscular tube that conveys food from the pharynx to the stomach.
- Is 10 inches (25 cm) long.
- Is divided into three parts, i.e., cervical, thoracic and abdominal.
- *Extent:* Begins as continuation of pharynx in the neck at the lower border of the cricoids cartilage (C6 vertebra) to the cardiac end of the stomach in the abdomen (opposite T 11 vertebra).
- *Course:*
  - In its cervical part it descends behind the trachea and in front of the bodies of the vertebrae.
  - It then passes down through the superior and posterior mediastinum.
  - Enters the abdomen by passing through the opening in the diaphragm (T 10 vertebral level).
  - After a short course in the abdomen (2 cm) opens in the cardiac end of stomach.
- *Curvatures:* Oesophagus presents two lateral and two anteroposterior curvatures.
  - *Lateral curvatures:*
    - Upper convex towards the left.
    - Lower convex towards the right.
  - *Anteroposterior curvatures:*
    - Cervical curvature – convex forwards.
    - Thoracic curvature – concave forwards.
- *Constrictions:* Oesophagus has four constrictions: (Fig. 23.2)
  - *1st constriction:* At the beginning of oesophagus (15 cms from incisor teeth).
  - *2nd constriction:* Where the arch of aorta crosses it (22 cms from incisor teeth).
  - *3rd constriction:* Where the left bronchus crosses it (27 cms from incisor teeth).
  - *4th constriction:* Where it passes through the diaphragm (40 cm from incisor teeth).

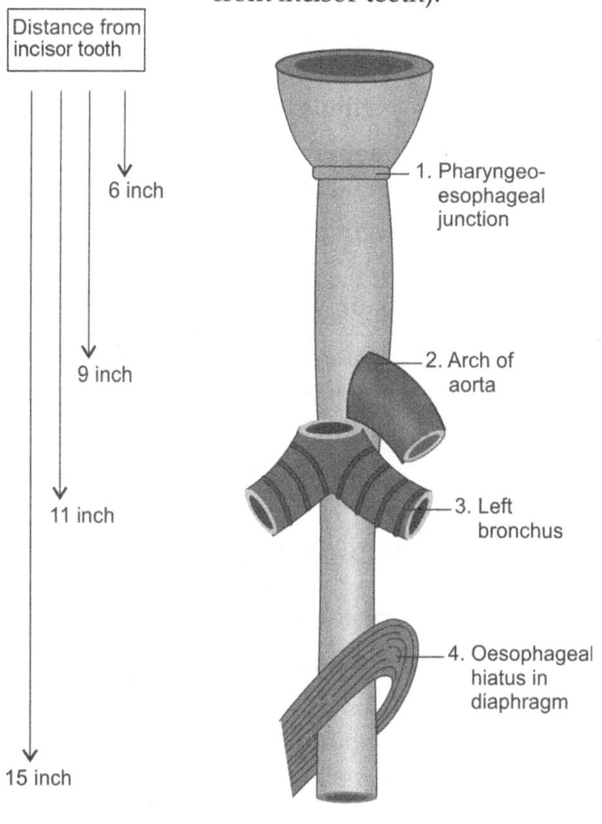

Fig. 23.2: Constrictions of oesophagus

- The knowledge of the constrictions of oesophagus is important for passage of Ryle's tube, inserted in stomach for gastric analysis and gastric feeding.
- At these sites the swallowed foreign bodies are most likely to become impacted and strictures may occur after swallowing corrosive fluids.

- ***Arterial supply:***
  - *Cervical part:* Oesophageal branches of inferior thyroid artery.
  - *Thoracic part:* Oesophageal branches of descending thoracic aorta.
  - *Abdominal part:* Oesophageal branches of left gastric artery.
- ***Venous drainage:***
  - *Cervical part:* Into inferior thyroid veins.
  - *Thoracic part:* Into azygous and hemiazygous veins.
  - *Abdominal part:* Into hemiazygous vein (tributary of inferior vena cava) and into left gastic vein (tributary of portal vein).

  * Abdominal part of oesophagus is the site of portocaval anastomosis.
- ***Lymphatic drainage:***
  - *Cervical part:* Into deep cervical nodes.
  - *Thoracic part:* Into posterior mediastinal nodes draining into supraclavicular nodes.
  - *Abdominal part:* Into left gastric nodes.

  * Hard fixed supraclavicular nodes may be palpated in patients with advanced oesophageal cancer.
- ***Applied anatomy:***
  - *Oesophageal varices:* Are dilated submucosal veins in the lower esophagus. They occur most often as a consequence of portal hypertension commonly due to cirrhosis. Lower end of oesophagus is one of the site of portocaval anastomosis. In case of portal hypertension due to back pressure in portal circulation, the collateral channels of portocaval anastomosis open up, become dilated and tortuous to form oesophageal varices which may rupture to cause hematemesis (vomiting of blood).
  - Radiologically barium swallow may show marked backward displacement of the oesophagus caused by the enlargement of left atrium in mitral stenosis.
  - *Achalasia cardia:* Results from spasm of sphincter at the lower end of oesophagus. It causes dysphagia, i.e., inability to swallow.

b. **Thoracic duct:** It is the largest lymph duct that drains lymph from all the parts of the body except:
   - Right half of head and neck.
   - Right half of thoracic cavity and right lung.
   - Right upper limb.
   - ***Beginning:*** Begins at the upper end of cisterna chyli (at lower border of T12 vertebra).
   - ***Course: (Fig. 23.3)***
     - Enters posterior mediastinum by passing through the aortic opening of the diaphragm lying between azygous vein on right side and descending aorta on the left side.
     - Ascends up in the posterior mediastinum on the right side of the median plane.
     - Crosses from right to left side behind the oesophagus and in front of the 5th thoracic vertebra.
     - Ascends in the superior mediastinum along the left of the oesophagus.
     - Passes through inlet of thorax and enters root of the neck.
     - In the neck it curves laterally in front of vertebral vessels and behind the carotid sheath.

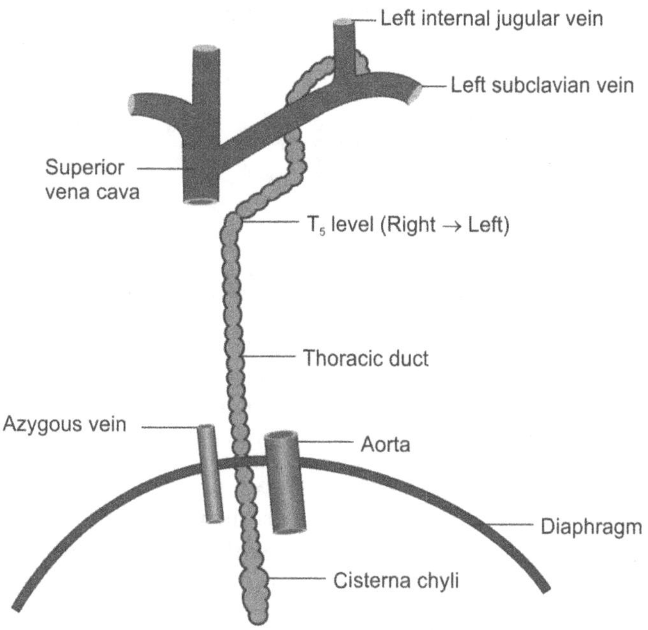

Fig. 23.3: Course of thoracic duct

- ***Termination:*** Drains into the junction of left internal jugular and left subclavian veins.
- ***Tributaries:***
  - Cisterna chyli located in front of L1 and L2 vertebra. It receives lymph from:
    - Intestinal lymph trunk.
    - Two lumbar lymph trunks.
  - Lymphatics from the lower posterior intercostals nodes.
  - Left bronchomediastinal lymph trunk.
  - Left jugular lymph trunk.
  - Left subclavian lymph trunk.

> Thoracic duct may get torn as a result of fracture of thoracic vertebrae and result in chylothorax.

c. **Thoracic part of sympathetic trunk:**

- ***Thoracic part of sympathetic chain descends in front of:***
  - The neck of the 1st rib.
  - Heads of 2nd-10th ribs.
  - Bodies of 11th and 12th thoracic vertebrae.
- Continues as lumbar part of sympathetic chain by passing behind the medial arcuate ligament of the diaphragm.
- There are 11 ganglia in this part of sympathetic chain one for each thoracic spinal nerve except the first ganglion which usually fuses with the inferior cervical ganglion.
- The ganglion receive preganglione sympathetic fibers from the spinal cord via ventral ramii of the corresponding spinal nerves.
- ***The branches are:***
  - *Grey rami communicantes:* Carrying postganglionic branches to the ventral ramii of spinal nerves.
  - *Greater splanchnic nerve:* Carry preganglionic branches from 5th–9th ganglion which synapse in celiac ganglia. Its fibers synapse at the celiac ganglia. The fibers in this nerve modulate the activity of the enteric nervous system of viscera derived from foregut. They also provide the sympathetic innervation to the adrenal medulla.
  - *Lesser splanchnic nerve:* Carry preganglionic branches from the 10th and 11th ganglion. Its fibers synapse in the aorticorenal ganglion. The nerve modulates the activity of the enteric nervous system of the viscera derived from midgut.
  - *Least splanchnic nerve:* Carry preganglionic fibers from the 12th thoracic ganglion. Its fibers synapse in the renal ganglion.
  - Branches from 2nd-5th ganglion to deep cardiac and pulmonary and oesophageal plexsus.

24 CHAPTER JOINTS OF THORAX

1. **Name the joints of thoracic cage.**

Ans. Joints of thoracic cage:

a. *Manubriosternal Joint:*
   - Is a secondary cartilaginous joint.
   - Permits slight movements of the body of the sternum on the manubrium during respiration.

b. *Costovertebral Joints:*
   - Head of a typical rib articulates with its own vertebra, and also with the body of the next higher vertebra, to form two plane synovial joints separated by an intra-articular ligament.

c. *Costotransverse Joints:*
   - Tubercle of a typical rib articulates with the transverse process of the corresponding vertebra to form a synovial joint.
   - Capsular ligament is strengthened by three costotransverse ligaments (superior, inferior and lateral).
   - Articular facets on the tubercles of the upper 6 ribs are convex, and permit rotation of the rib neck for pump-handle movements of these ribs.
   - Articular surfaces of the 7th to 10th ribs are flat, permitting up and down gliding movements for the bucket-handle movements of the lower ribs.

d. *Chondrosternal Joints:*
   - First chondrosternal joint is a primary cartilaginous joint. It does not permit any movement.
   - 2nd to 7th costal cartilages articulate with the sternum by synovial joints.

e. *Costochondral Joints:*
   - Joints between the sternal end of ribs and the costal cartilages are primary cartilaginous joints. There is normally no movement at these joints.

f. *Interchondral Joints:*
   - 5th to 9th costal cartilages articulate with one another by synovial joints.
   - Tenth cartilage is united to the ninth by fibrous tissue.

25 CHAPTER

DIAPHRAGM

1. **Describe the diaphragm under the following headings:**
   a. **Gross features**
   b. **Origin**
   c. **Insertion**
   d. **Nerve supply**
   e. **Blood supply**
   f. **Actions of diaphragm**

Ans. a. **Gross features:**

- Diaphragm is a musculoaponeurotic portion between the thoracic and abdominal cavities.
- The peripheral part is muscular and the central part is aponeurotic.
- It is dome (bidomed) shaped.
- Thoracic surface is convex on right and left sides and depressed in the middle.
- The summits of the convexities are known as cupola.
- Right cupola is higher than the left.

b. **Origin:**

- ***Sternal:*** Two fleshy slips from the posterior surface of xiphoid process.
- ***Costal:*** From the inner surface of lower six ribs and their costal cartilages.
- ***Vertebral:***
  - *Right crus:* From the front of the bodies and intervertebral discs of upper three lumbar vertebra.
  - *Left crus:* From the front of the bodies and intervertebral discs of upper two lumbar vertebra.
- From medial arcuate ligament.
- From the lateral arcuate ligament.

c. **Insertion:**

- All the muscular fibers ascend upwards and converge medially toward the central tendon.

d. **Nerve supply:**

- ***Motor:*** By both left and right phrenic (C3, C4, C5) nerves.
- ***Sensory (proprioceptive):***
  - Central part by phrenic nerves.
  - Peripheral part by lower five intercostal nerves and subcostal (ventral ramii of T7-T12) nerves.

> Phrenic nerve lesion paralyses the corresponding half of the diaphragm. It may lead to paradoxical movement of the paralysed half of the diaphragm, resulting in poor oxygenation of blood.

e. **Blood supply:**

- Musculophrenic and pericardico-phrenic arteries (branches of internal thoracic artery).
- Lower 5-6 posterior intercosal arteries.
- Superior phrenic artery (last branch of descending thoracic aorta).
- Inferior phrenic artery (first branch of abdominal aorta).

f. **Actions of diaphragm:**

- It is the chief muscle of inspiration. When it contracts, it descends and increases the vertical diameter of thoracic cavity.
- It increases intra-abdominal pressure during expulsive acts like micturition, defecation, vomiting and parturition.
- Acts requiring forcible expulsion of the air from lungs like sneezing or laughing are preceded by a deep

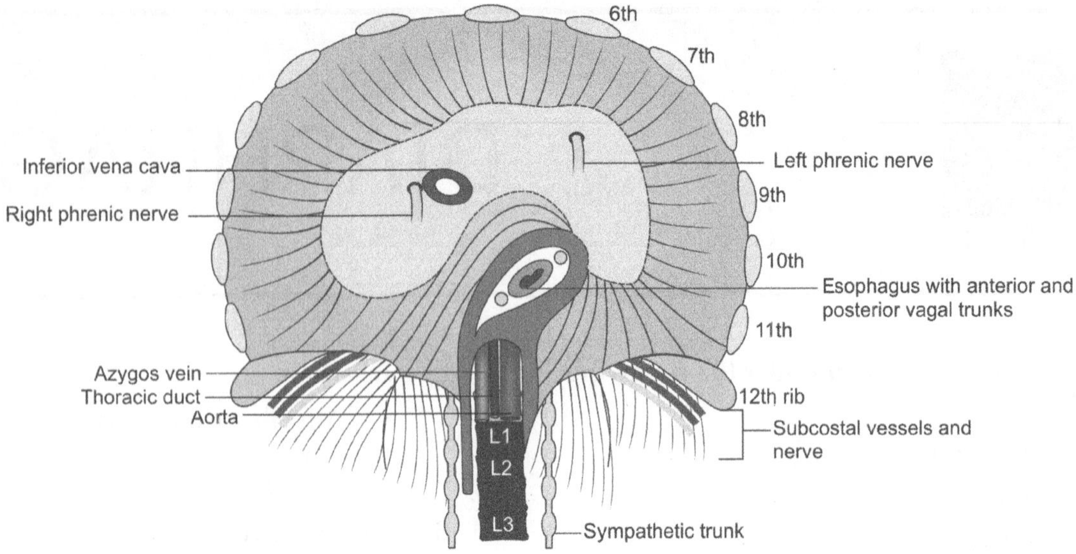

Fig. 25.1a: Diaphragm with its major openings

inspiration (contraction of diaphragm) by expiration.

- Fibers of right crus of diaphragm exercise a sphincteric control over esophageal opening.

2. **Name the major openings of the diaphragm and structures passing through them.**

Ans. The three major openings in the diaphragm: (Fig. 25.1a and Fig. 25.1b)

Inferior vena cava	*Esophageal*	*Aortic*	
Location	In the central tendon (2.5 cm to the right of the median plane	In the muscular part of the diaphragm (1.25 cm to the left of the median plane	Behind the median arcuate ligament
Shape	Quadrilateral	Elliptical	Oval
Vertebral level	8th thoracic vertebra	10th thoracic vertebra	12th thoracic vertebra
Structures passing	Inferior vena cava	Right phrenic nerve	Few lymph vessels from liver
Esophagus	Anterior and posterior vagal trunks, artery and corresponding veins	Esophageal branches of left gastric	Phreno-esophageal ligament
	Thoracic duct Azygous vein		Abdominal aorta

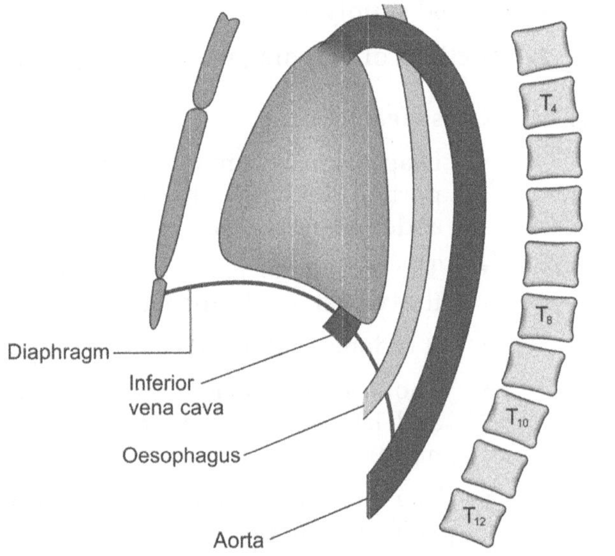

Fig. 25.1b: Vertebral level of major openings of diaphragm

- Walls of IVC are adherent to the diaphragmatic opening in the central tendon therefore, when diaphragm contracts during inspiration the vena caval opening dilates and more blood enters right atrium.
- During inspiration the esophageal opening is constricted (sphincteric action of right crus) and therefore inspiration and deglutition cannot take place simultaneously.

3. **Enumerate the minor opening of the diaphragm and the structures passing through them.**

Ans. Minor openings of the diaphragm:

- ***Between the sterna origin and 7th costal cartilage (Space of Larry):*** Transmits superior epigastric vessels.
- ***Between the costal origin from 7th and 8th costal cartilage:*** Transmits musculo-phrenic vessels.
- ***Piercing each crus:*** Greater and lesser splanchnic nerves.
- ***Behind medial arcuate ligament:*** Sympathetic trunk and sometimes least splanchnic nerve.
- ***Behind lateral arcuate ligament:*** Subcostal vessels and nerve.
- ***Left cupola in front of the central tendon is pierced by:*** Left phrenic nerve.

4. Describe briefly diaphragmatic hernias.

Ans. Diaphragmatic hernias: Are of two types:

- ***Congenital:*** Due to defects in the development of the diaphragm.
  - *Retrosternal hernia:* An abnormally large gap may be present between the sterna and costal origin of the diaphragm (Foramen of Morgagni). Abdominal viscera may be herniated through the gap.
  - *Posterolateral hernia:* Diaphragm fails to arise from the lateral arcuate ligament due to failure of closure of pericardiopleural canal. A triangular gap known as costovertebral trigone or Bochdalek's triangle persists. It is usually seen on the left side.
- ***Acquired:*** Occur through the dilated esophageal hiatus.
  - *Sliding hernia (Fig. 25.2a):* The gastroesophageal junction slides into the thorax through the lax hiatus. Normal angulation between the esophagus and stomach is lost, as a result the acidic contents from the stomach regurgitate into the esophagus. The cause could be:
    - Weakness of muscle around the esophageal hiatus.
    - Increased intra-abdominal pressure.
  - *Rolling or paraesophageal hernia (Fig. 25.2b):* Gastroesophageal junction remains in the normal position and the hernia sac containing the fundus projects into the thorax by the side of the esophagus.

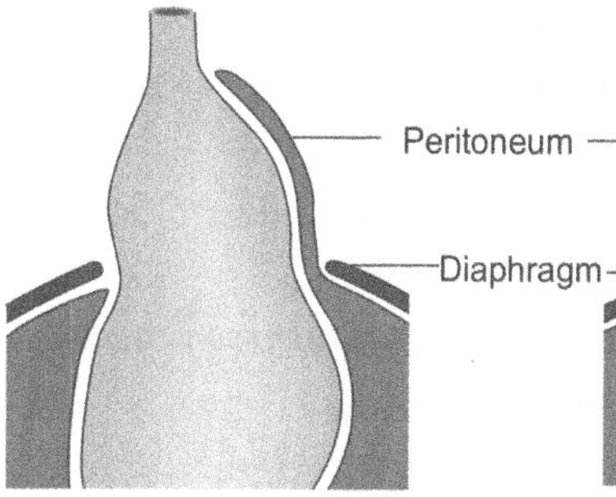

Fig. 25.2a: Sliding hernia

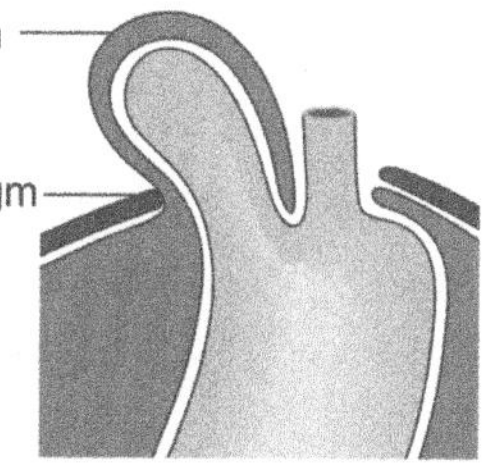

Fig. 25.2b: Rolling or paraesophageal hernia

26 CHAPTER ANTERIOR ABDOMINAL WALL

1. **Enumerate:**
   a. **Layers of anterior abdominal wall**
   b. **Topographic regions of abdomen with their contents**
   c. **Muscles of anterior abdominal wall, their origin, insertion and nerve supply**
   d. **Actions of muscles of anterior abdominal wall**
   e. **Structures present at transpyloric plane**

Ans. a. Layers of anterior abdominal wall are:

- Skin.
- *Superficial fascia:*
  - Outer fatty layer (Camper's fascia).
  - Inner membranous layer (Scarpa's fascia).
- *Muscles (arranged in three layers):*
  - External oblique.
  - Internal oblique.
  - Transversus abdominis.
- Fascia transversalis.
- Extraperitoneal tissue.
- Peritoneum (parietal layer).

> There is no deep fascia in the anterior abdominal wall.

b. Topographic regions of abdomen with their contents:

Abdomen is divided into nine regions using:

- ***Two horizontal planes:***
  - *Transpyloric plane:* Passes in front through the tips of the ninth costal cartilage and behind at the lower border of L1 vertebra.
  - *Subcostal plane:* Passes in front at the level of inferior margin of 10th rib and behind through the upper part of L3 vertebra.
- ***Two vertical planes:***
  - Right and left midclavicular planes. They pass through the midpoint of clavicle to the midinguinal point (midway between the anterior superior iliac spine).

> **Vertebral levels of important abdominal planes: (Fig. 26.1)**
> - ***Transpyloric plane***: Lower border of L1 vertebra.
> - ***Subcostal plane:*** Upper part of body of L3 vertebra.
> - ***Plane passing through the highest point of iliac crest:*** L4.
> - ***Intertubercular plane:*** Upper part of body of L5 vertebra.

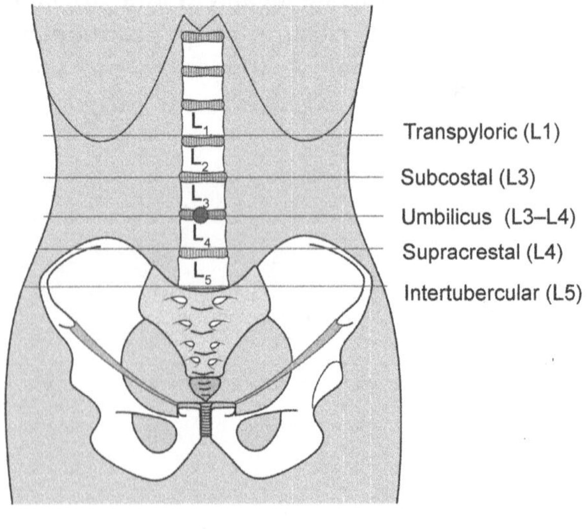

Fig. 26.1: Planes of abdomen

- The nine regions (Fig. 26.2) and their contents are:

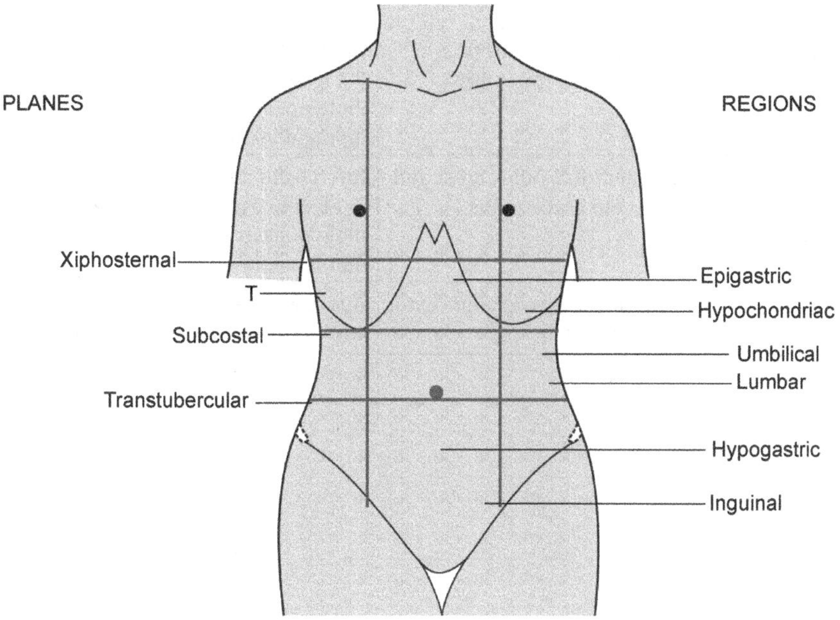

Fig. 26.2: Regions of anterior abdominal wall

Right hypochondrium	*Epigastrium*	*Left hypochondrium*
Right lobe of liver Gallbladder Right colic flexure Right suprarenal gland Upper part of right kidney	Pyloric part of stomach Liver Pancreas Duodenum Abdominal aorta	Spleen Tail of pancreas Stomach Left suprarenal gland Upper part of left kidney Left colic flexure
Right lumbar region	*Umbilical region*	*Left lumbar region*
Lower part of right kidney Ascending colon Part of duodenum Coils of jejunum	Stomach and greater omentum Transverse colon Coils of jejunum and ileum	Lower part of the kidney Descending colon Coils of jejunum
Right iliac region	*Hypogastrium*	*Left iliac region*
Terminal part of ileum Caecum with appendix Ascending colon Right ureter Right ovary (in females) Right spermatic cord (in males)	Urinary bladder (when distended) Coils of ileum Gravid uterus in pregnant mother	Pelvic colon Left ureter Left ovary (in females) Left spermatic cord (in males)

c. **Muscles of anterior abdominal wall, their origin, insertion and nerve supply (See table).**

Muscle	*Origin*	*Insertion*	*Innervation*	
External oblique	Lower 8 ribs	Linea alba, pubic crest and tubercle, anterior superior iliac spine and anterior half of iliac crest	Intercostal nerves 7-11, subcostal	Fig. 26.3a External oblique

Contd.

Contd.

Internal oblique	Thoracolumbar fascia, anterior 2/3rd of the iliac crest, lateral 2/3rd of the inguinal ligament	Lower 3rd or 4th ribs, linea alba, pubic crest	Intercostal nerves 7-11, subcostal, iliohypogastric and ilioinguinal nerves	Fig. 26.3b Internal oblique
Transversus abdominis	Lower 6 ribs, thoracolumbar fascia, anterior 3/4th of the iliac crest, lateral 1/3rd of inguinal ligament	Linea alba, pubic crest and pecten of the pubis	Intercostal nerves 7-11, subcostal, iliohypogastric and ilioinguinal nerves	Fig. 26.3c Transversus abdominis
Rectus abdominis	Pubis and the pubic symphysis	Xiphoid process and costal cartilages 5-7	Intercostal nerves 7-11 and subcostal nerve	Fig. 26.3d Rectus abdominis
Pyramidalis	Pubis, anterior to the rectus abdominis	Linea alba	Subcostal nerve	The pyramidalis is not always present

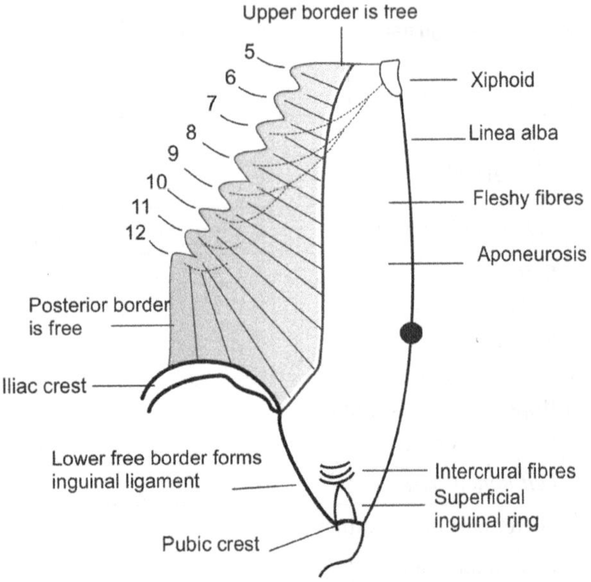

Fig. 26.3a: External oblique

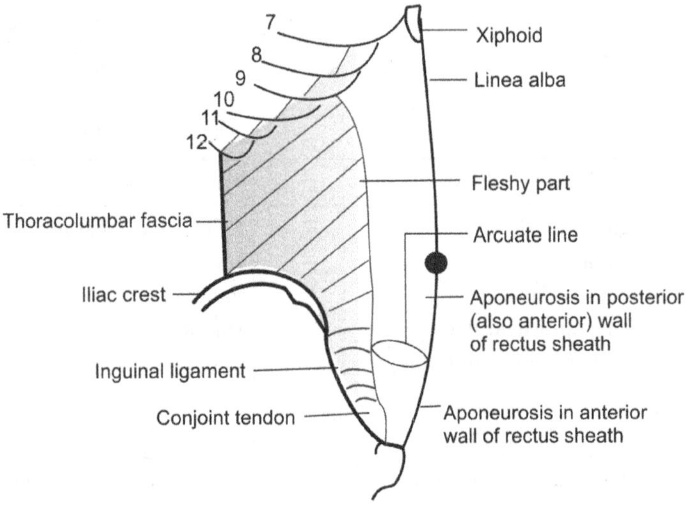

Fig. 26.3b: Internal oblique

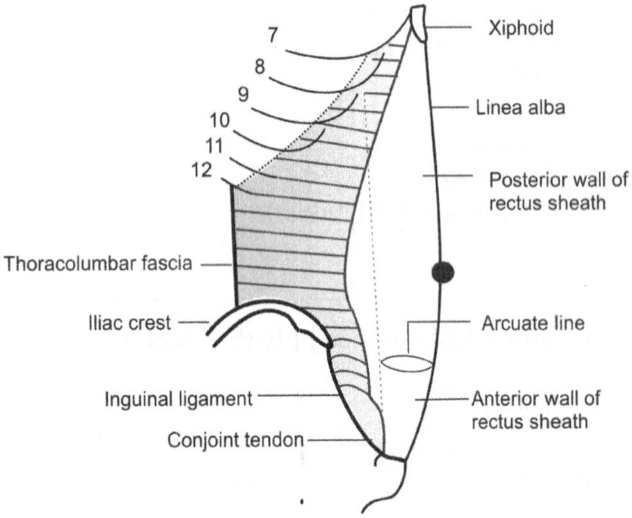

Fig. 26.3c: Transversus abdominis

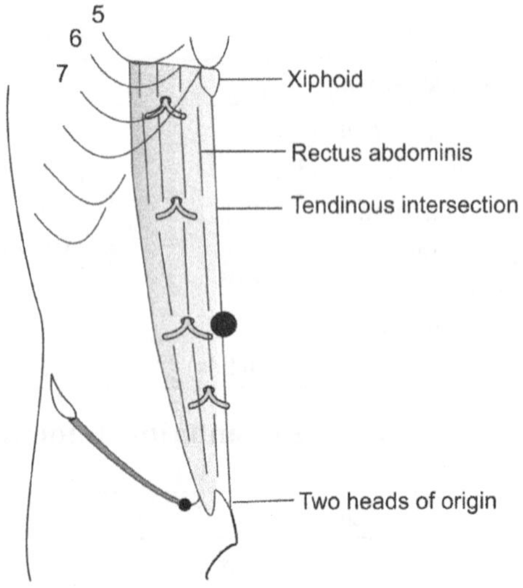

Fig. 26.3d: Rectus abdominis

d. **Actions of anterior abdominal wall muscles:**
   - Support and protect the abdominal viscera.
   - Help in forced expiration that occurs during coughing, sneezing, vomiting.
   - Increase the intra-abdominal pressure and thereby help in defecation, micturition (urination) and parturition (childbirth).
   - Flex the trunk laterally and rotate it to the opposite side (external oblique of one side and internal oblique of the opposite side.
   - Flex the trunk laterally – external and internal oblique muscles of the same side.
   - Flex the trunk laterally, the trunk anteriorly (rectus abdominis).

e. **Structures present at transpyloric plane:**
   - Pylorus of stomach.
   - Neck of pancreas.
   - Duodeno-jejunal flexure.
   - Fundus of gallbladder.
   - Hilum of kidneys.
   - Termination of spinal cord.
   - Origin of superior mesenteric artery.
   - Tip of ninth costal cartilage.

2. **Describe in brief:**
   a. **Linea alba**
   b. **Linea semilunaris**
   c. **Umbilicus**
   d. **Membranous layer of superficial fascia of anterior abdominal wall**

Ans. a. **Linea alba:** Is an avasular fibro tendinous raphe formed by the interlacing fibers of the aponeurosis of the three lateral muscles of anterior abdominal wall (external oblique, internal oblique and transversus abdominis) extending from the xiphoid process to pubic symphysis.

b. **Linea semilunaris:** A curved fibrous line at the lateral margin of the rectus sheath that extends from the tip of the ninth costal cartilage to the pubic tubercle.

c. **Umbilicus:**
   - Is a depressed scar in the midline of anterior abdominal wall, normally between the xhiphoid process and pubic symphysis or between L3 and L4 vertebra.
   - Represents the site of attachment of fetal end of umbilical cord.
   - Is innervated by T10 spinal segment.
   - Acts as a water-shed line with respect to lymph and venous flow.
   - Is one of the sites of portocaval anastomosis.

- **Fibrous bands attached to the inner aspect of umbilicus:**
  - ***Median umbilical ligament (Urachus):*** Remnant of allantois.
  - ***Medial umbilical ligaments:*** Remnant of umbilical arteries.
  - ***Ligamentum teres hepatis:*** Remnant of left umbilical vein.
- **Omphalocele:** Occurs due to failure of reduction of physiological herniation of midgut loop, herniated loops of small intestine are covered by aminion.
- **Congenital umbilical hernia:** Occurs due to herniation of loops of small intestine through imperfectly closed umbilicus. The herniated loop is covered by peritoneum.
- **Fecal fistula:** Occurs due to persistence and complete patency of vitellointestinal duct through which ileum communicates with the exterior.
- **Urinary fistula:** Patent urachus (connecting umbilicus to urinary bladder) may lead to dribbling of urine from the umbilicus.
- **Caput medusae:** In case of portal hypertension, the superficial veins radiating from the umbilicus (site of portocaval anastomosis) become dilated and tortuous.
- Referred pain in case of appendicitis is felt at umbilicus as both are supplied by the T_{10} spinal segment.

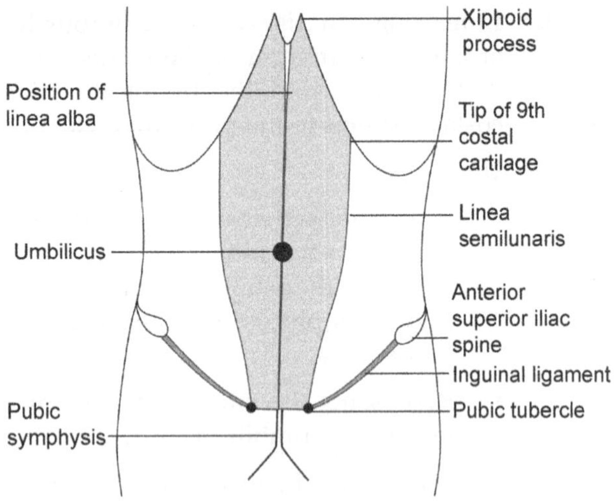

Fig. 26.4: Surface landmarks of anterior abdominal wall

d. **Superficial fascia of anterior abdominal wall:** In the lower part of the anterior abdominal wall (below the line passing through the midpoint between the umbilicus and pubic symphysis), the superficial fascia has two layers:

- Superficial fatty layer (Camper's fascia).
- Deep membranous layer (Scarpa's fascia) (Fig. 26.4).

> The superficial fatty layer is continuous with the superficial fascia of the rest of the body, the membranous layer which is devoid of fat and has more of elastic fibers.

Attachment of Scarpa's fascia:

- It passes over the inguinal ligament and is attached to the deep fascia of the thigh along an horizontal line (Holden's line approx 8 cm) passing laterally from the pubic tubercle.
- Medially, it passes downwards over the body of the pubis and becomes continuous with the superficial perineal fascia (Colle's fascia).
- It extends into the penis and scrotum (labia majora).
- The superficial perineal fascia is attached laterally to conjoint ischiopubic rami and posteriorly it is fused with the posterior border of perineal membrane.

> It is because of these attachments that in case of rupture of bulbar urethra the extravasation of urine may occur into the superficial perineal pouch, scrotum, penis and lower anterior abdominal wall deep to scarpa's fascia, but will not extend into the thigh due to attachment along Holden's line, pubic body, ischiopubic ramus (Fig. 26.5).

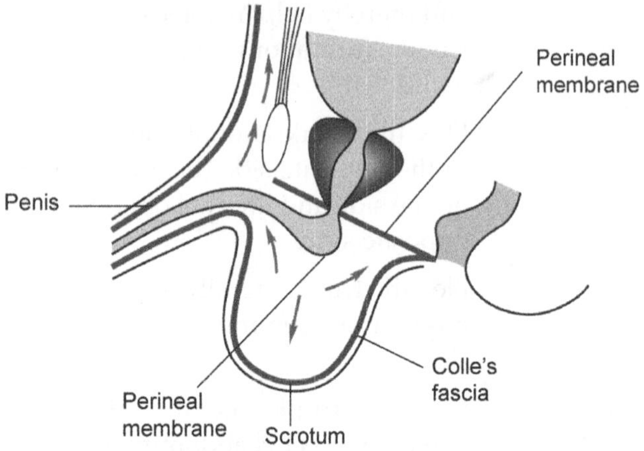

Fig. 26.5: Course of extravasated urine in case of rupture of bulbar urethra

3. **Draw labeled diagram of the following:**
   a. **Arteries supplying anterior abdominal wall**
   b. **Lymphatic drainage of anterior abdominal wall**
   c. **Cutaneous nerves supplying anterior abdominal wall**

Ans. a. **Arteries supplying anterior abdominal wall (Fig. 26.6).**
b. **Lymphatic drainage of anterior abdominal wall (Fig. 26.7).**
c. **Cutaneous nerves supplying anterior abdominal wall (Fig 26.8).**

4. **Describe rectus sheath under the following headings:**
   a. **Formation** b. **Contents**

Ans. Rectus sheath is an aponeurotic envelope for rectus abdominis and pyramidalis muscle. It is situated on either side of linea alba. It prevents the bow stringing of the rectus abdominis muscle when contracted. It also strengthens the anterior abdominal wall.

a. **Formation:** Rectus sheath has anterior and posterior walls and medial and lateral margins.

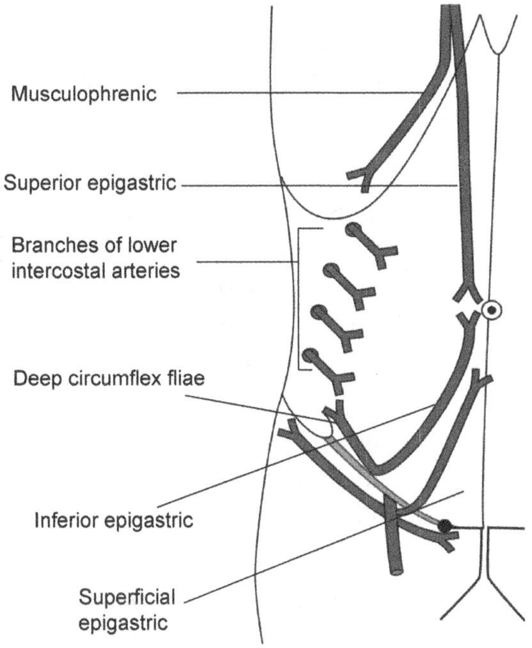

Fig. 26.6: Arteries of anterior abdominal wall

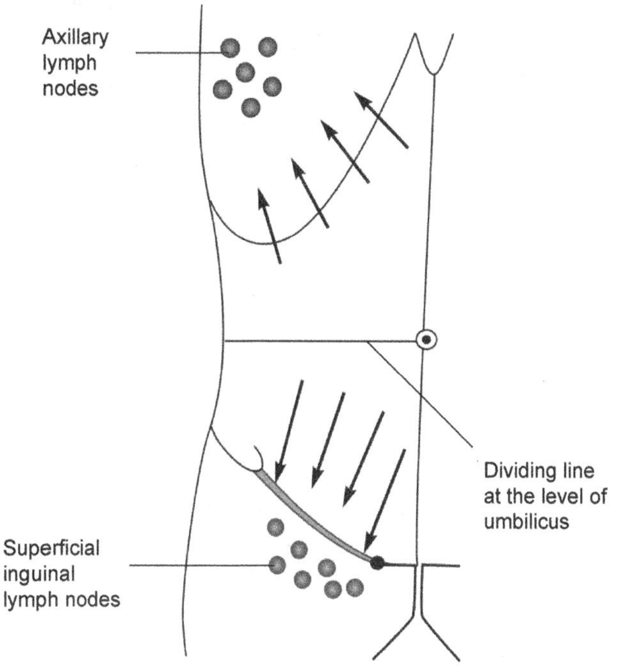

Fig. 26.7: Lymphatic drainage of anterior abdominal wall

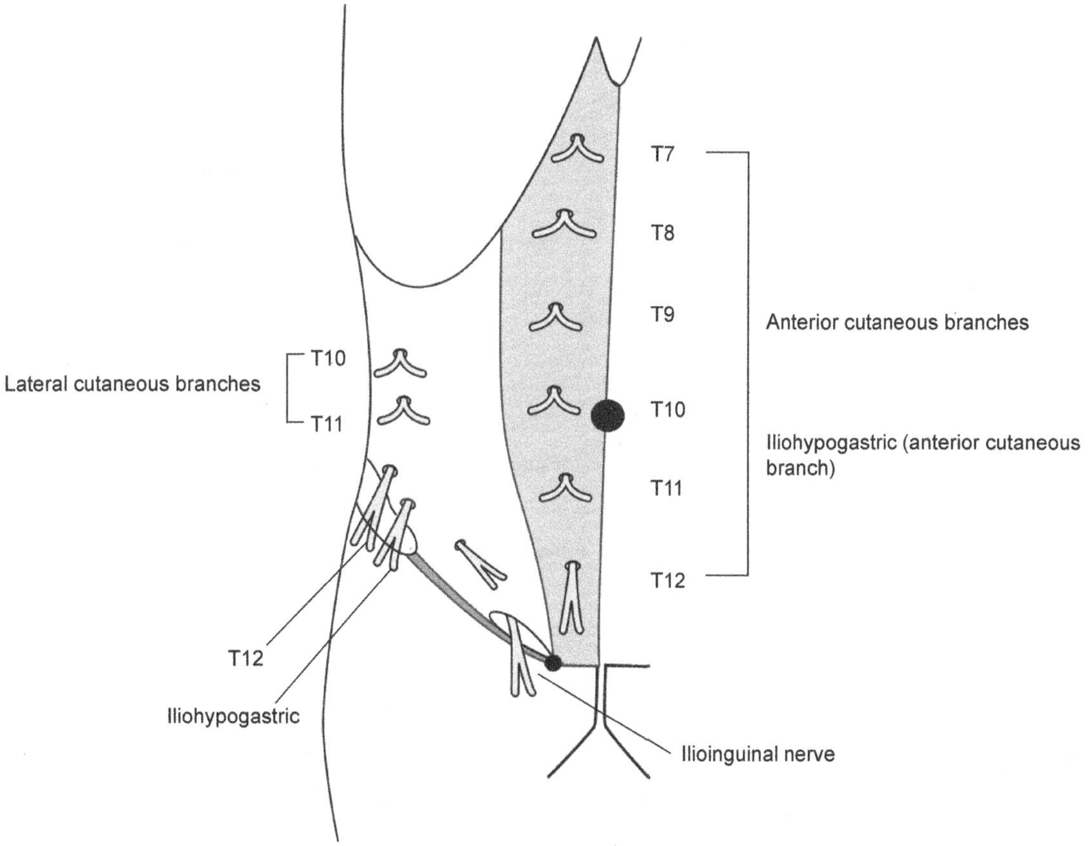

Fig. 26.8: Cutaneous nerves of anterior abdominal wall

– ***Anterior wall:*** It is complete but differs in thickness at different levels.
  - *Region above the costal margin:* Is thin and formed by aponeurosis of external oblique.
  - *Region from costal margin to midway between umbilicus and pubic symphysis:* Is thicker and is formed by the anterior lamella of aponeurosis of internal oblique with the aponeurosis of external oblique.
  - *Region between the midpoint of umbilicus and pubic symphysis to pubic symphysis:* Is thickest and is formed by the fusion of the aponeurosis of the three flat muscles of the abdomen.
  - * Anterior wall of the rectus sheath is adherent to the anterior surface of the rectus muscle along the three tendinous intersections.

– ***Posterior wall:***
  - *Region above the costal margin:* In this region, the posterior wall is deficient and the rectus abdominis rests directly on the 5th, 6th and 7th costal cartilages.
  - *From the costal margin to midway between umbilicus and symphysis pubis:* It is formed by the posterior lamella of aponeurosis of internal oblique with the aponeurosis of transverse abdominis.
  - *Region between the midpoint of umbilicus and pubic symphysis to pubic symphysis:* It is formed by fascia transversalis (Fig. 26.9a to d).

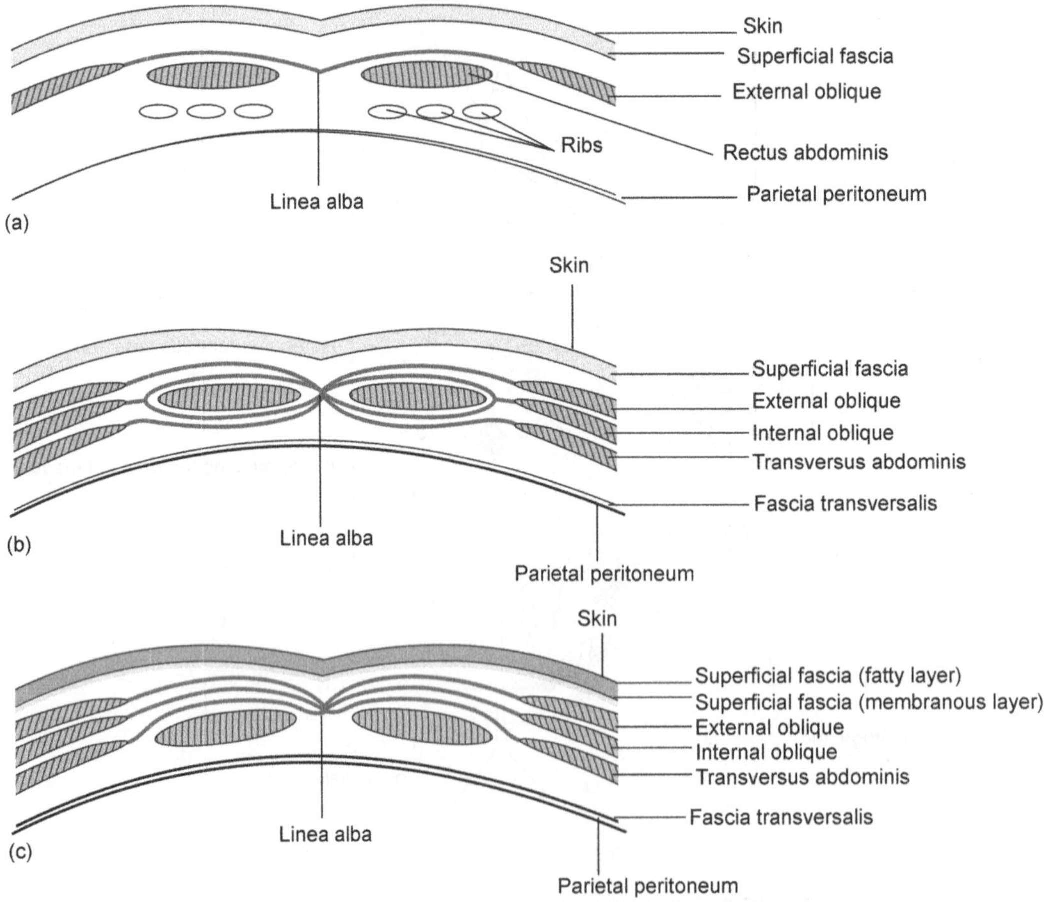

(d)

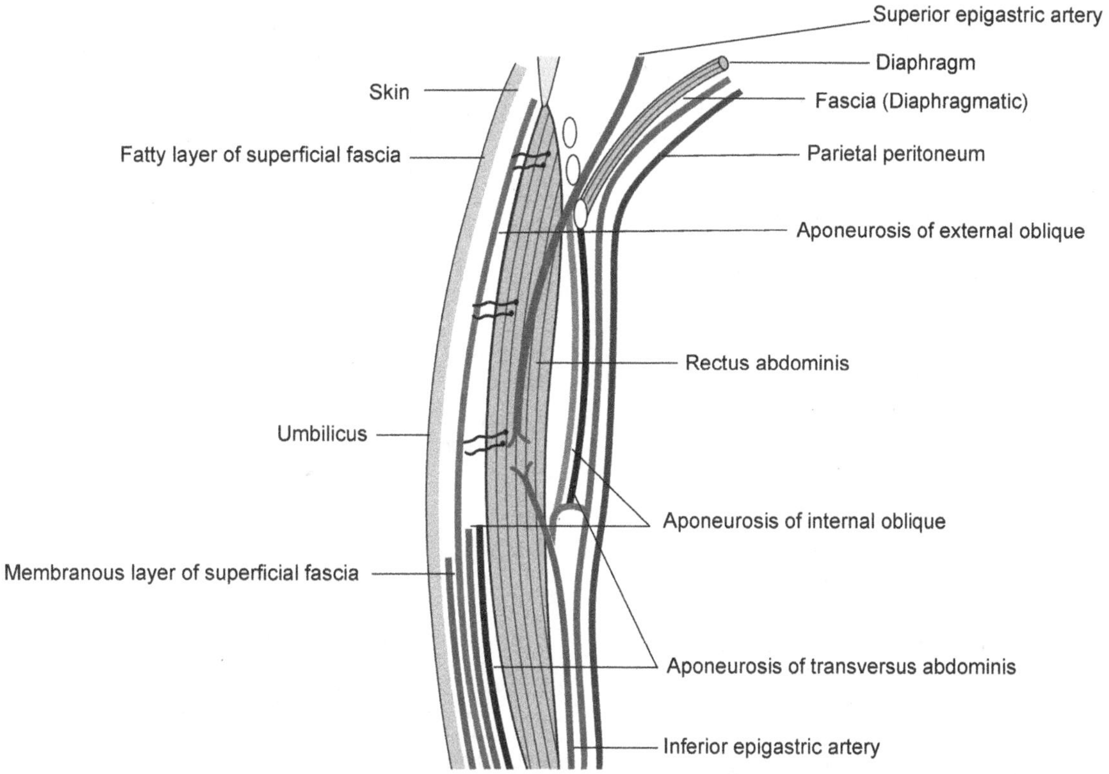

Fig. 26.9a,b,c and d: Rectus sheath (a) Above the costal margin (b) From the costal margin to midway between umbilicus and symphysis pubis (c) Between the midpoint of umbilicus and pubic symphysis to pubic symphysis (d) Rectus sheath

- Superior to the costal margin, the posterior wall of the rectus sheath is deficient because the transversus abdominis muscle passes internal to the costal cartilages and the internal oblique muscle is attached to the costal margin. Hence, superior to the costal margin, the rectus muscle lies directly on the thoracic wall.
- A crescentic border called the *arcuate line* marks the inferior limit of the posterior wall of the rectus sheath. It is usually midway between the umbilicus and the pubic crest.

b. **Contents:**

- *Muscles:*
  - Rectus abdominis.
  - Pyramidalis.
- *Blood vessels:*
  - Superior epigastric.
  - Inferior epigastric.
- *Nerves:*
  - Terminal parts of lower 5 intercostals.
  - Subcostal.

5. **Describe briefly the following:**
   a. **Cremaster muscle and cremasteric reflex**
   b. **Conjoint tendon**
   c. **Inguinal ligament**

Ans. a. **Cremaster muscle:**

- It is derived from the lower arched fibers of internal oblique. It consists of a series of loops of muscle fibers around the spermatic cord. The medial ends of loops are attached to the pubic tubercle and pubic crest.
- It is supplied by sympathetic fibers from L1 and L2 spinal segments through the genital branch of genitofemoral nerve.
- Its contraction pulls the spermatic cord and the testis upwards towards the superficial inguinal ring which helps to plug the superficial inguinal ring.

Cremasteric reflex: Upon stroking the skin of the upper medial aspect of the thigh, there is reflex contraction of the cremaster muscle leading to elevation of the testis. The afferent fibers pass along the ilioinguinal nerve (L1) which supplies the skin of the medial aspect of proximal thigh. The efferent limb is formed by the genital branch of genitofemoral nerve (L1, L2) which supplies the cremaster muscle.

b. **Conjoint tendon (falx inguinalis):**
   - Is formed by the fusion of aponeurotic fibers of internal oblique and transversus abdominis muscles.
   - It forms the medial half of the posterior wall of the inguinal canal and strengthens the canal opposite the superficial inguinal ring.
   - Is attached to the pubic crest and medial part of the pectineal line (pectin pubis).

> In old age weakening of the conjoint tendon predisposes the occurrence of direct inguinal hernia.

c. **Inguinal ligament:**
   - Is formed by the lower free border of the aponeurosis of the external oblique muscle.
   - It extends from the anterior superior iliac spine to the pubic tubercle.

6. **Describe briefly the anatomy of the following abdominal incisions: (Fig. 26.10)**
   a. **Midline incision**
   b. **Paramedian incision**
   c. **Pararectus incision**
   d. **Subcostal incision**
   e. **Muscle split or grid iron approach to the appendix**

Ans. a. Midline incision: It is made through linea alba. Linea alba provides an almost bloodless line along which abdomen can be opened. The disadvantage is that it leads to postoperative weakness and herniation may occur.

b. **Paramedian incision:** Is placed 1–1½ inch lateral and parallel to the midline, the anterior wall of rectus sheath is opened, the rectus abdominis is displaced laterally and posterior wall of rectus sheath with the peritoneum is then incised.

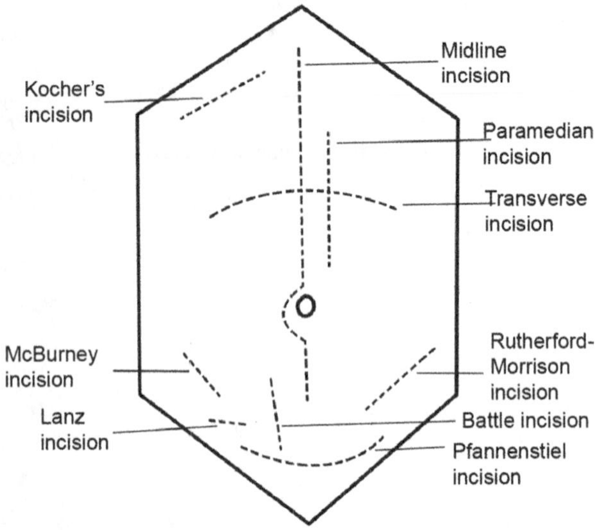

Fig. 26.10: Abdominal incisions

> Rectus abdominis should be retracted laterally to avoid injury to nerves that pierce the sheath laterally.

c. **Pararectus incision:** It is same as paramedian incision adjacent to rectus muscle.

d. **The subcostal (Kocher) incision:** Is used on the right side for gallbladder surgery and on the left, for exposure of spleen. The skin incision begins at the midline and extends parallel to and 1 inch below the costal margin.

e. **Muscle split or grid iron incision:** A transverse incision in the line of the skin crease 1 inch above and forward from the anterior superior iliac spine or an oblique incision centered at Mc Burney's point along the line from anterior superior iliac spine to umbilicus. The aponeurosis of external oblique is incised obliquely downwards and medially (in the line of its fibers). The internal oblique and the transverse muscles are then split in the line of their fibers and retracted without dividing their fibers. On closing the incision, these muscles snap together, leaving almost undamaged anterior abdominal wall.

7. **Describe inguinal canal under the following headings:**
   a. **Definition**
   b. **Location and extent**
   c. **Boundaries**
   d. **Inlet and outlet**
   e. **Contents**
   f. **Protective mechanism**

Ans. a. Definition (Fig. 26.11): It is an oblique intermuscular space in the anterior abdominal wall for the passage of spermatic cord in males and the round ligament of the uterus in the females.

b. Location:

- It lies ½ inch above and parallel to the medial half of the inguinal ligament.
- In adults the canal is directed downwards, forwards and medially.
- In newborn the canal is directed straight forward.

Extent:

- It is about 4 cm long and extends from deep inguinal ring to the superficial inguinal ring.

c. Boundaries:

- ***Anterior wall:*** Is formed by:
  - Skin.
  - Superficial fascia.
  - Aponeurosis of external oblique.
  - In lateral 1/3rd by fleshy fibers of internal oblique.
- ***Posterior wall:*** Is formed by:
  - Transversalis fascia.
  - *Medial ½* – In front of fascia transversalis by conjoint tendon.
  - *Medial 1/4th* – In front of conjoint tendon by reflected part of inguinal ligament.
- ***Roof:***
  - Arched fibers of internal oblique.
  - Arched fibers of transverse abdominis.
- ***Floor:***
  - Grooved upper surface of inguinal ligament.
  - Medially, upper surface of lacunar ligament.

d. Inlet and outlet:

- ***Inlet – Deep inguinal ring:***
  - Is an oval shaped opening in fascia transversalis.
  - Is situated ½ inch above the midinguinal point.
  - Is lateral to the inferior epigastric artery.

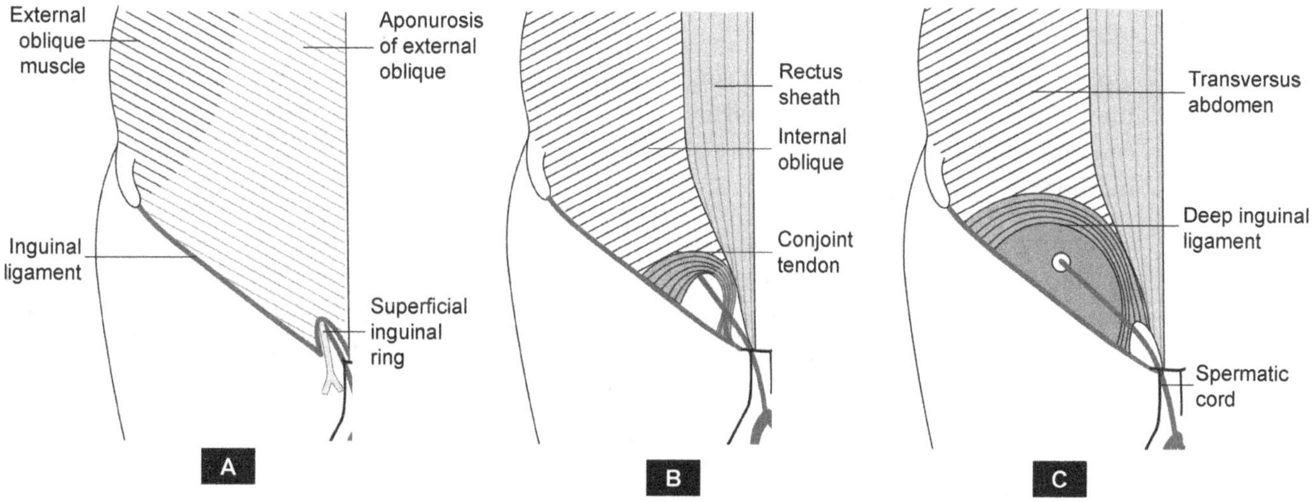

Fig. 26.11: Inguinal canal

- Structures passing through are:
  - Spermatic cord in males and round ligament of uterus in females.
  - Genital branch of genito-femoral nerve.
- *Outlet – Superficial inguinal ring:*
  - Is a triangular gap in the aponeurosis of external oblique, above and lateral to the pubic crest.
  - Structures passing through are:
    - Spermatic cord in males and round ligament of uterus in females.
    - Ilioinguinal nerve.

e. **Contents:**

- *In males:* Spermatic cord and ilioinguinal nerve.
- *In females:* Round ligament of uterus and ilioinguinal nerve.

> Ilioinguinal nerve does not enter the canal through deep inguinal ring but does so by piercing internal oblique muscle and comes out through the superficial inguinal ring.

f. **Protective mechanism:**

- Opposite the deep inguinal ring the anterior wall of the canal is strengthened by the fleshy fibres of internal oblique muscle.
- Opposite the superficial inguinal ring the posterior wall is strengthened by conjoint tendon and reflected part of inguinal ligament.
- Obliquity of the canal produces a flap-valve mechanism. During increased intra-abdominal pressure the posterior wall comes in contact with anterior wall and the canal is obliterated.
- Contraction of arched fibers of internal oblique and transversus abdominis brings roof in approximation to floor like a shutter (Keith's shutter mechanism).
- In males during increased intra-abdominal pressure cremaster muscle contracts which pulls up spermatic cord and plugs superficial inguinal ring (Ball-valve mechanism).

8. **Describe inguinal hernias under the following headings:**

a. **Definition**

b. **Types**

c. **Coverings**

Ans.

a. **Inguinal hernia (Definition):** Protrusion of abdominal viscera (e.g., intestinal loops) into the inguinal canal is termed inguinal hernia.

b. **Types:** There are two types of inguinal hernias:

- Direct inguinal hernia.
- Indirect inguinal hernia.
- *Indirect inguinal hernia/Oblique inguinal hernia:*
  - It passes through the deep inguinal ring into the inguinal canal, it may emerge through the superficial inguinal ring and descend into the scrotum.
  - When the hernia reaches the scrotal sac, it is complete and when it remains in the canal and does not pass through the superficial inguinal ring it is said to be incomplete.
  - This type of hernia is more common than the direct inguinal hernia.

- It can be congenital (due to patent processus vaginalis) or acquired (due to increased intra-abdominal pressure as during weight lifting.
- It lies lateral to the inferior epigastric artery.

- *Direct inguinal hernia:*
  - It pushes its way into the inguinal canal directly forwards through the posterior wall of the inguinal canal through the Hesselbach's triangle.
  - The neck of the hernia sac lies medial to the inferior epigastric artery.

Hesselbach's Triangle: It is located above the medial half of the inguinal ligament (Fig. 26.12).

- ***Base:*** Inguinal ligament.
- ***Laterally:*** Inferior epigastric artery.
- ***Medially:*** Lateral border of rectus abdominis.
- ***Apex:*** Where the inferior epigastric artery meets the lateral border of rectus abdominis.
- ***Floor:*** Conjoint tendon and fascia transversalis.
- The triangle is divided by obliterated umbilical artery into medial and lateral parts.

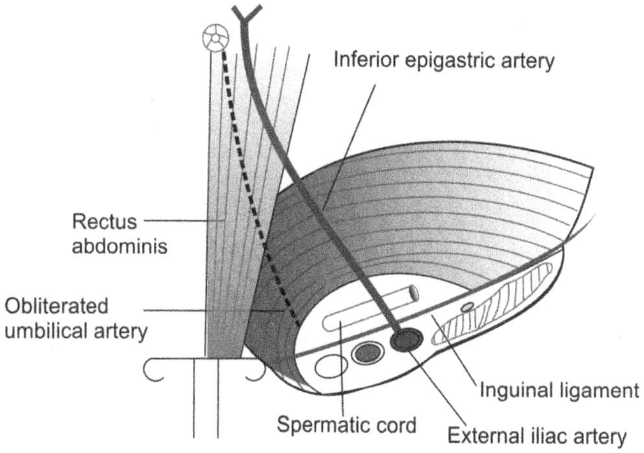

Fig. 26.12: Hesselbach's triangle

- ***Differences between direct and indirect inguinal hernias: (Fig. 26.13a and 26.13b)***

	Indirect inguinal hernia	*Direct inguinal hernia*
1.	Viscus enters the inguinal canal through	Viscus enters the canal by pushing forward the posterior deep inguinal ring wall of the inguinal canal through Hesselbach's triangle
2.	Neck of the hernia sac lies lateral to artery	Neck of the hernia sac lies medial to the inferior epigastric artery
3.	Occurs in young people	Occurs in old age
4.	Congenital – occurs due to persistent processus vaginalis	Acquired–Occurs due to weakness of muscles for-ming posterior wall of inguinal canal

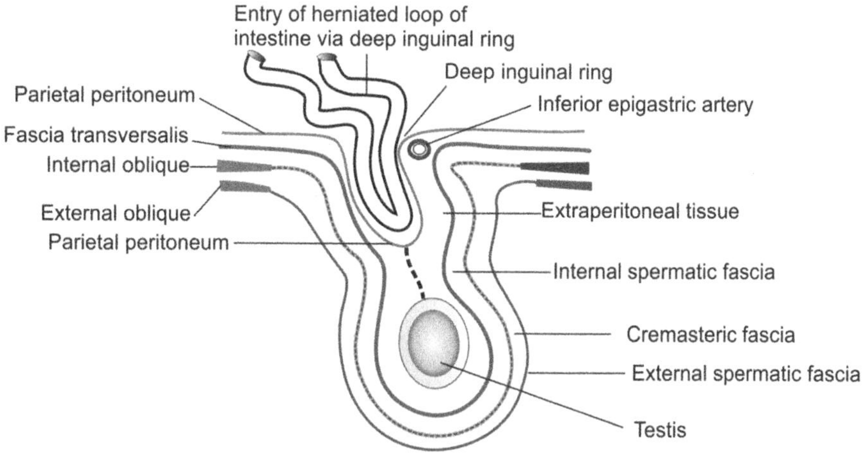

Fig. 26.13a: Indirect inguinal hernia

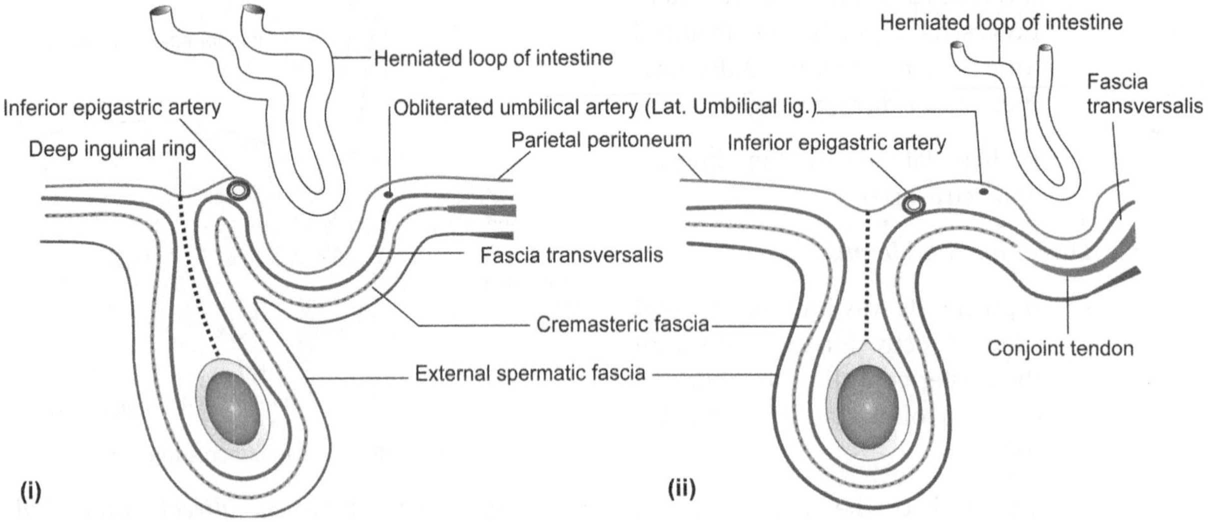

Fig. 26.13b: Direct inguinal hernia: (i) Lateral direct inguinal hernia (ii) Medial direct inguinal hernia

c. Coverings of hernia sac in direct and indirect inguinal hernias

Indirect inguinal hernia	*Direct inguinal hernia*
• Skin	• Skin
• Superficial fascia	• Superficial fascia
• External spermatic fascia from external oblique aponeurosis	• External spermatic fascia from external oblique apo-neurosis
• Cremaster muscle and fascia from internal oblique	• Cremaster muscle and fascia (in lateral direct hernia)/ conjoint tendon (in medial direct hernia)
• Internal spermatic fascia from fascia transversalis	• Fascia transversalis
• Extraperitoneal tissue	• Extraperitoneal tissue

27 CHAPTER PERITONEUM

1. **Describe peritoneum under the following headings:**
   a. **Definition**
   b. **Layers**
   c. **Folds of peritoneum**
   d. **Functions of peritoneum**

Ans. a. **Definition:** Peritoneum is double layered serous membrane lined by simple squamous epithelium which lines the wall of abdominopelvic cavity and ensheath some of the abdominal viscera.

> Peritoneum covering the ovary is lined by cuboidal cells.

b. **Layers:** The peritoneum consists of two layers:

- ***Outer parietal layer:***
  - It lines the inner surface of the walls of abdominopelvic cavity from which it is separated by extraperitoneal tissue.
  - Is derived from somatopleural layer of the lateral plate mesoderm.
  - Is innervated by somatic nerves and is therefore pain sensitive.
- ***Inner visceral layer:***
  - Covers the outer surface of the some of the abdominal and pelvic viscera (forms the serosa of the wall of the viscera).
  - Is derived from splanchnopleural layer of the lateral plate mesoderm.
  - Is innervated by autonomic nerves and is therefore pain insensitive.

> The two layers of the peritoneum are separated from each other by a potential space, peritoneal cavity. The peritoneal cavity contains thin film of serous fluid which is secreted by the lining squamous cells of peritoneum.

c. **Folds of peritoneum:**

- They connect viscera to the abdominal wall (The visceral peritoneum becomes continuous with the parietal layer along these peritoneal folds).
- They also extend between the viscera.
- Peritoneal folds provide mobility to the viscera.
- They provide passage to nerves and vessels.
- They are named according to the organs they are associated with:
  - ***Omentum:*** Folds of peritoneum associated with stomach:
    - Greater omentum.
    - Lesser omentum.
  - ***Mesentery:*** Peritoneal fold that ensheathes the small intestine and attach it to posterior abdominal wall.
  - ***Mesocolon:*** The peritoneal folds that suspend certain parts of large intestine.
- Transverse mesocolon.
- Sigmoid or pelvic mesocolon.
  - ***Ligaments:*** All other folds of peritoneum that connect viscera to abdominal wall or to each other.
    - *Coronary and triangular ligaments:* Connect liver to diaphragm.

- *Falciform ligament:* Connecting liver to anterior abdominal wall.
- *Gastrophrenic ligament:* Between stomach and diaphragm.
- *Gastrosplenic ligament:* Between stomach and spleen.
- *Lienorenal ligament:* Between spleen and left kidney.

d. **Functions of peritoneum:**
- Allows smooth movement of viscera.
- Protect vicera as it contains phagocytic cells which guard against infection.
- Absorption of fluids into the capillaries as peritoneum is semipermeable membrane.
- ***Dialysis:*** Metabolites like urea can be removed from the blood by artificially circulating fluid through the peritoneal cavity.
- Storage of fat.
- ***Healing of wounds:*** Mesothelial cells can transform themselves into fibroblast and promote healing of wounds.

2. **Enumerate:**
   a. **Intraperitoneal organs**
   b. **Retroperitoneal organs**

Ans. a. **Intraperitoneal organs:** Organs completely surrounded by peritoneum:
- Stomach.
- Liver.
- Spleen.
- 1st part of duodenum.
- Jejunum and ileum.
- Appendix.
- Transverse and sigmoid colon.

b. **Retroperitoneal organs:** Located behind the peritoneum:
- Most of the duodenum.
- Pancreas.
- Kidneys and suprarenal glands.
- Ureter.
- Ascending and descending colon.
- Rectum.

3. **Draw labeled diagram of the following:**
   a. **Vertical disposition of peritoneum**
   b. **Transverse section of abdomen at the level of epiploic foramen showing horizontal disposition of peritoneum**
   c. **Transverse section of abdomen at the level of L4 vertebra (below umbilicus) showing horizontal disposition of peritoneum**

Ans. a. **Vertical disposition of peritoneum (Fig. 27.1).**

b. **Transverse section showing horizontal disposition of peritoneum at the level of epiploic foramen (Fig. 27.2).**

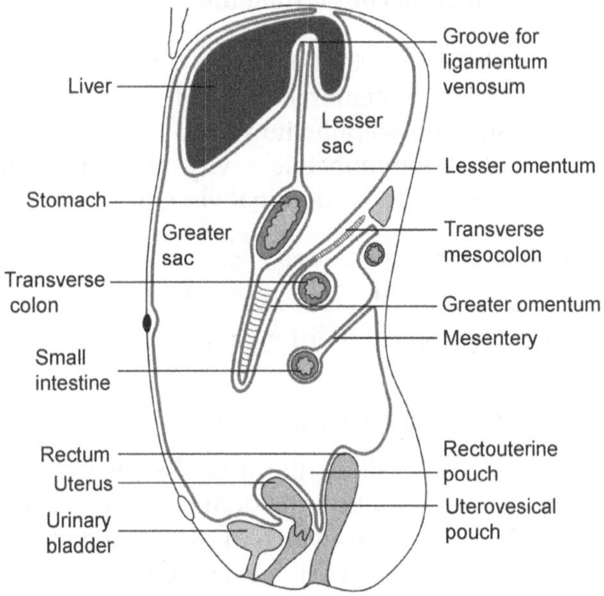

Fig. 27.1: Vertical disposition of peritoneum

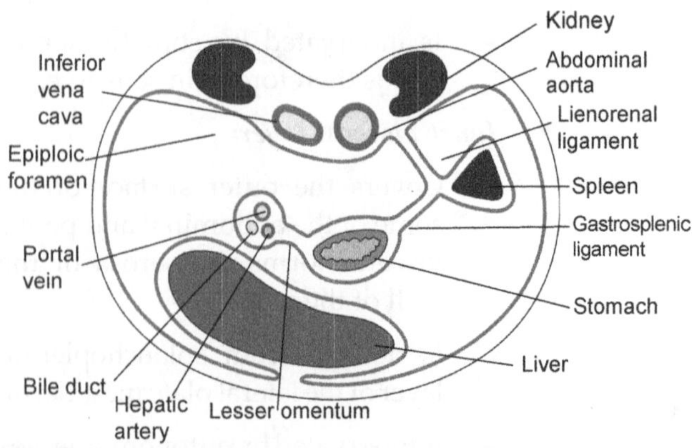

Fig. 27.2: Transverse section showing horizontal disposition of peritoneum at the level of epiploic foramen

c. Transverse section of abdomen at the level of L4 vertebra showing horizontal disposition of peritoneum in the infracolic compartment (Fig. 27.3).

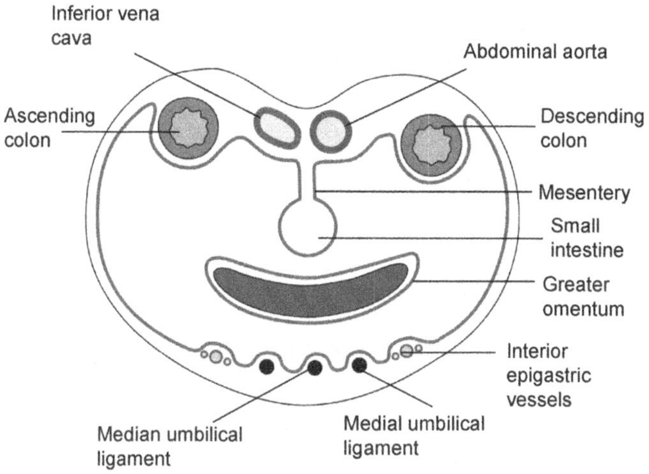

Fig. 27.3: Transverse section of abdomen at the level of L4 vertebra showing horizontal disposition of peritoneum in the infracolic compartment

4. **What are the subdivisions of peritoneal cavity?**

Ans. The peritoneal cavity is a potential space between the parietal and visceral layers of peritoneum. Normally, it contains a thin film of serous fluid secreted by peritoneum which lubricates the adjoining surface of viscera and prevents friction during movements.

> All the organs are extraperitoneal, some of the organs invaginate the closed serous sac of peritoneum and are covered by visceral (inner) layer of peritoneum which separates them from the peritoneal cavity.

The two subdivisions of peritoneal cavity are:

- **Larger greater sac.**
- **Smaller lesser sac** communicate with each other via epiploic foramen:
  - *Greater sac* is the main art of the cavity that extends from the diaphragm to the pelvis. It is further subdivided into:
    - *Supracolic compartment:* Occupies the upper anterior part of abdominal cavity above the transverse colon.
    - *Infracolic compartment:* Occupies the lower abdominopelvic cavity below the transverse colon.
    - *Lesser sac* also known as *omental bursa* is a diverticulum of the greater sac mainly located behind the stomach and lesser omentum.

5. **Write short notes on:**
   a. **Lesser sac**
   b. **Epiploic foramen**
   c. **Subphrenic spaces**
   d. **Peritoneal recesses in relation to duodenum**
   e. **Intersigmoid recess**

Ans. a. Lesser sac is the smaller part of the peritoneal cavity that lies behind stomach and lesser omentum. It allows expansion and mobility of stomach. The sac has:

- 2 walls – anterior and posterior.
- 4 borders–superior, inferior, right and left.
- 3 recesses–superior, inferior and splenic.
- 1 opening–epiploic foramen opens into greater sac (Fig. 27.4).
- ***Anterior wall*** is formed by (from above downwards):
  - Posterior layer of lesser omentum.
  - Posterior surface of stomach covered by peritoneum.
  - Anterior two layers of greater omentum.
- ***Posterior wall*** consists of (from above downwards):
  - Peritoneum covering the structures forming stomach bed.
  - Transverse mesocolon.
  - Transverse colon.
  - Posterior two layers of greater omentum.
- ***Superior border*** is formed by the peritoneum extending from the caudate lobe of liver to the diaphragm.
- ***Inferior border*** is formed by junction of anterior two layers of greater omentum with its posterior two layers.
- ***Right border*** is formed by (from above downwards):
  - Is deficient above as epiploic foramen is present here.

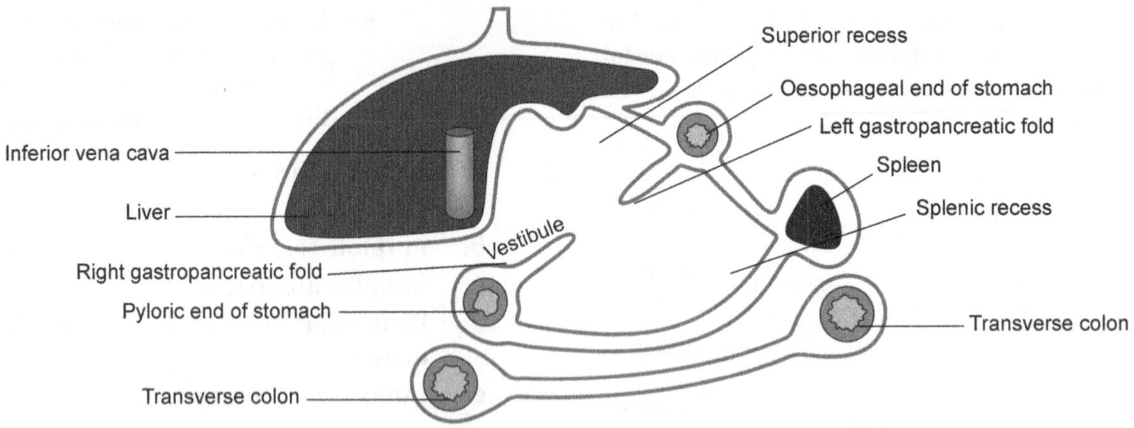

Fig. 27.4: Lesser sac (After removal of its anterior wall)

- Peritoneum reflected from posterior surface of proximal part of duodenum to the head of pancreas.
- Right border of greater omentum.

- ***Left border is formed by*** (from above downwards):
  - Gastrophrenic ligament.
  - Gastrosplenic and lienorenal ligament.
  - Left border of greater omentum.
- ***Subdivisions of lesser sac are:*** Lesser sac is divided into five parts:
  - *Vestibule:* Part of lesser sac immediately to the left of epiploic foramen. It is a constricted area between the left gastropancreatic fold of peritoneum (produced by left gastric artery) and right gastropancreatic fold (raised by common hepatic artery).
  - *Body:* Lies behind the lesser omentum and stomach.
  - *Superior recess:* Part behind the caudate lobe of liver.
  - *Splenic recess:* Between the gastrosplenic and lienorenal ligaments.
  - *Inferior recess:* Between the folds of greater omentum (is obliterated in adults).

The lesser sac may get filled with fluid as a result of perforation of gastric ulcer on the posterior wall of stomach or from an inflamed pancreas to form pseudopancreatic cyst.

b. **Epiploic foramen/Foramen of Winslow: (Fig. 27.5)**

- Is the communication between the greater and lesser sac.
- Is located at the level of the T12 vertebra.
- Its boundaries are:
  - ***Anteriorly:*** Free edge of lesser omentum containing within its layers:
    - Bile duct (in front and to the right).
    - Hepatic artery (in front and to the left).
    - Portal vein (behind).
  - ***Posteriorly:*** Inferior vena cava covered by peritoneum.
  - ***Superiorly:*** Caudate process of liver.
  - ***Inferiorly:*** 1st part of duodenum.

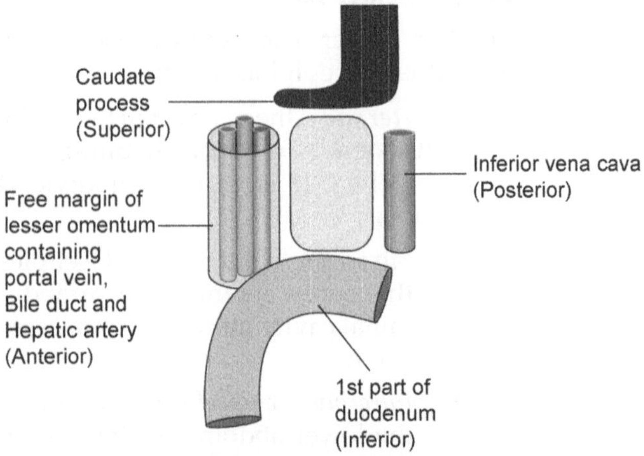

Fig. 27.5: Epiploic foramen

A loop of intestine may be herniated through the epiploic foramen into the lesser sac. If the herniated loop is strangulated the reduction is not possible through epiploic foramen as none of its boundaries can be incised due to important relations. The alternate approach is along the cleavage between the greater omentum and transverse mesocolon. The bowl has to be deflated to withdraw the loop through the epiploic foramen.

c. **Subphrenic spaces:** Are potential spaces in close proximity to the liver and are below the diaphragm. Ligaments of the liver limit them. There are three spaces on the right side and three on the left:
   - ***Right and left subdiaphragmatic spaces (Right and left anterior intra-peritoneal):***
     - They are present between the diaphragm and liver.
     - Are separated from each other by falciform ligament.
     - Are intraperitoneal.
   - ***Right and left subhepatic spaces (right and left posterior intraperitoneal):***
     - They lie below the diaphragm.
     - *Right subhepatic space* is also known as *Morison's hepatorenal pouch.* Its boundaries are: (Fig. 27.6)
       - Superior: Inferior layer of coronary ligament.
       - Anterior: Visceral surface of right lobe of liver.
       - Posterior: Parietal peritoneum covering right suprarenal gland and right kidney.
       - The space opens inferiorly into the paracolic gutter, through which it communicates with pelvic cavity.
       - To the left, it communicates with the lesser sac via epiploic foramen.

Morison's pouch is the most common site of abscess formation, postoperatively as it is the most dependent space in the supine position. The abscess may form here secondary to appendicitis, cholecystitis.

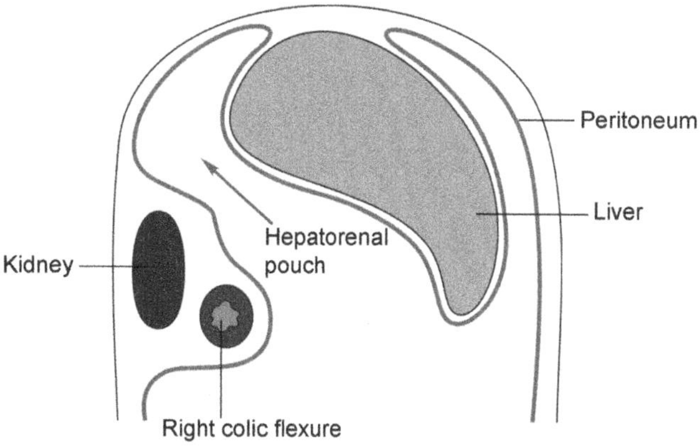

Fig. 27.6: Morison's hepatorenal pouch

     - *Left subhepatic space* is also known as *lesser sac* (described earlier).
   - ***Right extraperitoneal space:***
     - Lies between the bare area of liver and the diaphragm.
   - ***Left extraperitoneal space:***
     - Is in front of diaphragm, left suprarenal gland and kidney and behind the bare area of stomach.

d. **Peritoneal recesses in relation to duodenum:** Five peritoneal recesses are encountered around the fourth part of duodenum. These may be the site of internal hernia as these may trap a small loop of intestine. The recesses are: (Fig. 27.7)
   - Superior duodenal recess–To the left of the terminal part of duodenum.
   - Inferior duodenal recess–To the left of the terminal part of duodenum.
   - Retroduodenal recess–Behind the fourth part of the duodenum.
   - Duodenojejunal recess–At dudeno-jejunal junction.
   - Paraduodenal recess–Is guarded by a paraduodenal *vascular fold containing inferior mesenteric vein.*

e. **Intersigmoid recess: (Fig. 27.8)**
   - Lies behind the apex of inverted V-shaped attachment of pelvic meso-colon.
   - ***Left ureter lies in its posterior wall.***

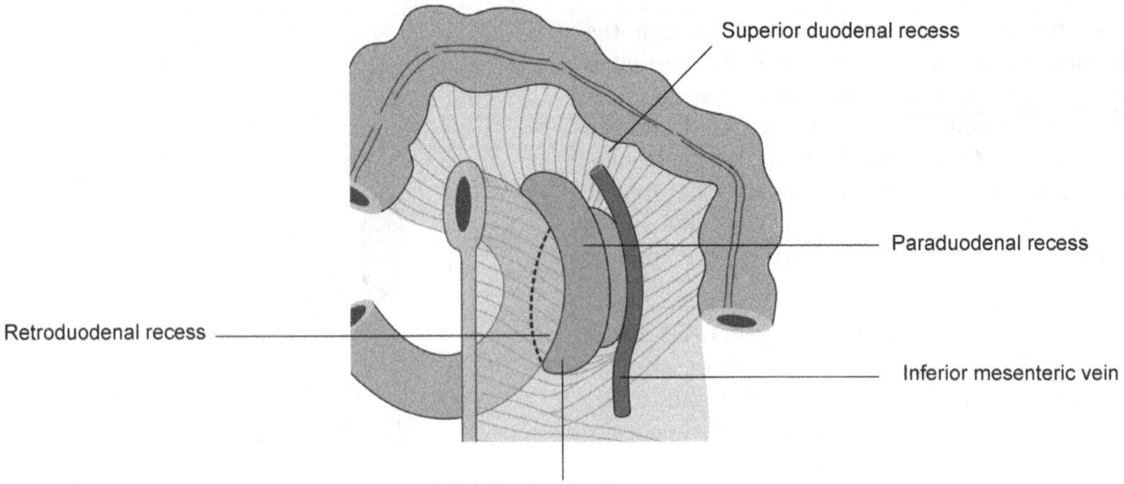

Fig. 27.7: Duodenal recesses

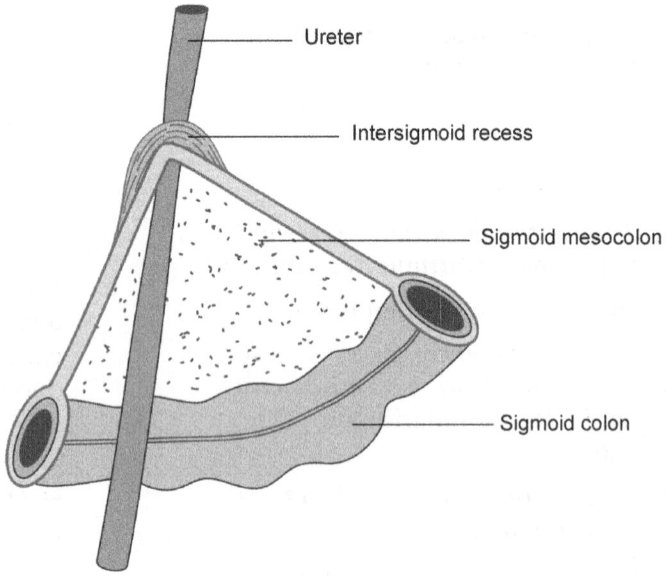

Fig. 27.8: Intersigmoid recess

28 CHAPTER STOMACH

1. **Enumerate:**
   a. **Abdominal regions occupied by the stomach**
   b. **Gross features of stomach**
   c. **Arteries supplying stomach**
   d. **Venous drainage of stomach**
   e. **Structures forming stomach bed (posterior relations)**
   f. **Peritoneal folds and ligaments attached along the lesser and greater curvature**

Ans. a. **Abdominal regions occupied by the stomach are:**
- Epigastric.
- Left hypochondriac.
- Umbilical.

b. **Gross features of stomach: (Fig. 28.1)**
- *Two ends:* Cardiac and pyloric.
- *Two surfaces:* Anterosuperior and posteroinferior.
- *Two curvatures:* Lesser and greater.
- *Four parts:* Fundus, body, pyloric antrum and pyloric canal.

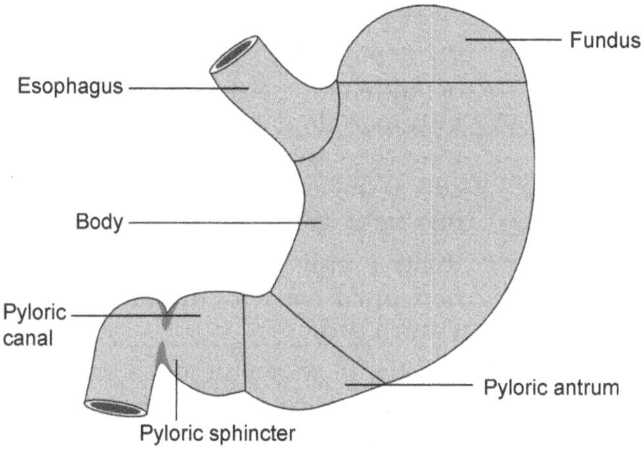

Fig. 28.1: Parts of stomach

> **Vertebral levels of:**
> - Cardiac orifice – T11 (1" to the left of median plane).
> - Pyloric orifice – L1 (1/2" to the right of median plane).

c. **Arteries supplying stomach:** Branches of celiac trunk supply stomach (Fig. 28.2).
- *Along the lesser curvature:*
  - Left gastric (from celiac trunk).
  - Right gastric (from hepatic artery - > celiac trunk).
- *Along the greater curvature:*
  - Short gastric arteries (from splenic artery - > celiac trunk).
  - Left gastroepiploic artery (from splenic artery - > celiac trunk).
  - Right gastroepiploic artery (from gastroduodenal - > hepatic - > celiac trunk).

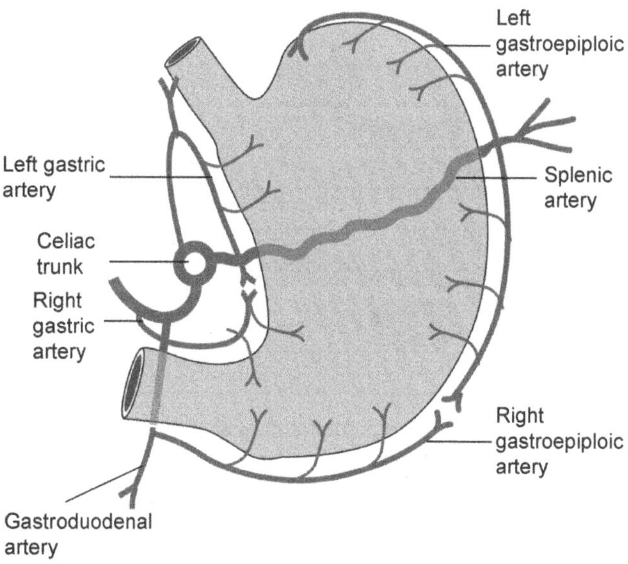

Fig. 28.2: Arterial supply of stomach

d. **Venous drainage of stomach: (Fig. 28.3)**

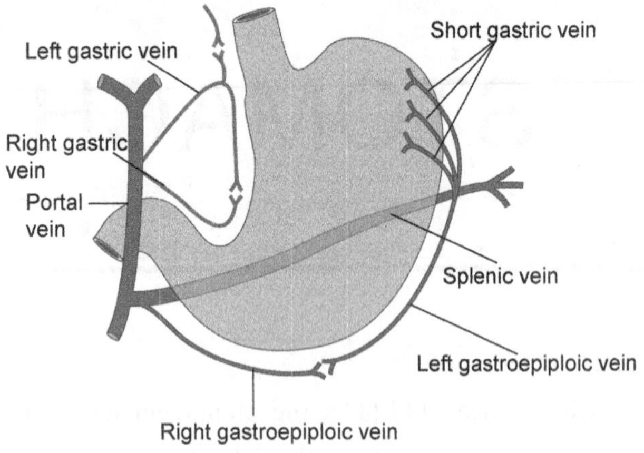

Fig. 28.3: Venous drainage of stomach

e. **Structures forming stomach bed: (Fig. 28.4)**

- Diaphragm
- Left suprarenal gland
- Left kidney
- Splenic artery
- Pancreas
- Transverse colon
- Splenic flexure of colon

(Diaphragm to splenic flexure of colon: Are separated from stomach by lesser sac)

- Spleen – is separated from stomach by greater sac.

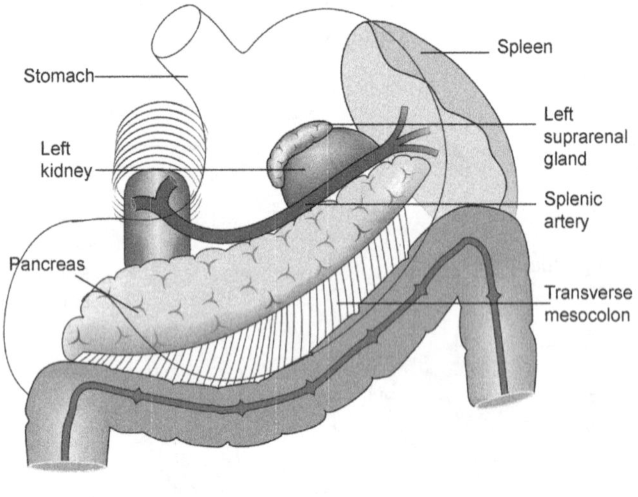

Fig. 28.4: Structures forming stomach bed

f. **Peritoneal folds and ligaments attached along the lesser and greater curvature: (Fig. 28.5)**

- *Lesser curvature:* Lesser omentum.
- *Greater curvature:*
  - Gastrophrenic ligament.
  - Gastrosplenic ligament.
  - Greater omentum.

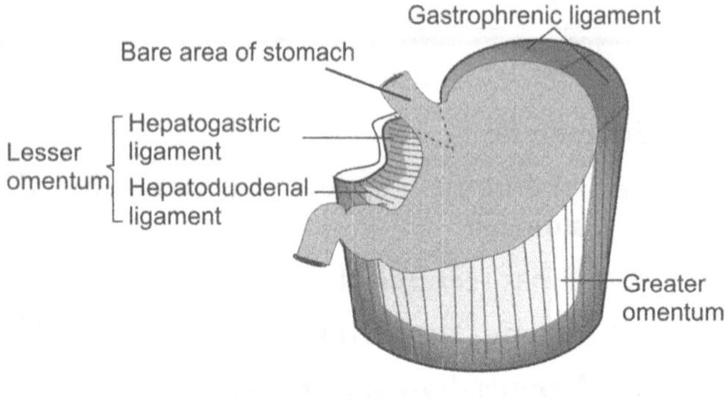

Fig. 28.5: Peritoneal folds and ligaments attached along the lesser and greater curvature

2 **What is gastric canal? What is its clinical significance?**

Ans. The mucosal folds (rugae) are arranged longitudinally on either side of the lesser curvature to form the gastric canal. The canal allows rapid passage of fluids along the lesser curvature and therefore it is irritated most by the swallowed liquids and hence it is most common site for occurrence of peptic ulcer.

3. **Describe briefly:**

a. **Lymphatic drainage of stomach**

b. **Nerve supply of stomach**

Ans. a. Lymphatic drainage of stomach: (Fig. 28.6)

- Lymph vessels accompany the blood vessels of the stomach.
- To explain the lymphatic drainage of different parts of stomach, an imaginary line is drawn that extends from the cardiac notch to the greater curvature and divides the stomach into right 1/3rd and left 2/3rd.
- Right part is further divided by a horizontal line into upper 2/3rd and lower 1/3rd.
- The lymphatics from the above mentioned region drains into the following lymph nodes:

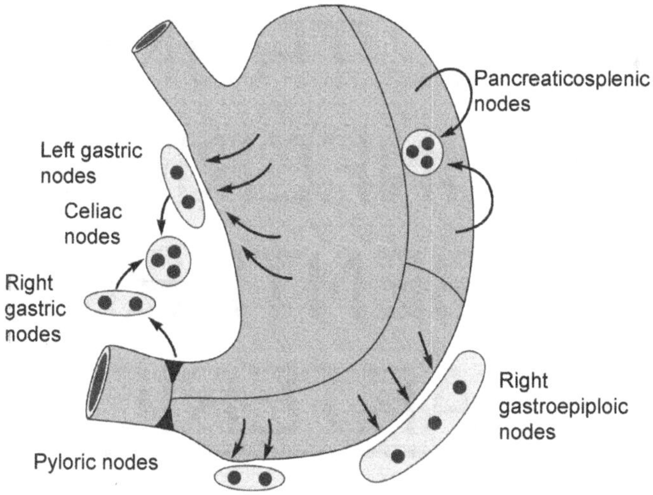

Fig. 28.6: Lymphatic drainage of stomach

- ***Pancreaticosplenic lymph nodes:*** From the left 2/3rd lymphatics pass to these lymph nodes via gastrosplenic and lienorenal ligaments.
- ***Para cardiac lymph nodes:*** Cardiac end and the adjoining area.
- ***Left gastric lymph nodes:*** Upper 2/3rd of right 1/3rd of stomach.
- ***Right gastroepiploic lymph nodes:*** Lower 1/3rd of right 2/3rd of stomach.
- ***Pyloric and hepatic lymph nodes:*** Pyloric part of stomach.
- Efferents from all the above lymph nodes terminate into *celiac group of preaortic nodes.*

> Carcinoma of the stomach may spread into the esophagus, but not into the duodenum because at the cardiac end the gastric lymph vessels are connected to the lymphatic vessels of esophagus, whereas at the pyloric end the lymphatics are not continuous with the lymphatics of duodenum due to the presence of connective tissue septum in the submucosa of pyloric end.

b. **Nerve supply of stomach:** Stomach is innervated by autonomic nervous system.

Sympathetic	*Parasympathetic*
Preganglionic fibers from T6-T10 spinal segment (via greater splanchnic nerves)	Preganglionic fibers from left and right vagus
Postganglionic fibers from celiac ganglia	Postganglionic fibers from ganglion in submucosal and myenteric plexuses
Vasomotor	Secretomotor
Motor to the pyloric sphincter	Inhibitor to pyloric sphincter
Inhibitor to the rest of the musculature	Motor to the musculature
Carry pain sensation	Carry sensation of hunger and nausea

> Gastric pain is referred to the epigastric region (due to innervation by T6-T10 spinal segments)

29 CHAPTER

CELIAC TRUNK, SUPERIOR & INFERIOR MESENTERIC ARTERIES

1. **Enumerate the ventral branches of abdominal aorta.**

Ans. There are three ventral branches of abdominal aorta:

- **Celiac trunk:** Supplies all the organs derived from the foregut.
- **Superior mesenteric artery:** Supplies all the organs derived from the midgut.
- **Inferior mesenteric artery:** Supplies all the organs derived from the hindgut.

2. **Write in a tabulated form the origin, branches and structures supplied by celiac trunk, superior and inferior mesenteric arteries.**

Ans. See the following Table.

3. **Draw labeled diagram showing:**
   a. **Branches of celiac trunk**
   b. **Branches of superior mesenteric artery**
   c. **Branches of inferior mesenteric artery**

Ans. a. Branches of celiac trunk (Fig. 29.1).

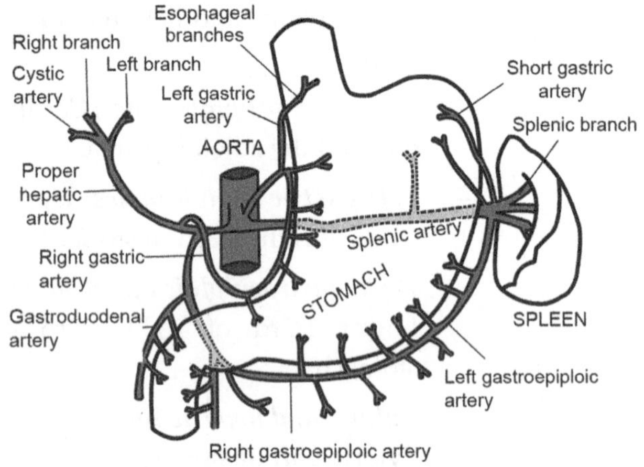

Fig. 29.1: Celiac trunk

Table: Celiac trunk, superior and inferior mesenteric arteries

	Vertebral level of origin	*Branches*	*Structures supplied*
Celiac trunk	T12	• Left gastric • Common hepatic artery • Splenic	• Lower end of esophagus • Stomach • Duodenum up to the opening of hepatopancreatic duct • Liver • Extrahepatic biliary apparatus • Spleen
Superior mesenteric artery	L1	• Inferior pancreaticoduodenal • Jejunal and ileal • Ileocolic • Middle colic • Right colic	• Duodenum distal to the opening of bile duct • Jejunum and ileum • Appendix • Ascending colon • Right 2/3rd of transverse colon
Inferior mesenteric artery	L3	• Left colic • Sigmoidal arteries	• Left 1/3rd of the transverse colon • Descending colon • Sigmoid colon

b. **Branches of superior mesenteric artery (Fig. 29.2).**

c. **Branches of inferior mesenteric artery (Fig. 29.3).**

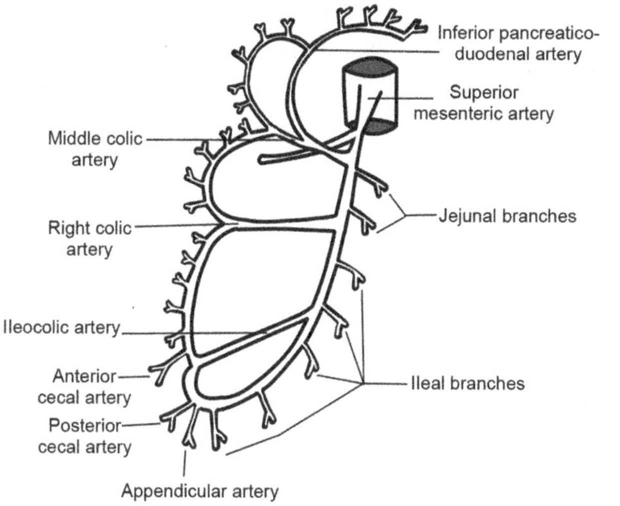

Fig. 29.2: Superior mesenteric artery

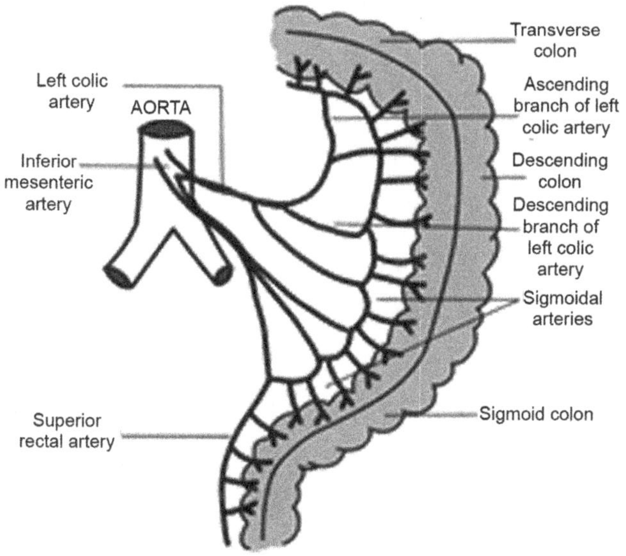

Fig. 29.3: Inferior mesenteric artery

4. **Enumerate the branches of:**
   a. **Splenic artery**
   b. **Common hepatic artery**

Ans. a. Branches of splenic artery:

- Splenic branches (5-6).
- Pancreatic branches.
- *Branches to stomach:*
  - Short gastric arteries (5-6).
  - Left gastroepiploic artery.

b. **Branches of common hepatic artery:**

- *Gastroduodenal artery which divides into:*
  - Superior pancreaticoduodenal artery.
  - Right gastroepiploic artery.
- Right gastric artery.
- Right and left hepatic arteries.

5. **Describe briefly the marginal artery of Drummond.**

Ans. Marginal artery of Drummond: (Fig. 29.4)

- Runs along the concave margin of three sided loop formed by large intestine.
- It extends from the ileocecal junction to the rectosigmoid junction.

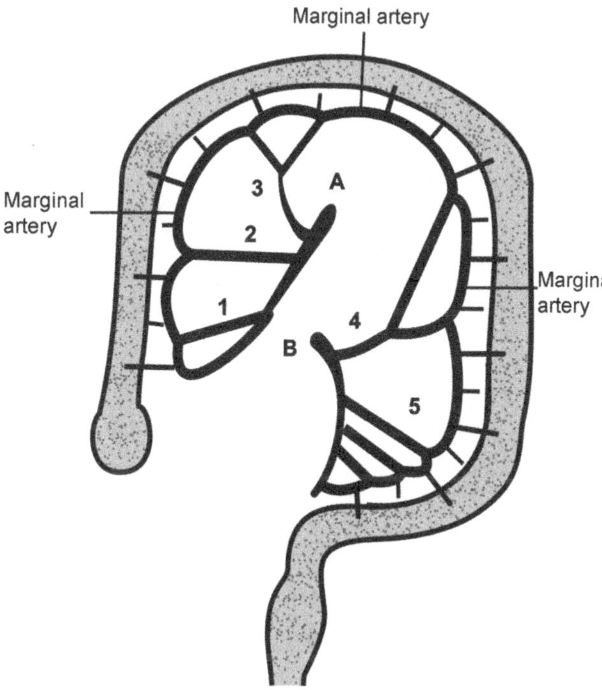

A. Superior mesenteric artery B. Inferior mesenteric artery
1. Ileocolic 2. Right colic 3. Middle colic 4. Left colic
5. Sigmoid arteries

Fig. 29.4: Marginal artery

- Is formed by anastomosis between the main arteries supplying large intestine (ileocolic, right colic, middle colic) (branches of superior mesenteric artery) and left colic and sigmoidal arteries (branches of inferior mesenteric artery).
- For it arise vasa recta, the terminal arteries that supply large intestine.
- Is capable of supplying the large intestine even if one of the large feeding trunk is severed.

The weakest point of anastomosis in the marginal artery is the region of left colic flexure (area where branches of superior mesenteric and inferior mesenteric artery anastomose, i.e., left branch of middle colic and ascending branch of left colic respectively).

30 CHAPTER SPLEEN

1. Describe spleen under the following headings:

a. Location

b. Size and shape

c. External features

d. Relations

Ans. Spleen is the largest lymphoid organ.

a. Location:

- Is located in the left hypogastrium between the fundus of stomach and diaphragm.
- Lies opposite to 9th - 11th ribs.
- Its long axis is parallel to the 10th rib.

b. Shape: Is tetrahedral/ovoid in shape.

Size: Length – 12 cm, Width – 7 cm, Thickness – 3 cm, Weight – 150-200 gms.

- Normal spleen is not palpable. Only when it enlarges twice its normal size, it can be palpated under the left costal margin on inspiration.
- Splenomegaly (enlarged spleen); Causes include malaria, typhoid fever, hemolytic anemia.

c. External features: Spleen has:

- *Two surfaces:* Diaphragmatic and visceral.
- *Three borders:* Superior, inferior and intermediate.
- *Two ends:* Anterior and posterior.

d. Relations:

- ***Relations of diaphragmatic surface:*** Is related to left costodiaphragmatic recess, left lung, diaphragm and 9th to 11th rib (Fig. 30.1).

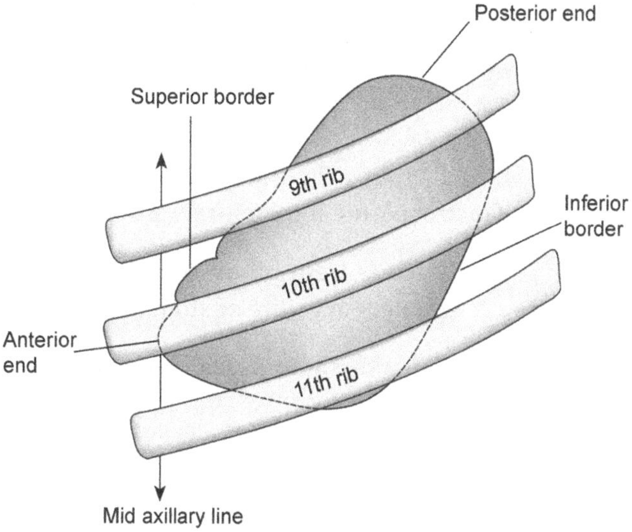

Fig. 30.1: Diaphragmatic surface of spleen

- ***Relations of visceral surface:*** It is related to the following viscera:
  - Stomach.
  - Left kidney.
  - Left colic flexure.
  - Pancreas.
  - Visceral surface bears hilum through which splenic vessels enter the spleen. Lienorenal and gastrosplenic ligaments are attached to the hilum (Fig. 30.2).

2. Name the peritoneal folds attached to the hilum and their contents.

Ans. Two peritoneal folds are attached to the hilum of spleen.

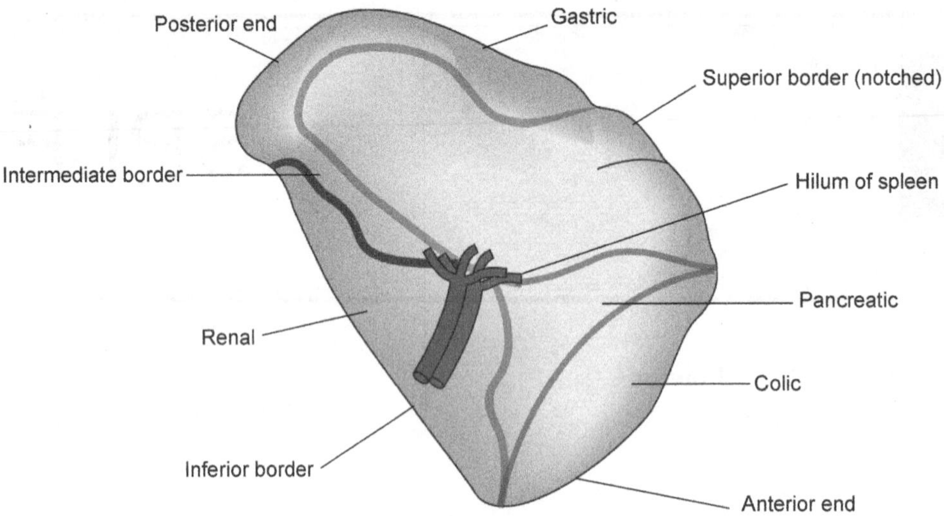

Fig. 30.2: Visceral surface of spleen showing visceral impressions

- **Gastrosplenic ligament: (Fig. 30.3)**
  - Extends from hilum of spleen to the greater curvature of stomach.
  - Contains short gastric arteries.
- **Lienorenal ligament:**
  - Extends from the hilum of spleen to the left kidney.
  - Contains splenic vessels and tail of pancreas.

- The close relationship of the tail of pancreas to the hilum of spleen and splenic vessels has to be kept in mind during splenectomy as it may be easily wounded. Enzymes released from the severed pancreas may digest the surrounding tissues. Secondly, the tail contains maximum number of Islet of Langerhan's and injury to it may cause diabetes mellitus.
- **Accessory spleens:** May occur near the hilum, in the tail of pancreas, omentum, mesentery of small intestine, ovary or testis. While performing splenectomy all accessory spleen should be located and excised, otherwise the symptoms of the disease will persist.

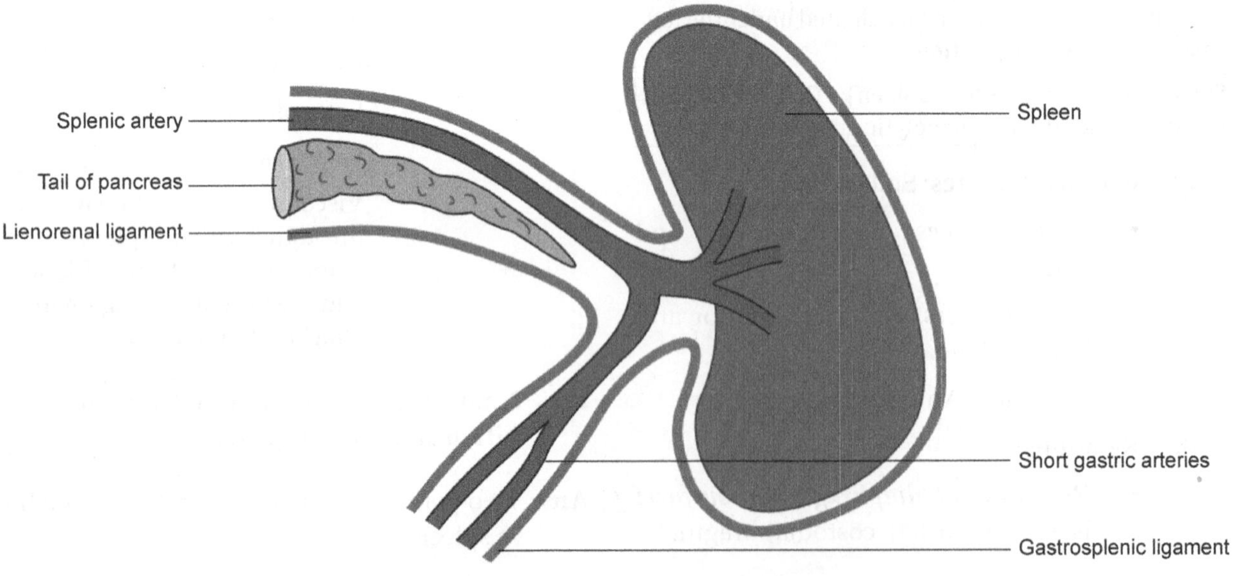

Fig. 30.3: Gastrosplenic and lienorenal ligaments

31 CHAPTER DUODENUM

1. **Describe briefly:**
   a. **Gross features of duodenum**
   b. **Relations of the four parts of duodenum**
   c. **Anterior of the second part of duodenum**
   d. **Arterial supply of duodenum**

Ans. a. **Gross features of duodenum: (Fig. 31.1)**

- Is the shortest, widest and more or less fixed proximal part of the small intestine.
- Is 25 cm or 10" (equivalent to 12 fingers) in length.
- Extends from the pyloric end of the stomach to duodenojejunal flexure.
- Lies above the umbilicus at the level of L1-L3 vertebrae.
- Forms a 'C' shaped curve surrounding the head of the pancreas.
- Only first 1" has attachment of peritoneal folds (lesser and greater omentum), rest is retroperitoneal.
- *Is divided into four parts:*
  - *First part* – From pyloric end to superior duodenal flexure (5 cm or 2").
  - *Second part* – From superior duodenal flexure to inferior duodenal flexure (7.5 cm or 3").
  - *Third part* – From inferior duodenal flexure to the front of aorta (10 cm or 4").
  - *Fourth part* – From the front of aorta to duodenojejunal flexure (2.5 cm or 1").

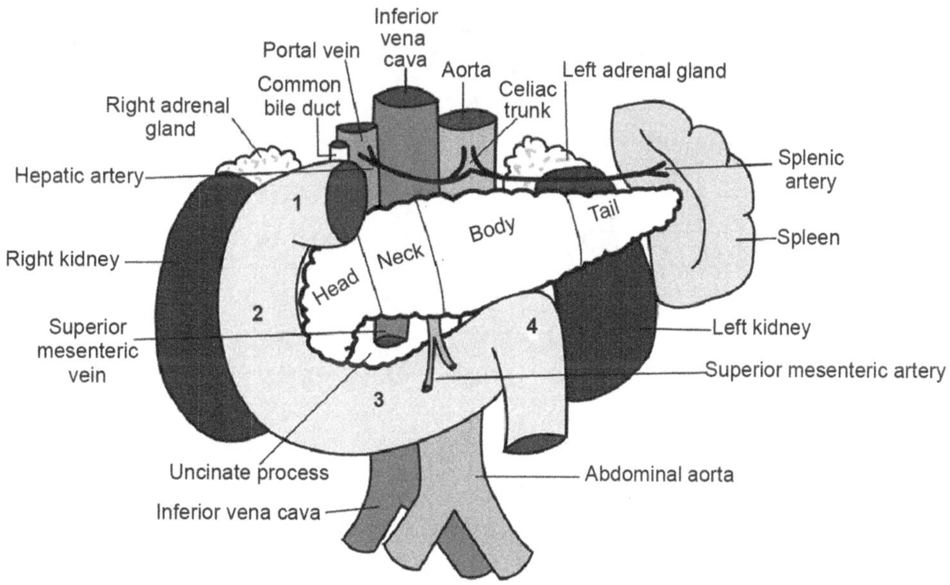

Fig. 31.1: Gross features of duodenum

b. i. Relations of first part of the duodenum: (Fig. 31.2a and Fig. 31.2b)

- *Anterior:*
  - Quadrate lobe of the liver.
  - Neck and body of the gallbladder.
- *Posterior:*
  - Bile duct, portal vein and gastroduodenal artery.
  - Behind all these inferior vena cava.
- *Superior:*
  - Epiploic foramen.
  - Horizontal part of hepatic artery.
- *Inferior:*
  - Head and neck of the pancreas.

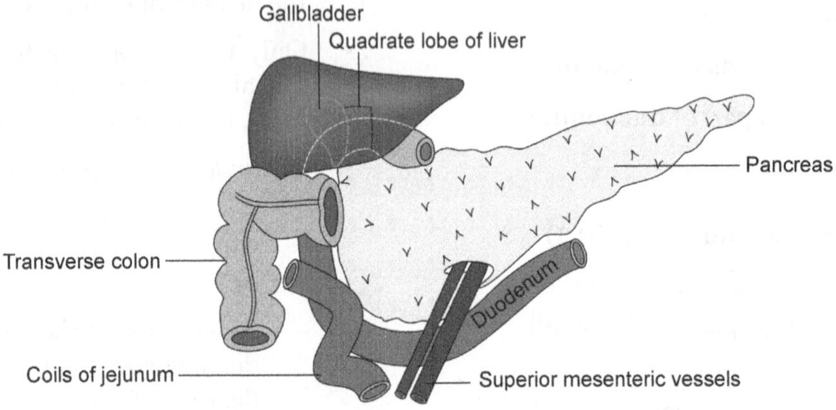

Fig. 31.2a: Anterior relations of duodenum

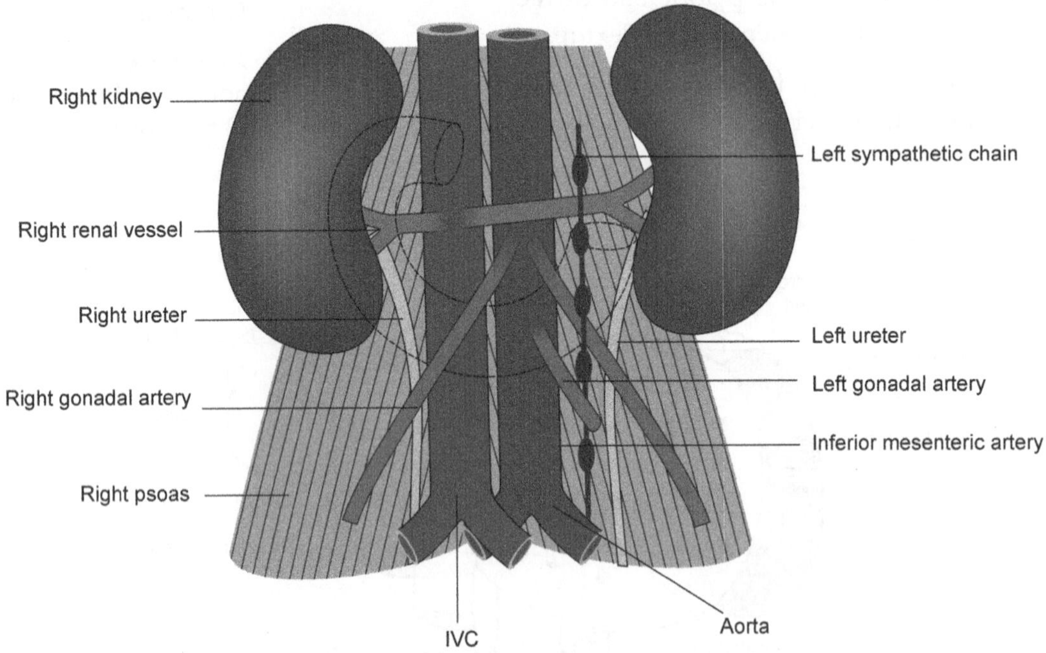

Fig. 31.2b: Posterior relations of 2nd, 3rd, 4th part of duodenum

Characteristic features of first part of the duodenum:

- Most movable part.
- Is supplied by end arteries.
- Is devoid of circular folds.
- Is most commonly affected by peptic ulcer.

Duodenal cap: A triangular radiopaque shadow known as duodenal cap is observed in the first part of the duodenum after the barium meal. It is produced because the first part is kept patent due to the protrusion of the pylorus and gets filled by barium meal. Any deformity in the duodenal cap will indicate mainly peptic ulcer.

ii. **Relations of the second part of duodenum:**

- *Anterior:*
  - Right lobe of liver.
  - Transverse colon.
  - Coils of jejunum.
- *Posterior:*
  - Right kidney (near the hilum).
  - Inferior vena cava.
  - Right psoas major.
- *Lateral:*
  - Right colic flexure.
- *Medial:*
  - Head of pancreas.
  - Bile duct.
  - Main and accessory pancreatic duct.

Anterior of the second part of duodenum: Two elevations are present along the posteromedial aspect.

- ***Major duodenal papilla:*** Is a conical elevation situated 8-10 cm from the pyloric end of the stomach. Ampulla of Vater (formed by union of bile duct and main pancreatic duct) opens on its summit. The opening is guarded by sphincter of Oddi.
- ***Minor duodenal papilla:*** Is a small conical elevation about 2 cm above the major duodenal papilla and accessory pancreatic duct opens on its summit.

iii. **Relations of third part of duodenum:**

- *Anterior:*
  - Superior mesenteric vessels.
  - Root of mesentery.
- *Posterior:*
  - Right psoas major.
  - Right ureter.
  - Right gonadal vessels.
  - Inferior vena cava.
  - Abdominal aorta and origin of inferior mesenteric artery.
- *Superior:* Head of pancreas.
- *Inferior:* Coils of jejunum.

iv. **Relations of fourth part of duodenum:**

- *Anterior:*
  - Transverse colon and mesocolon.
  - Stomach.
- *Posterior:*
  - Left crus of diaphragm.
  - Left psoas major and left sympathetic chain.
  - Left renal vessels.
  - Left gonadal vessels.
  - Inferior mesenteric vein.
- *Right:* Uncinate process of pancreas.
- *Left:* Left kidney and ureter.
- *Superior:* Body of the pancreas.

Suspensory ligament of treitz:

- Is a fibromuscular band that extends from the posterosuperior surface of duodenojejunal flexure to the right crus of the diaphragm.
- Upper 1/3rd consists of striated muscle, middle third of elastic fibers and lower third of smooth muscle.

d. **Arterial supply of duodenum: (Fig. 31.3)**

- Above the level of opening of bile duct, duodenum is supplied by superior pancreaticoduodenal artery and below by inferior pancreaticoduodenal artery.

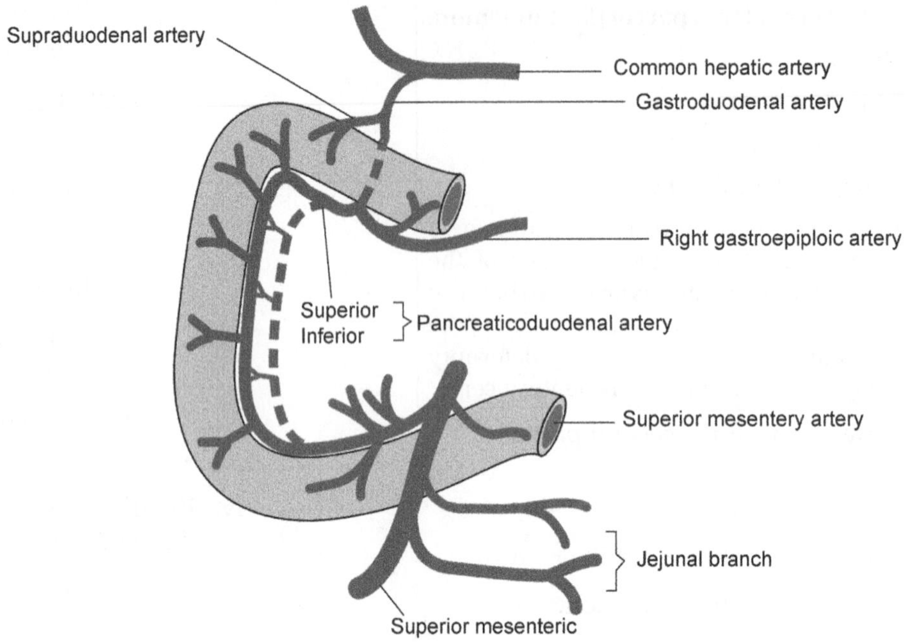

Fig. 31.3: Arterial supply of duodenum

- ***First part of duodenum receives additional supply from:***
  - Right gastric artery.
  - Supraduodenal artery (branch of hepatic artery).
  - Retroduodenal artery (branch of gastroduodenal artery).
  - Right gastroepiploic artery.

> Duodenum develops from both foregut and midgut, therefore it is supplied by the branches of arteries of foregut (celiac trunk) and midgut (superior mesenteric).

32 CHAPTER JEJUNUM AND ILEUM

1. **Enumerate:**
   a. **Differences between jejunum and ileum**
   b. **Contents of mesentery**
   c. **Structures crossed by the root of mesentery**

Ans. a. **Differences between jejunum and ileum:** See the following Table.

b. **Contents of mesentery:**
- Coils of jejunum and ileum.
- Jejunal and ileal branches of superior mesenteric artery.
- Mesenteric lymph nodes.
- Intestinal lymph vessels.
- Nerve plexus.
- Extraperitoneal loose connective tissue.
- Fat.

c. **Structures crossed by root of mesentery: (Fig. 32.1)**
- Mesentery is a fold of peritoneum that suspends jejunum and ileum from the posterior abdominal wall.
- Its attached margin (to posterior abdominal wall) is called root of the mesentery.
- The root is approx. 15 cm long.
- It extends from the left side of the L2 vertebra to the right sacroiliac joint.
- Structures crossed by the root of the mesentery from above downwards are:
  - Third part of duodenum.
  - Abdominal aorta.
  - Inferior vena cava.
  - Right gonadal vessels.
  - Right ureter.
  - Right psoas major muscle.

Feature	*Jejunum*	*Ileum*
Location	Usually occupies umbilical region	Occupies hypogastric and pelvic regions
Length	Proximal 2/5th of small intestine except duodenum	Distal 3/5th of small intestine
Caliber	Wider	Narrower
Wall thickness	Thicker	Thinner
Vascularity	More vascular	Less vascular
Plicae circulares	Closely set	Widely separated
Peyer's patches (aggregated lymphoid follicles)	Scanty	Numerous
Mesentery		
Distribution of fat	Less	More
Number of arcades	1-2	3-4
Vasa recta	Longer and fewer	Shorter and numerous

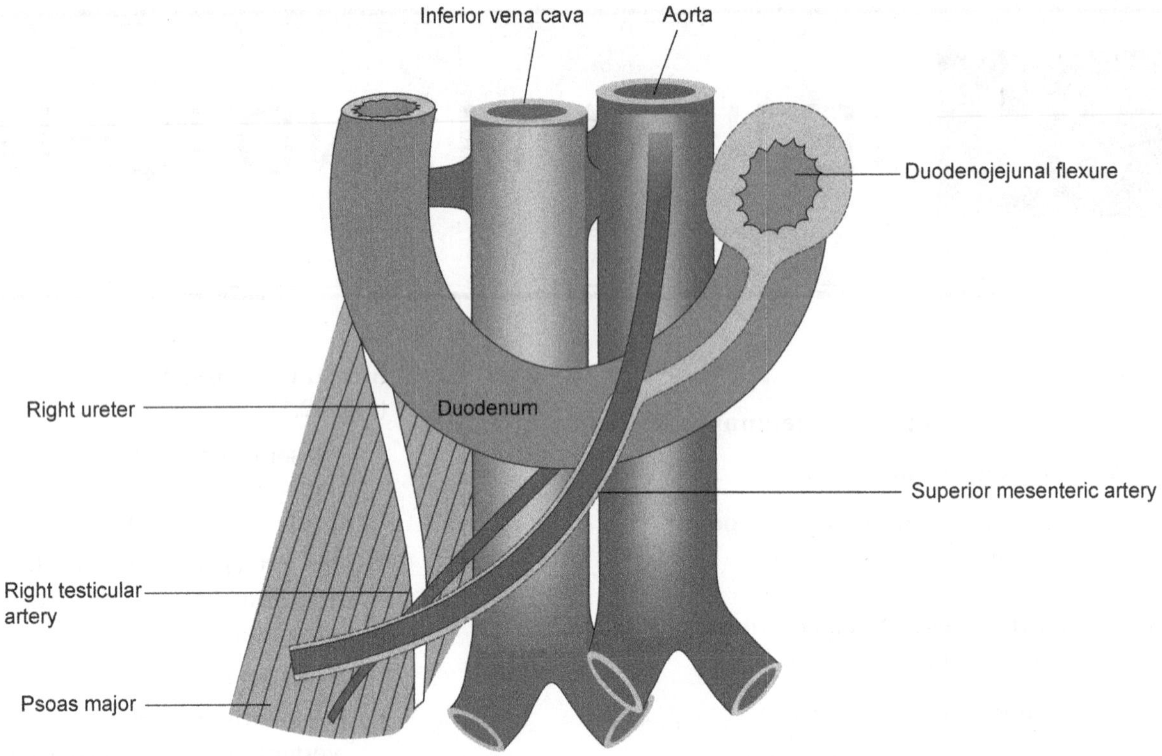

Fig. 32.1: Structures crossed by the root of the mesentery

2. **Which branch of abdominal aorta supplies jejunum and ileum?**

Ans. Superior mesenteric artery:

- 12-15 jejunal and ileal arteries arise from the left side of superior mesenteric artery to supply jejunum and ileum.
- Within the mesentery they branch and anastomose to form arterial arcades from the terminal arcades vasa recta arise that supply jejunum and ileum (Fig. 32.2).

> - ***Meckel's diverticulum:*** Is a blind diverticulum from the antimesenteric border of ileum.
> - Is located about two feet from ileocaecal junction.
> - Is a remnant of vitellointestinal duct.

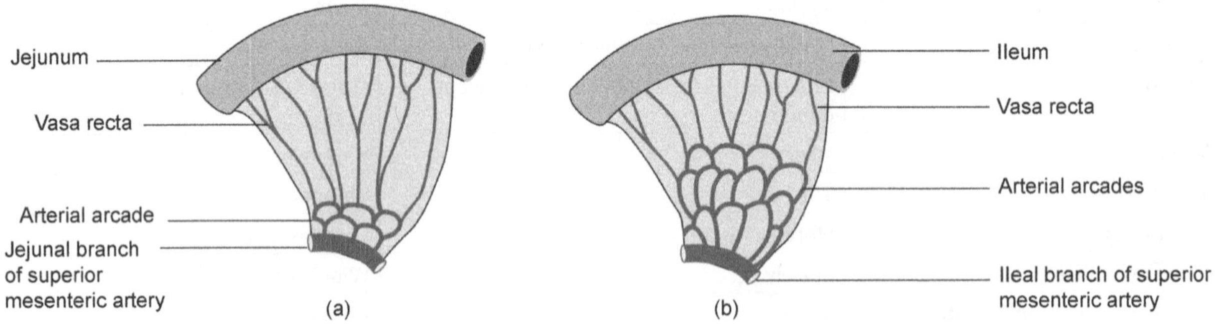

Fig. 32.2: Blood supply of (a) Jejunum (b) Ileum

33 CHAPTER

LIVER AND EXTRAHEPATIC BILIARY APPARATUS

1. **Describe the following features of liver:**

   a. **Location** b. **Shape**

   c. **Weight** d. **Gross features**

Ans. Liver is the largest gland of the body. It consists of both exocrine (secretes bile into ducts) and endocrine (secretes plasma proteins, heparin and glucose from glycogen into the blood) parts.

a. **Location:** It occupies whole of right hypochondrium, upper part of epigastrium and left hypochondrium (up to left midclavicular line).

b. **Shape:** Wedge shaped.

c. **Weight:** Average 1.5 kg (ratio of body weight: weight of live-in adults: 1/36, in newborn: 1/18 Liver is large in newborn due to the haemopoietic activity).

d. **Gross features:**

- *Liver has 5 surfaces:* Anterior, posterior, superior, inferior, right lateral.
- *Only one prominent border:* Inferior border.

- Liver is highly vascular.
- It has high regenerative power–surgical removal of 2/3rd of liver is compatible with life.

2. **What are anatomical and physiological/surgical lobes of liver?**

Ans. Anatomically the liver is divided into two lobes: Right and left (Fig. 33.1 and Fig. 33.2).

Demarcation:

- *Anteriorly and Superiorly:* Attachment of falciform ligament.
- *Inferiorly:* Fissure for ligamentum teres hepatis.
- *Posteriorly:* Fissure for ligamentum venosum.

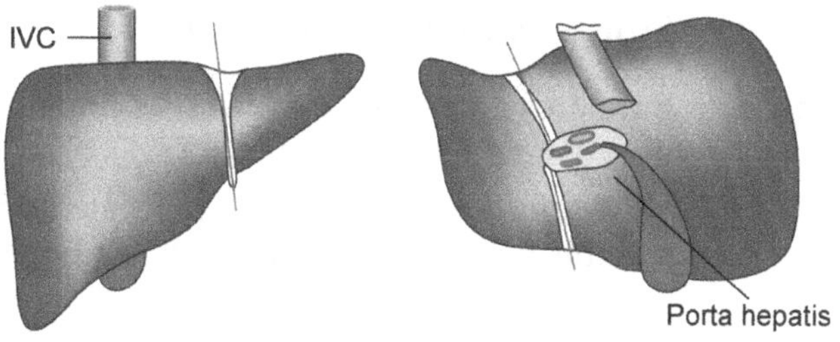

Fig. 33.1a: Anatomical lobes of liver

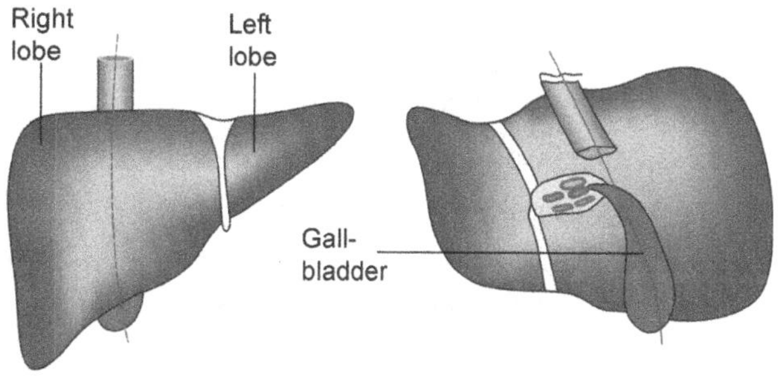

Fig. 33.1b: Physiological lobes of liver

Physiologically the liver is divided into right and left lobes on the basis of distribution of hepatic artery, portal vein and hepatic duct (i.e., right lobe receives blood from the right branches of hepatic artery and portal vein and pours bile into right hepatic duct).

Demarcation:

- *Anterosuperiorly:* The plane passes along the line joining the cystic notch to the groove for IVC.
- *Inferiorly:* Through fossa for gallbladder.
- *Posteriorly:* Through the middle of the caudate lobe.

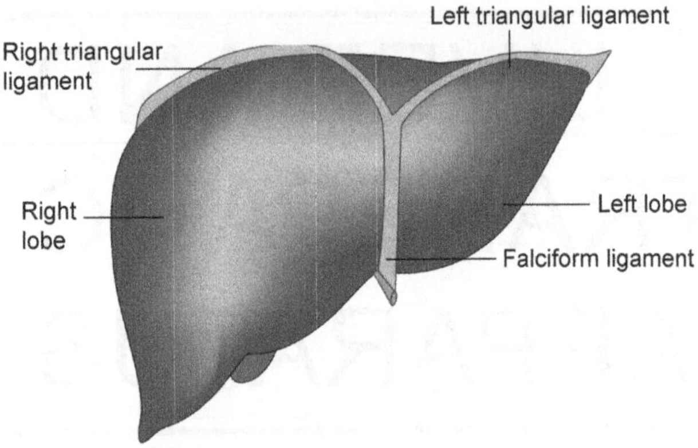

Fig. 33.2: Anterior surface of liver

3. **Enumerate:**
   a. **Bare areas of liver**
   b. **Ligaments and peritoneal folds attached liver**
   c. **Structures in the porta hepatis**

Ans. a. **Bare areas of liver:** Are the areas that are not covered by peritoneum.

- ***Main bare area of liver:*** Is located on the posterior surface. Its boundaries are:
  - *Base:* Groove for inferior vena cava.
  - *Apex:* Right triangular ligament.
  - *Sides:* Superior and inferior layers of coronary ligaments.
- Groove for inferior vena cava.
- Fossa for gallbladder.
- Fissures for ligamentum teres hepatis and ligamentum venosum.
- Porta hepatis.

b. **Ligaments of liver:**

- ***True ligaments:***
  - Ligamentum teres hepatis (obliterated left umbilical vein), extends from umbilicus to left branch of portal vein.
  - Ligamentum venosum (obliterated ductus venosus), extends from left branch of portal vein to inferior vena cava.
- ***False ligaments:***
  - Falciform ligament.
  - Coronary ligament.
  - Right and left triangular ligament.
  - Lesser omentum.

c. **Structures in the porta hepatis:**

- Common hepatic duct – anteriorly
- Heptic artery – in the middle
- Portal vein – posteriorly

} at porta hepatis the hepatic duct, hepatic artery and portal vein divide into right and left branches

- Autonomic nerve fibers (sympathetic from celiac plexus and parasympathetic from vagus).
- Lymph vessels and nodes.

4. **Draw labeled diagram to show:**
   a. **Visceral relations to the inferior surface of liver**
   b. **Segments of liver**

Ans. a. See Figure 33.3.

b. See Figure 33.4.

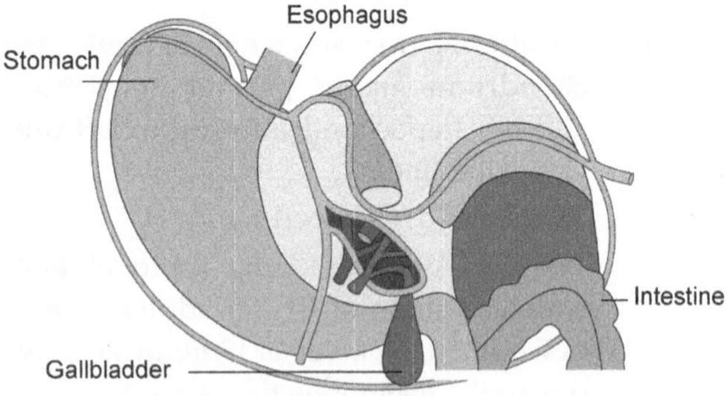

Fig. 33.3: Visceral surface of liver

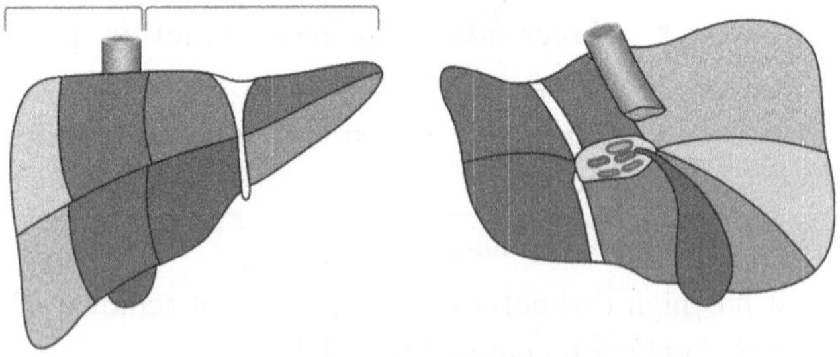

Fig. 33.4: Segments of liver

5. **What are the components of extrahepatic biliary apparatus?**

Ans. **Components of extrahepatic biliary apparatus:**
   a. Right and left hepatic ducts.
   b. Common hepatic duct.
   c. Gallbladder and cystic duct.
   d. Common bile duct.

6. **Draw labeled diagram showing components of extrahepatic biliary apparatus.**

Ans. Components of extrahepatic biliary apparatus (Fig. 33.5).

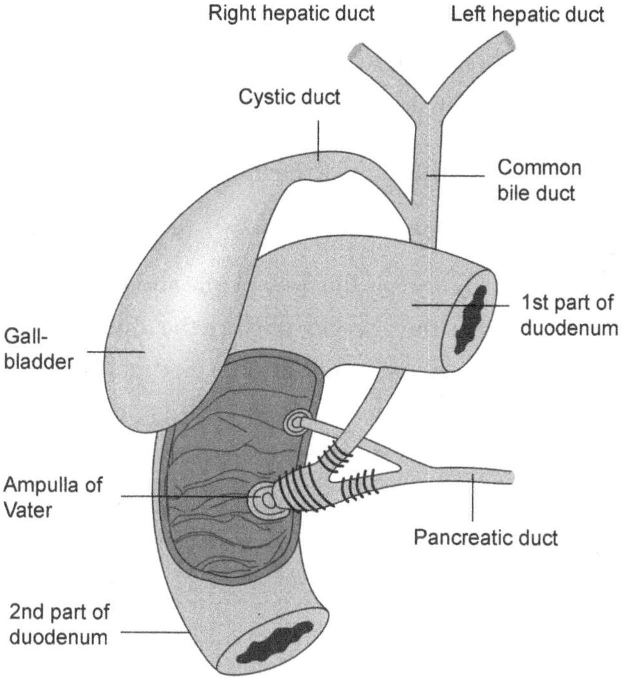

Fig. 33.5: Components of extrahepatic biliary apparatus

7. **Describe in brief:**
   a. **Gallbladder and cystic duct**
   b. **Common bile duct**

Ans. a. **Gallbladder and cystic duct:**

- It is a pear shaped fibromuscular sac that stores the bile.
- It lies in the gallbladder fossa on the inferior surface of right lobe of liver.
- ***Function:***
  - It stores bile.
  - It absorbes water and electrolyte and thus concentrates the bile.
- ***Measurements:***
  - 7-10 cm.
  - 3 cm in its widest part.
  - 30-50 ml.
- ***Parts:*** It has three parts:
  - *Fundus:* Is the lower free expanded part covered by peritoneum on all the sides.
  - *Body:* Is the major part of gallbladder extending from fundus to neck.
  - *Neck:* Is the upper narrow part which end in cystic duct.

Hartmann's pouch: Is a small recess that projects downwards from the right side of neck of gallbladder.

- It is supplied by cystic branch of right hepatic artery which passes through the Calot's triangle (Fig. 33.6).

Calot's triangle: Is an important landmark for localization of cystic artery which lies in the triangle. Its boundaries are:

- **Superiorly:** Inferior surface of liver.
- **Left:** Common hepatic duct.
- **Right:** Cystic duct.

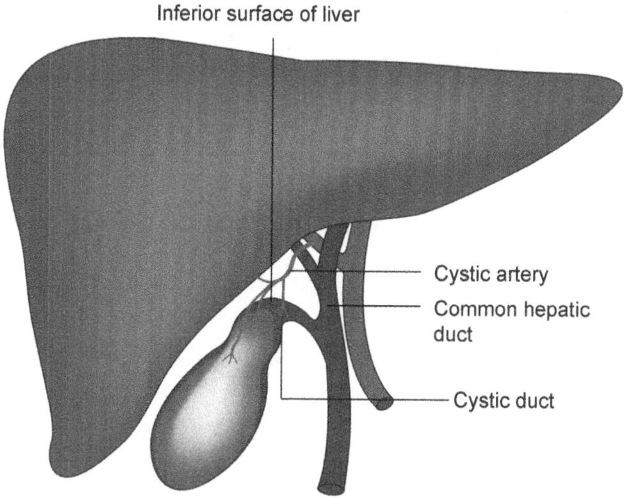

Fig. 33.6: Calot's triangle

b. **Common bile duct:**

- It is approximately 8 cm long and 6 mm wide.
- It is formed by union of common hepatic duct and cystic duct.
- It is divided into 4 parts according to its course:
  - *Supraduodenal:* Above the first part of duodenum, runs in the free margin of lesser omentum.

- *Retroduodenal:* It is behind the first part of duodenum.
- *Infraduodenal:* It is below the first part of duodenum and behind the head of pancreas.
- *Intraduodenal:* It is passing through the wall of duodenum along with the main pancreatic duct.

8. Referred pain in cholecystitis is referred to tip of right shoulder.

Ans. The inflammation of the gallbladder may cause irritation of the subdiaphragmatic parietal peritoneum which is supplied by phrenic nerve (root value – C3, 4, 5) and the pain may be referred to the skin over the tip of the right shoulder as it is supplied by supraclavicular nerve (C3, C4).

9. What is Murphy's sign?

Ans. A positive Murphy's sign is seen in acute cholecystitis. It is elicited by firmly placing a hand at the costal margin in the right upper abdominal quadrant and asking the patient to breathe deeply. If the gallbladder is inflamed, the patient will experience pain and catch their breath as the gallbladder descends and contacts the palpating hand.

10. What is biliary dyskinesia?

Ans. Musculature of gallbladder wall and sphincter of Oddi (controls the flow of bile and pancreatic juice into the second part of the duodenum) have reciprocal innervation, i.e., if gallbladder contracts, sphincter relaxes. If this mechanism is disrupted it is called biliary dyskinesia.

> Gangrene of gallbladder is uncommon in occlusion of cystic artery because of rich secondary blood supply from the liver bed (gallbladder fossa).

34 CHAPTER PANCREAS

1. **Describe pancreas under the following headings:**
   - a. **Gross features**
   - b. **Parts and relations**
   - c. **Pancreatic ducts**
   - d. **Arterial supply of pancreas**
   - e. **Applied anatomy**

Ans. a. Gross features:

- Pancreas is a soft lobulated composite gland which consists of both exocrine and endocrine parts.
- It is roughly retort shaped.
- Its dimensions are: ***Length:*** 12-15 cm, ***Breadth:*** 3-4 cm, ***Thickness:*** 1.5-2 cm, ***Weight:*** 80-90 gms.
- It extends from concavity of duodenum to the hilum of spleen.
- It is retroperitoneal.
- It occupies posterior part of epigastrium and left hypochondriac regions (at the level of L1 and L2).

b. Parts and relations:

- ***Head:*** It is the right enlarged part of the pancreas lodged in the duodenal curvature formed by 1st, 2nd and 3rd parts of duodenum. From its lower portion a hook like process called *uncinate process projects* directed towards left.
  - *Relations:*
    - Anterior: Gallbladder, pylorus with 1st part of duodenum, transverse colon, coils of jejunum.
    - Posterior: Inferior vena cava, bile duct, right middle suprarenal, renal and gonadal arteries.
- ***Neck:*** It is the constricted part at the junction of head and body of pancreas.
  - *Relations:*
    - Anterior: Pylorus and lesser sac, gastroduodenal artery.
    - Posterior: Formation of portal vein.
- ***Body:*** Is the elongated tapering portion lies obliquely across the posterior abdominal wall. It is triangular in section and has:

  3 borders: Superior, anterior and inferior.

  Anterior border provides attachment to transverse mesocolon.

  3 surfaces: Anterior, posterior and inferior.
  - *Relations:*
    - Anterior surface: Stomach separated by lesser sac.
    - Posterior surface:

      Aorta and origin of superior mesenteric artery.

      Left crus of diaphragm.

      Left kidney and suprarenal gland.

      Left renal vessels.

      Splenic vein.
    - Inferior surface: Duodenojejunal flexure, coils of jejunum and left colic flexure.

- *Tail:* Narrow end that lies between the two layers of lieno-renal ligament (along with splenic vessels).

> Tail of pancreas contains maximum number of islets of Langerhans. While performing splenectomy care has to be taken to preserve the tail while ligating splenic vessels.

c. **Pancreatic ducts:** Exocrine part of the pancreas pours its secretions through two ducts, the main pancreatic duct and accessory pancreatic duct.

- **Main pancreatic duct (Wirsung's duct):**

Commences from the tail of the pancreas

↓

Passes through the body

↓

Passes through the lower part of head

↓

Pierces posteromedial wall of 2nd part of duodenum

↓

Joins bile duct and forms Ampulla of Vater

↓

Opens on the summit of major duodenal papilla (8-10 cm from the pylorus)

- **Accessory pancreatic duct (Duct of Santorini):**

Commences from uncinate process

↓

Passes upwards and towards right

↓

Crosses the main pancreatic duct

↓

Opens in 2nd part of duodenum on minor duodenal papilla (2 cm above the major duodenal papilla)

Parts and ducts of pancreas

d. **Arterial supply of pancreas: (Fig. 34.1)**

- *Head:* Is supplied by superior and inferior pancreaticoduodenal arteries.
- *Neck body and tail:* Are supplied by pancreatic branches of splenic artery.

e. **Applied anatomy:**

- *Annular pancreas:* Is a congenital defect, where the second part of duodenum is surrounded by head of pancreas. It causes narrowing and obstruction of the lumen of duodenum.
- *Cancer of head of pancreas:* It may cause jaundice due to pressure upon bile duct which passes behind the head of pancreas. It may also cause portal hypertension due to pressure on portal vein.
- *Inflammation of pancreas* called *pancreatitis* is often associated with collection of fluid in the lesser sac.
- *Accessory pancreatic tissue:* May be present in the walls of the stomach, duodenum, jejunum or Meckel's diverticulum.

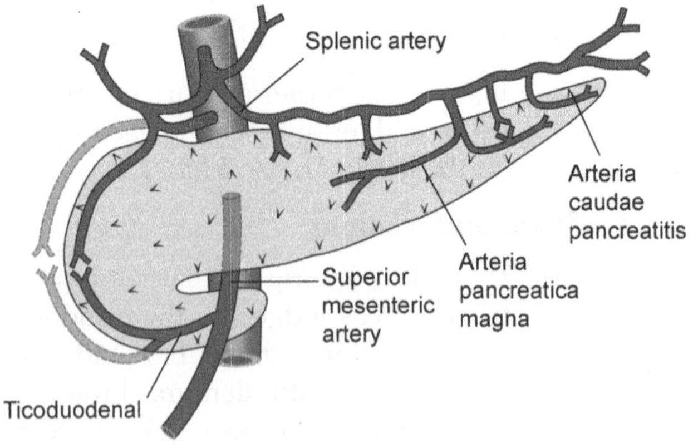

Fig. 34.1: Arterial supply of pancreas

35 CHAPTER

LARGE INTESTINE

1. What are the different parts of large intestine?

Ans. Large intestine begins at ileocaecal junction and ends at anus. The length is 6 feet and is subdivided into the following parts: (Fig. 35.1)

a. Caecum and Appendix.

b. Ascending colon.

c. Transverse colon.

d. Descending colon.

e. Sigmoid colon.

f. Rectum.

g. Anal canal.

Most parts of the large intestine are retroperitoneal except appendix, transverse colon and sigmoid colon.

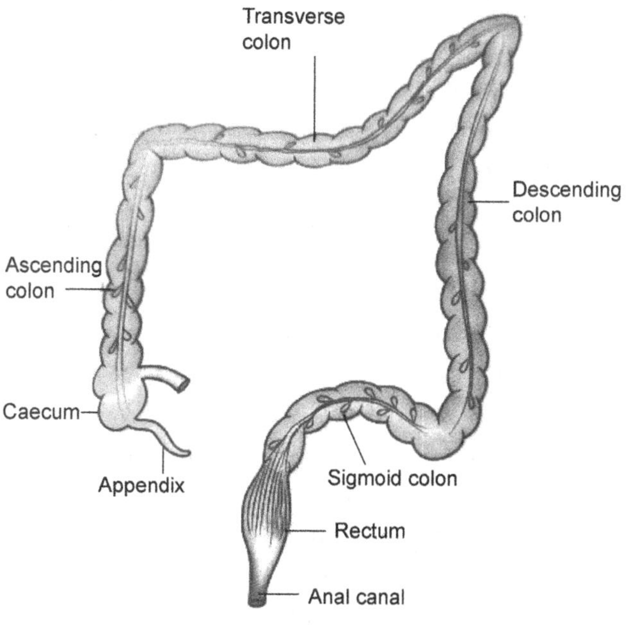

Fig. 35.1: Parts of large intestine

2. Enumerate the cardinal features of large intestine.

Ans. Cardinal features of large intestine are: (Fig. 35.2)

a. Presence of taenia coli – ribbon like bands formed by longitudinal muscle (begin from base of appendix and extend till the end of sigmoid colon.

b. Presence of sacculations/haustrations.

c. Presence of appendices epiploicae peritoneal pouches containing fat are absent in caecum, appendix and rectum.

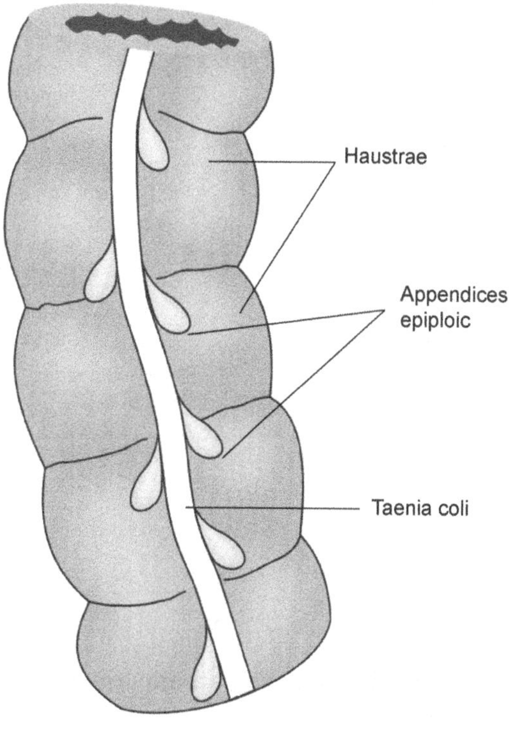

Fig. 35.2: Cardinal features of large intestine

3. Enumerate the differences between the small and large intestine.

Ans. See Table 35.1.

Table 35.1: Differences between the small and large intestine		
Features	*Small Intestine*	*Large Intestine*
Length	6-7 metres	1.5 metres
Caliber	Narrower	Wider
Taenia coli	Absent	Present
Sacculations	Absent	Present
Appendices epiploicae	Absent	Present
Villi	Present	Absent
Plicae circulars	Present	Absent
Peyer's patches	Present in ileum	Absent
Crypts of liberkuhn	Crypts contain absorptive cells and Paneth cells	Crypts contain numerous goblet cells, few absorptive cells and no Paneth cells

4. **Draw labeled diagram showing posterior relations of cecum.**

Ans. See Figure 35.3.

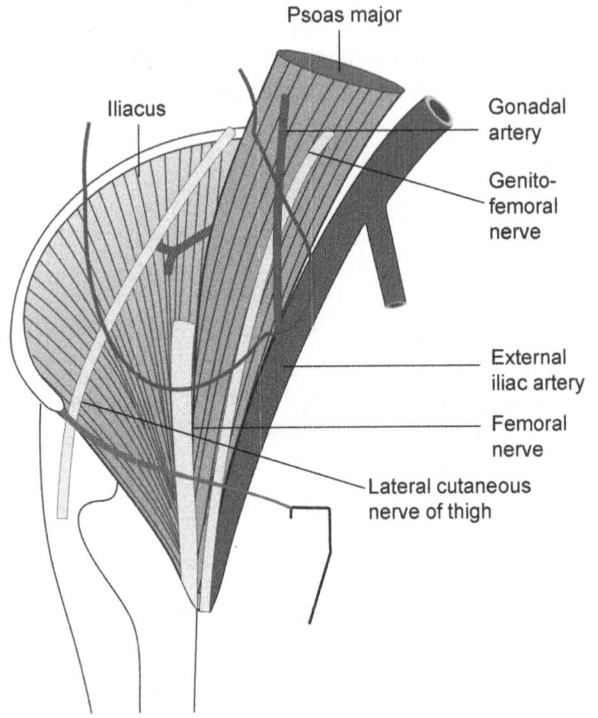

Fig. 35.3: Posterior relations of cecum

5. **Describe the parasympathetic innervations of the colon.**

Ans. Parasympathetic supply to the large intestine is derived from two sources:

- **Vagus nerve:** Supplies the part of the colon derived from the midgut (ascending colon and right 2/3rd of the transverse colon).
- **Pelvic splanchnic nerves (S2, S3, S4):** Supplies the colon that develops from hindgut (left 1/3rd of transverse colon, descending colon and sigmoid colon).

> Hirschsprung's disease or congenital megacolon is a condition in which there is congenital absence of parasympathetic neurons in a segment of colon (mostly sigmoid colon). This results in absence of peristalsis in that particular segment leading to dilatation of colon proximal to the affected segment due to accumulation of feces.

6. **Describe briefly the various positions of appendix.**

Ans. Vermiform appendix is a narrow tubular structure attached to the posteromedial wall of cecum, about 2 cm below the ileocecal valve. Its length varies from 2-20 cms (average 9 cm). The position of appendix is variable. The various positions are: (Fig. 35.4)

a. **Retrocecal (12 o'clock):** Appendix is located behind the cecum. This is the most common position.

b. **Splenic (2 o'clock):** Appendix lies in relation to terminal ileum. It may lie either anterior to ileum (pre-ileal) or posterior to ileum (post-ileal).

c. **Promonteric (3 o'clock):** Appendix is directed towards the sacral promontory.

d. **Pelvic (4 o'clock):** Appendix points towards the pelvic brim.

e. **Subcecal/midinguinal (6 o'clock):** Appendix lies below the cecum and points towards the mid-inguinal point.

f. **Paracolic/paracecal (11 o'clock):**

- The pain of appendicitis is referred to the umbilicus as both are supplied by T10 spinal segment.
- Tenderness at McBurney's point is the cardinal sign of acute appendicitis (Fig. 35.5 and Fig. 35.6).

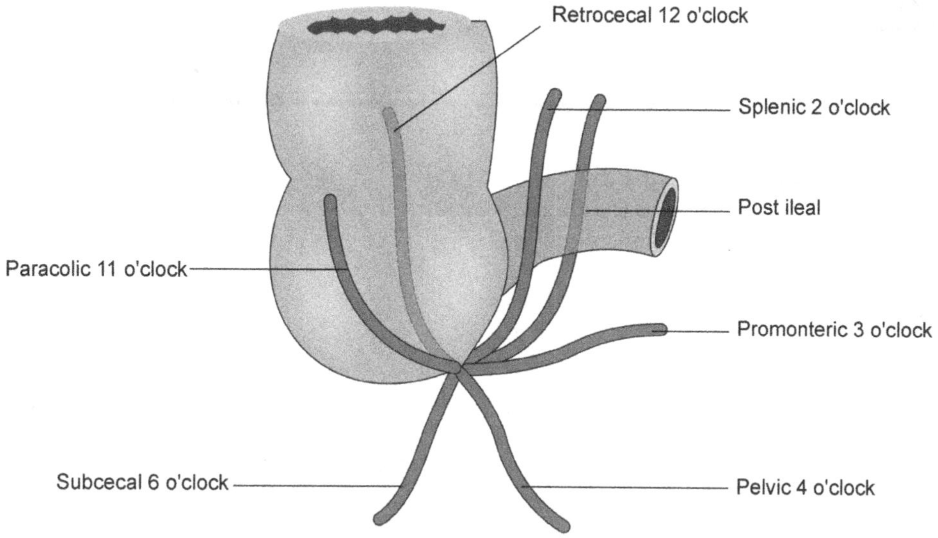

Fig. 35.4: Various positions of appendix

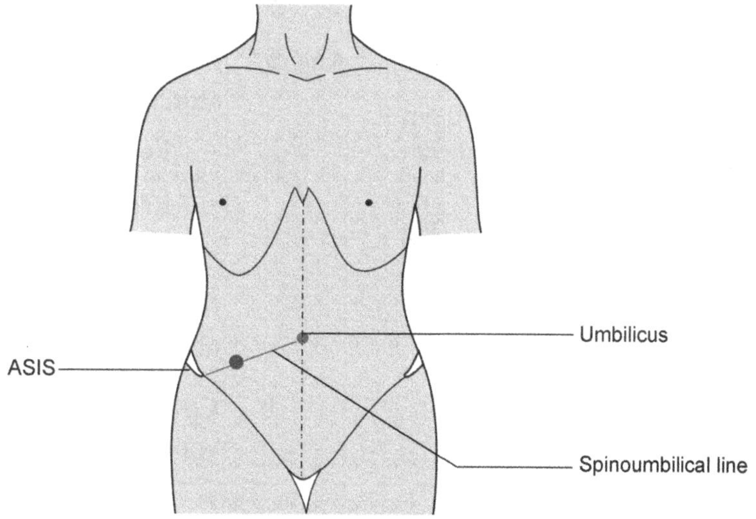

Fig. 35.5: McBurney's point

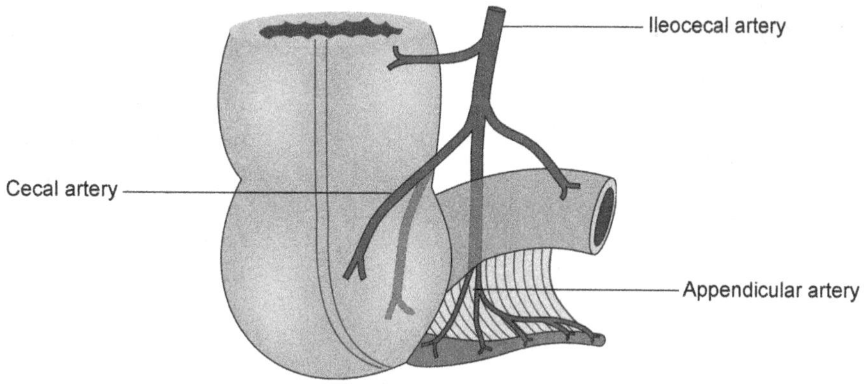

Fig. 35.6: Arterial supply of appendix

36 CHAPTER KIDNEYS

1. **Describe the following features of kidney:**
   a. **Location and extent**
   b. **Shape and size**
   c. **Gross features**

Ans. a. **Location:** Kidneys are located retroperitoneally on the posterior abdominal wall on either side of vertebral column.

Extent: T12 – L3 vertebra (right kidney is slightly lower than the left).

> Transpyloric plane (lower border of L1 verterbra) passes through the upper part of the hilum of right kidney and lower part of the hilum of left kidney.

b. **Shape:** Bean shaped. **Weight:** 130-170 gm. **Size:** Length – 11 cm, Breadth – 6 cm, Thickness – 3 cm.

c. **Gross features:** Each kidney has: (Fig. 36.1)

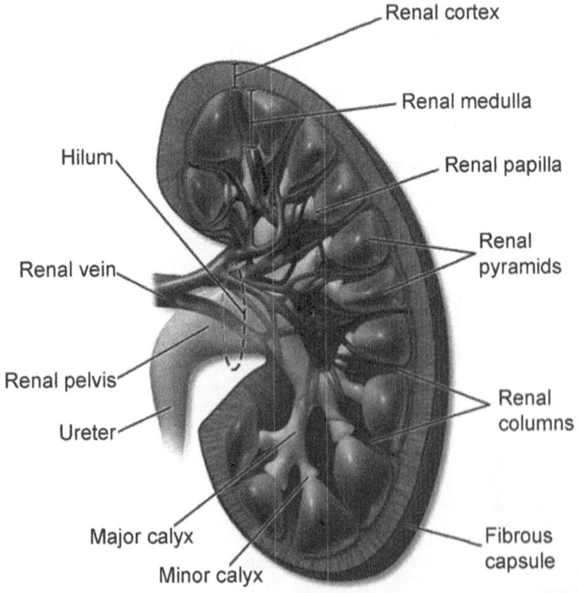

Fig. 36.1: Gross features of kidney

- *Two surfaces:* Anterior and posterior.
- *Two poles:* Upper and lower (Upper pole is nearer to the median plane).
- *Two borders:* Lateral and medial (Medial border presents a vertical cleft in the middle called hilum).

2. **Enumerate:**
   a. **Structures passing through the hilum**
   b. **Coverings of kidney**

Ans. a. **From anterior to posterior the following structures pass through the hilum:**

- Renal vein.
- Renal artery.
- Pelvis of ureter.

(Lymphatics and nerves (sympathetic) also pass through the hilum).

b. **Coverings of kidney:** From within outwards are:

- *Fibrous capsule:* Covers the entire organ, lines the renal sinus and covers the walls of major and minor calyces and pelvis of ureter.
- *Perinephric fat:* Is abundant alone the borders of the kidney and extends through the hilum into the renal sinus.
- *Renal fascia/Fascia of Gerota:* Is a fibroareolar sheath which surrounds the kidney and perirenal fat. It consists of two layers–anterior and posterior.

- *Above:* The two layers fuse at the upper pole and resplit to enclose the suprarenal gland and then blends with the subdiaphragmatic fascia.
- *Laterally:* Both the layers fuse and become continuous with the fascia transversalis.
- *Medially:* Anterior layer merges with the connective tissue surrounding aorta and inferior vena cava.

Posterior layer is continuous with the psoas fascia. Along the medial border of the kidney the two layers are connected to each other by a connective tissue septum.

- *Below:* The two layers do not fuse and extend downwards along the ureter. Anterior layer merges with extraperitoneal tissue of iliac fossa and the posterior layer with fascia iliaca.

> Perirenal effusion does not extend superiorly, laterally or medially as the two layers of renal fascia are either fused or connected by a septum (medially), however it can track down inferiorly as the two layers remain separate.

Paranephric fat: It is a layer of fat present outside the renal fascia. The fat in this layer is more abundant posteriorly between the thoracolumbar fascia and renal fascia.

3. **Draw labeled diagram of the following:**
   a. **Coverings of kidney**
   b. **Anterior relations of right and left kidneys**
   c. **Posterior relations of right and left kidneys**
   d. **Macroscopic features of kidney (coronal section)**

Ans. a. **See Figure 36.2a and 36.2b.**
b. **See Figure 36.3a.**
c. **See Figure 36.3b.**
d. **See Figure 36.4.**

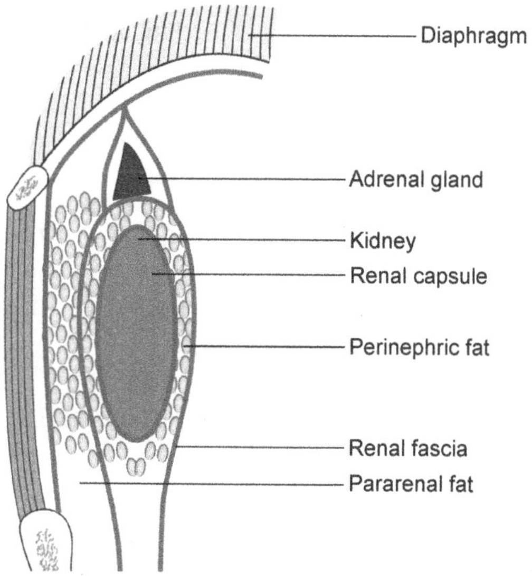

Fig. 36.2a: Coverings of kidney (sagittal section)

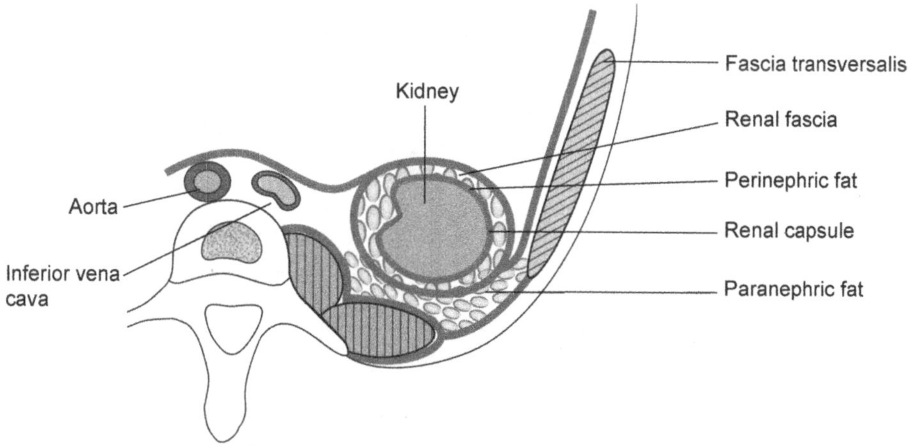

Fig. 36.2b: Coverings of kidney (transverse section)

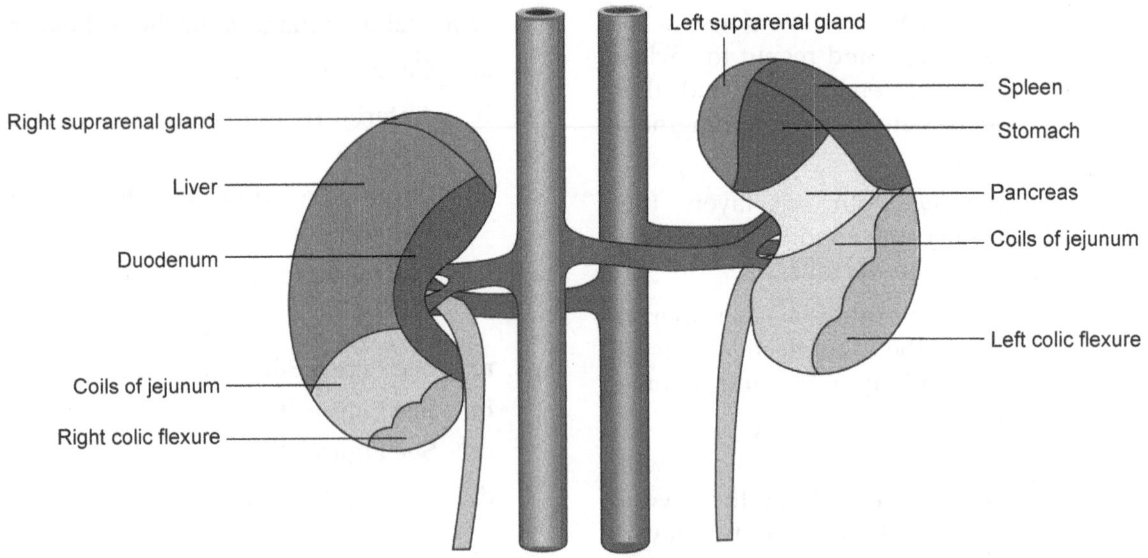

Fig. 36.3a: Anterior relations of kidney

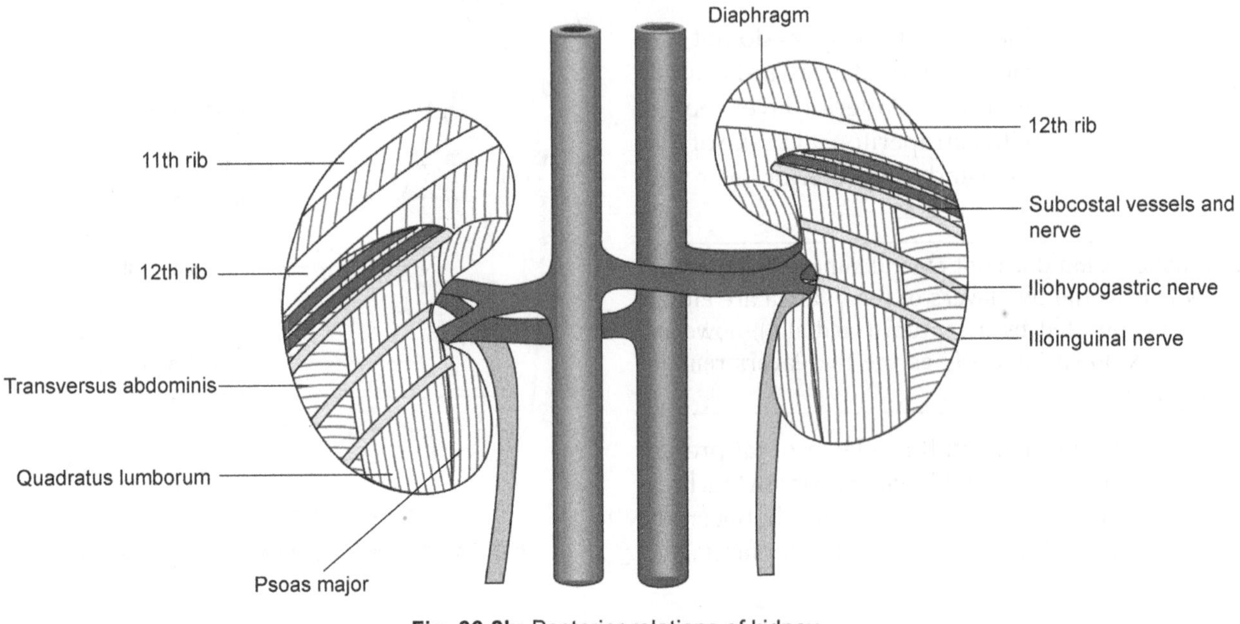

Fig. 36.3b: Posterior relations of kidney

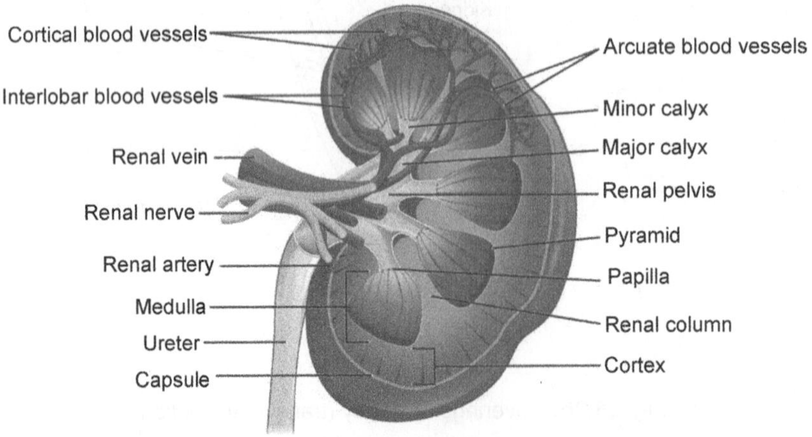

Fig. 36.4: Macroscopic features of kidney

37 CHAPTER

URETERS

1. Describe ureter under the following headings:

a. Extent and parts

b. Course

c. Arterial supply

d. Nerve supply

Ans. Ureter is a muscular tube that conveys urine by peristaltic movement from the renal pelvis to urinary bladder. It is retroperitoneal.

a. **Extent and parts:** It begins at the lower end of the renal pelvis (pelviureteric junction) at the lower pole of the kidney and ends by opening into the urinary bladder. It is approx. 25 cm long. Is divided into two parts:

- Abdominal.
- Pelvic.

b. **Course: (Fig. 37.1)**

- It descends in front of psoas major muscle along the tips of transverse processes of lumbar vertebrae.
- It crosses the pelvic inlet at the bifurcation of common iliac artery and enters pelvic cavity.
- It then runs downwards and backwards on the lateral pelvic wall along the anterior margin of greater sciatic notch to reach ischial spine.
- It turns forwards and medially and passes above the pelvic diaphragm to reach the posterosuperior angle of base of urinary bladder.
- It pierces wall of the urinary bladder and runs obliquely through its muscular coat and opens in the cavity of urinary bladder at the upper angle of the trigone of bladder.

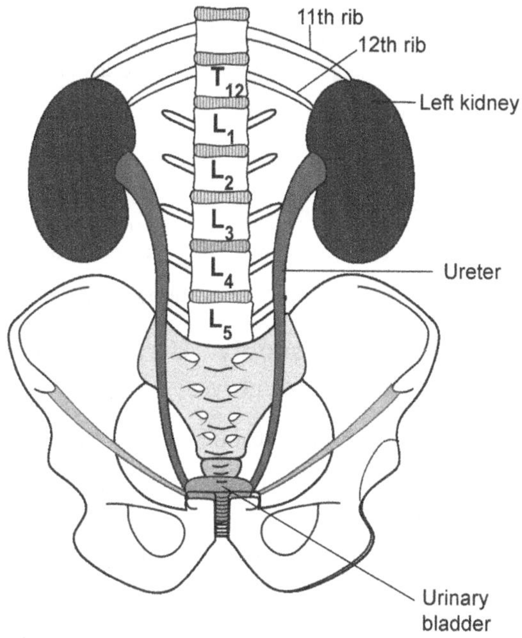

Fig. 37.1: Course of ureter

c. **Arterial supply: (Fig. 37.2)**

- ***Abdominal part:*** From:
  - Renal artery – upper part.
  - Abdominal aorta – middle part.
  - Testicular/ovarian artery – lower part.
- ***Pelvic part:*** From:
  - Common iliac artery.
  - Inferior vesicle artery (in males).
  - Uterine artery (in females).

Abdominal part of ureter receives blood supply from the medially related arteries and the pelvic part from the laterally related arteries, therefore, too much mobilization of abdominal part to lateral side and pelvic part towards medial side during removal of ureteric calculus should be avoided, so that blood supply is not interrupted.

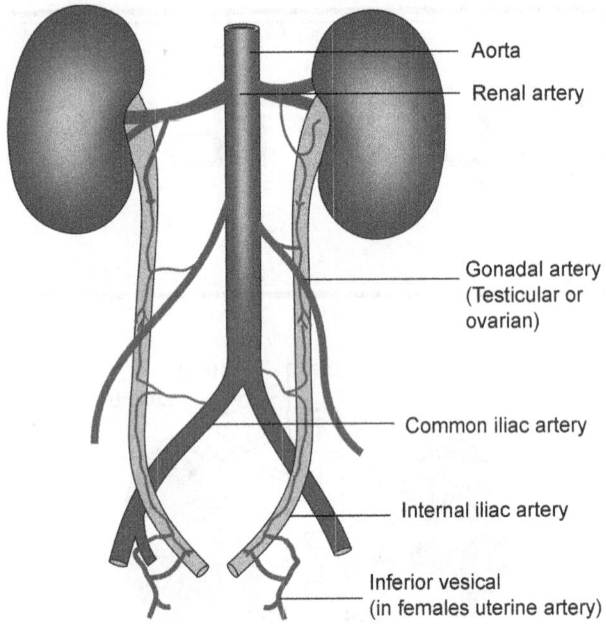

Fig. 37.2: Arterial supply of ureter

d. **Nerve supply:** Ureter is supplied by autonomic nerves.

- Sympathetic – T12 – L2.
- Parasympathetic – S2, S3, S4.

2. **Enumerate the sites of constrictions of ureter.**

Ans. There are three constrictions in the course of the ureter:

a. Pelviureteric junction.

b. At the pelvic inlet.

c. As it enters into the urinary bladder.

Relationship of the constrictions of ureter to the bony landmarks:

- 1st constriction – Near tip of transverse process of L2 vertebra.
- 2nd constriction – Overlying sacroiliac joint.
- 3rd constriction – Medial to the ischial spine.

Ureteric calculus is likely to lodge at one of these sites. This may lead to ureteric colic is referred to anterior abdominal wall according to the part of ureter where the stone is impacted.

Part of ureter where stone is impacted	*Nerve supply*	*Area of referred pain*	
Upper part	Lesser splanchnic nerve and T12 spinal segment	Lumbar region	Loin To Groin
Middle part	Lumbar splanchnic nerves (L1,L2 spinal segments)	Inguinal and pubic region	
Lower part	Pelvic splanchnic nerves (S2,S3,S4 spinal segments)	Perineum	

3. **Enumerate the important relations of:**

a. **Relations of abdominal part of ureter**

b. **Relations of pelvic part of ureter**

Ans. a. Relations of abdominal part of ureter:

- ***Anterior relations:***

Right ureter	*Left ureter*
Third part of duodenum	Left colic vessels
Root of mesentery with superior mesenteric vessels	Left testicular/ovarian vessels
Iliocolic and right colic vessels	Sigmoidal vessels
Right testicular/ovarian vessels	Apex of pelvic mesocolon

- ***Posterior relations (common on both the sides):***
  - Psoas major muscle.
  - Genitofemoral nerve.
  - Beginning of external iliac artery.

b. Relations of pelvic part of ureter:

In males	*In females*
a. Posterolateral part (in contact with lateral pelvic wall)	**a. Posterolateral part (in contact with lateral pelvic wall)**
Posteriorly: Internal iliac vessels, lumbosacral trunk and sacroiliac joint	***Posteriorly:*** Internal iliac vessels, lumbosacral trunk and sacroiliac joint
Anteriorly: Covered by peritoneum	***Anteriorly:*** Covered by peritoneum, forms posterior boundary of ovarian fossa*
Laterally: Obturator nerve and vessels, inferior vesical vessels and middle rectal vessels	***Laterally:*** Obturator nerve and vessels, uterine and vaginal vessels and middle rectal vessels
b. Anteromedial part (lies in extraperitoneal tissue on the floor of pelvic cavity)	**b. Anteromedial part (lies in extraperitoneal tissue on the floor of pelvic cavity)**
Superiorly: Parietal peritoneum	***Superiorly:*** Broad ligament of uterus, uterine artery lies above in front and then crosses it to lie medial to it**
Inferiorly: Levator ani muscle	***Inferiorly:*** Lateral cervical ligament
Near its termination: Crossed by ductus deferens (from lateral to medial)	***Near its termination:*** Lateral fornix of vagina and the anterior wall of vagina

* In this position, ureter is likely to be injured if clamped along with ovarian vessels.

** In this position, the ureter is liable to be injured during surgery for removal of uterus as it may be mistakenly claimed along with uterine vessels.

CHAPTER 38

SUPRARENAL GLAND

1. **Describe suprarenal glands under the following headings:**
   a. **Location**
   b. **Shape and measurements**
   c. **Gross features**
   d. **Relations**
   e. **Blood supply**

Ans. Suprarenal glands are paired endocrine glands that secretes number of steroid hormones.

a. **Location:** Upper poles of kidneys.

b. **Shape and measurements:**
   - *Shape:* Right gland-pyramidal Left – cresentric/semilunar.
   - *Length:* 5 cm.
   - *Breadth:* 3 cm.
   - *Thickness:* 1 cm.
   - *Weight:* 5 gm.

c. **Gross features:**
   - Right gland has an apex, base, three borders (anterior, medial, lateral) and two surfaces (anterior and posterior).
   - Left gland has two ends (upper and lower), two borders (medial and lateral), two surfaces (anterior and posterior).

d. **Relations:**
   - ***Right gland:***
     – *Anterior surface* – Inferior vena cava and right lobe of liver.
     – *Posterior surface* – Right crus of diaphragm (above) and kidney (below).
   - ***Left gland:***
     – *Anterior surface* – Stomach, splenic artery and pancreas.
     – *Posterior surface* – Left crus of diaphragm (medial) and kidney (lateral).

e. **Blood supply:**
   - ***Each gland is supplied by three arteries: (Fig. 38.1)***
     – Superior suprarenal artery – Branch of inferior phrenic artery.
     – Middle suprarenal artery – Branch of abdominal aorta.
     – Inferior suprarenal artery – Branch of renal artery.
   - ***Each gland is drained by a single vein:***
     – Right suprarenal vein drains into inferior vena cava.
     – Left suprarenal vein drains into left renal vein.

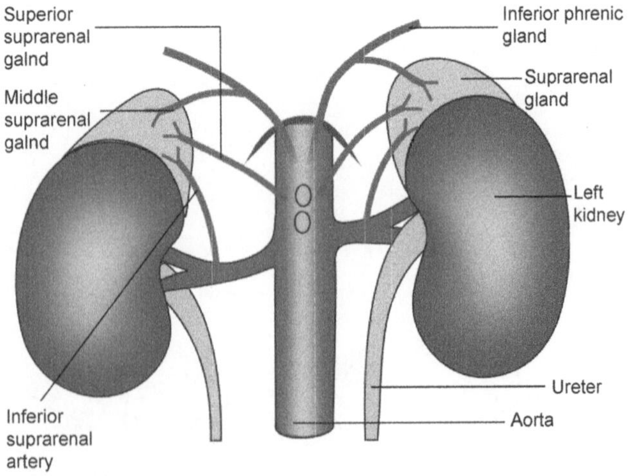

Fig. 38.1: Arterial supply of suprarenal glands

39 CHAPTER POSTERIOR ABDOMINAL WALL

1. Enumerate the components of posterior abdominal wall.

Ans. Posterior abdominal wall is made up of three bony and four muscular structures.

- **The bones are:**
  - Bodies of the lumbar vertebrae.
  - Sacrum.
  - Iliac fossae.
- **Muscles are: (Fig. 39.1)**
  - Diaphragm (posterior part).
  - Quadratus lumborum.
  - Psoas major.
  - Iliacus.

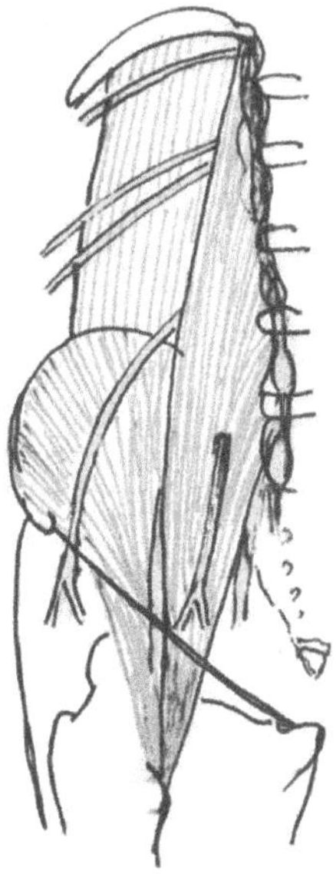

Fig. 39.1: Muscles and nerves of posterior abdominal wall

2. Describe briefly psoas major.

Ans. Psoas major is one of the muscles forming posterior abdominal wall.

- **Origin:** Transverse processes of all the lumbar vertebrae, sides of the bodies of lumbar vertebrae and the tendinous arch across the intervertebral discs between T12 and L5 vertebrae.
- It passes downwards and laterally at the margin of the pelvic brim, continues as a tendon in front of the hip joint beneath the inguinal ligament.
- **Insertion:** Is inserted along with iliacus into the lesser trochanter of the femur.
- **Action:** Flexion at hip joint (flexes the thigh or alternatively flexes the trunk, e.g., in sitting up from the lying position).
- **Psoas sheath:** Psoas muscle is enclosed in psoas sheath derived from lumbar fascia (Fig. 39.2).

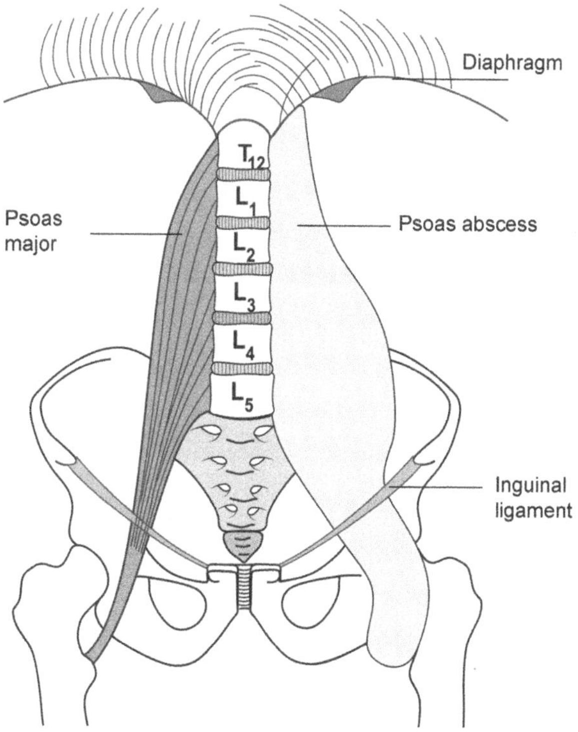

Fig. 39.2: Psoas muscle and abscess

Psoas abscess (Fig. 39.2): Pus may enter psoas sheath either from a tuberculous infection of lumbar vertebrae or from thoracic vertebrae via posterior mediastinum and behind the medial arcuate ligament. It may then spread down along psoas sheath deep to inguinal ligament into the femoral triangle where it produces a swelling. Occasionally, if neglected it may track along the femoral vessels along the femoral vessels to subsartorial canal and eventually in the popliteal fossa.

3. Draw labeled diagram of the lumbar plexus.

Ans. Lumbar plexus: (Fig. 39.3)

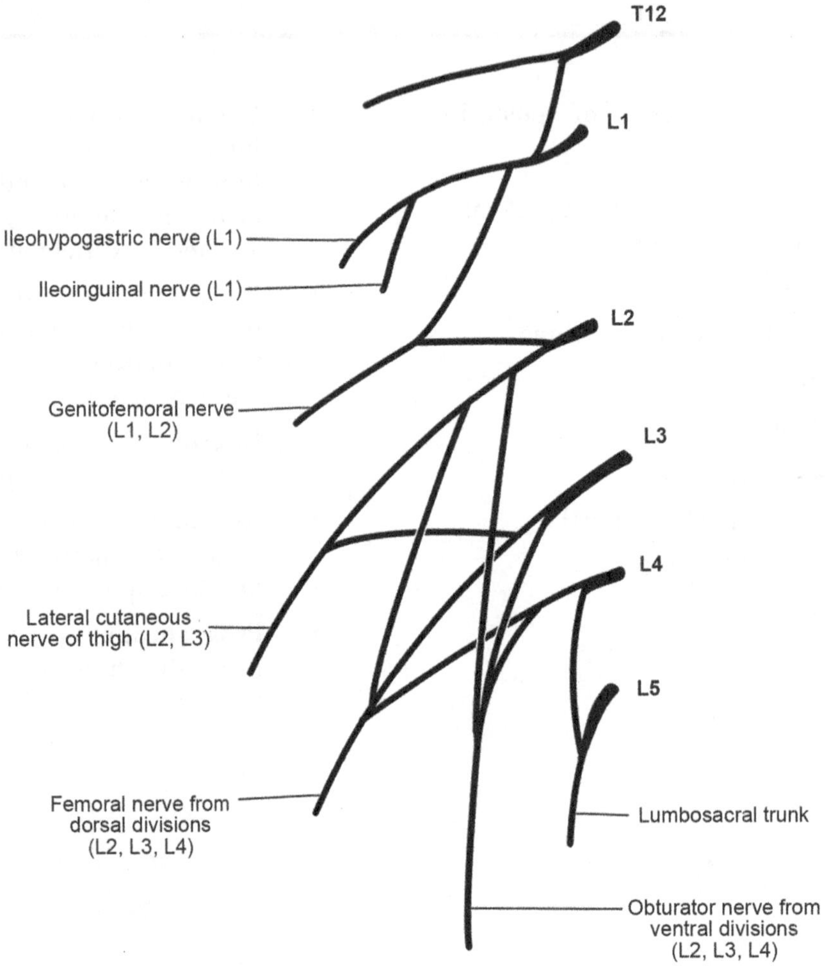

Fig. 39.3: Lumbar plexus

40 CHAPTER

ABDOMINAL AORTA, INFERIOR VENA CAVA & PORTAL VEIN

1. Describe the abdominal aorta under the following headings:

a. Extent **b. Relations**

c. Branches

Ans. a. **Extent:**

- It begins at the level of 12th thoracic aorta (as continuation of descending thoracic aorta).
- End at the level of disc between L5 and S1.

b. **Relations:**

- *Anterior:*
  From above downwards:
  - Celiac plexus.
  - Body of pancreas and splenic vein.
  - Left renal vein.
  - Third part of duodenum.
- *Posterior:*
  - Bodies of upper four lumbar vertebrae.
  - Intervertebral discs.
  - Anterior longitudinal ligament.
- *Right:*
  - Inferior vena cava.
  - Right sympathetic trunk.
  - Right crus of diaphragm.
  - Azygous vein and cysterna chyli.
- *Left:*
  - Left crus of diaphragm.
  - Fourth part of duodenum.
  - Left sympathetic trunk.
  - Inferior mesenteric vessels.

c. **Branches (Fg. 40.1):** Are divided into three groups:

- ***Ventral splanchnic branches and unpaired:***
  - *Celiac trunk:* Supplies structures derived from the foregut.
  - *Superior mesenteric artery:* Supplies structures derived from the mid-gut.
  - *Inferior mesenteric artery*: Supplies structures derived from the hind-gut.
- ***Lateral splanchnic branches are paired:***
  - Inferior phrenic artery.
  - Middle suprarenal artery.
  - Renal artery.
  - Gonadal artery (testicular or ovarian).
- ***Dorsal somatic branches:***
  - Four pairs of lumbar arteries.
  - Median sacral artery.
- ***Terminal branches:*** Two common iliac arteries.

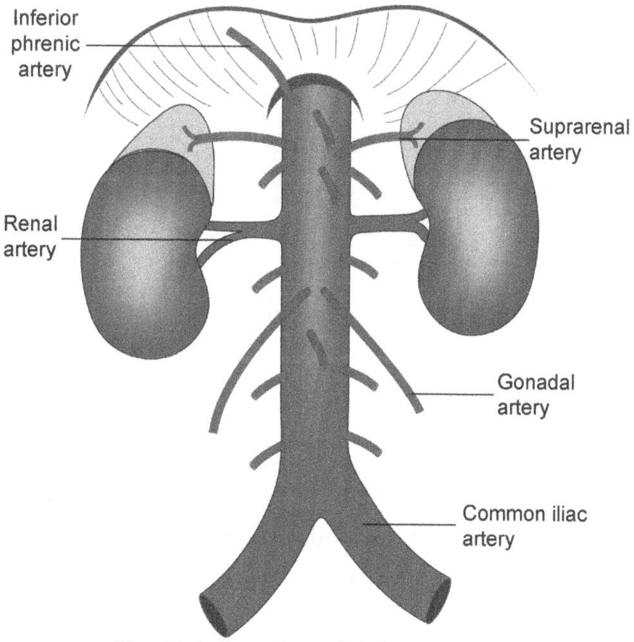

Fig. 40.1: Branches of abdominal aorta

2. **Describe inferior vena cava (IVC) under the following headings:**
   a. **Extent**
   b. **Tributaries**

Ans. a. **Extent:** IVC begins in front of the body of fifth lumbar vertebra by joining of common iliac veins and ends by opening into right atrium at the level of 8th thoracic vertebra.

b. **Tributaries: (Fig. 40.2)**
- Two common iliac veins.
- 3rd and 4th lumbar veins (of both the sides).
- Right testicular (ovarian) vein.
- Right suprarenal vein.
- Inferior phrenic veins.
- Renal veins.
- 2-3 hepatic veins.

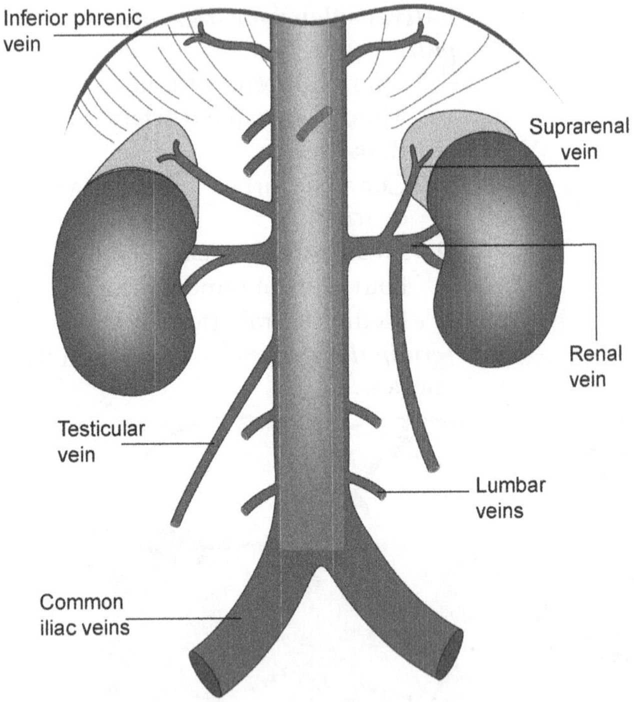

Fig. 40.2: Tributaries of inferior vena cava

3. **Describe portal vein under the following headings:**
   a. **Formation**
   b. **Course and relations**
   c. **Tributaries and branches**
   d. **Sites of portocaval anastomosis**

Ans. Portal vein drains blood to the liver from the abdominal part of the alimentary canal (excluding the anal canal), spleen, pancreas and the gallbladder and bile duct (Fig. 40.3).

a. **Formation:** Is formed by the union of superior mesenteric and splenic veins behind the neck of pancreas at the level of 2nd.

b. **Course:** Is 8 cm long and its course is divided into three parts:
- Infraduodenal.
- Retroduodenal.
- Supraduodenal.

Relations:
- ***Infraduodenal*** – *Anterior:* Neck of pancreas.
  Posterior: Inferior vena cava.
- ***Retroduodenal*** – *Anterior:* 1st part of duodenum, common bile duct, gastroduodenal artery.
  Posterior: Inferior vena cava.
- ***Infraduodenal*** – *Anterior:* Bile duct, hepatic artery.
  Posterior: Epiploic foramen.
- ***At porta hepatis:*** From before backwards:
  - Right and left hepatic ducts.
  - Right and left hepatic arteries.
  - Right and left branches of portal vein.

c. **Tributaries:**
- ***Formative:*** Splenic and superior mesenteric artery.
- ***Of the trunk:*** Right gastric, left gastric and occasionally superior pancreaticoduodenal.
- ***Of the branches:*** *Right branch:* Cystic vein. *Left branch:* Paraumbilical vein.

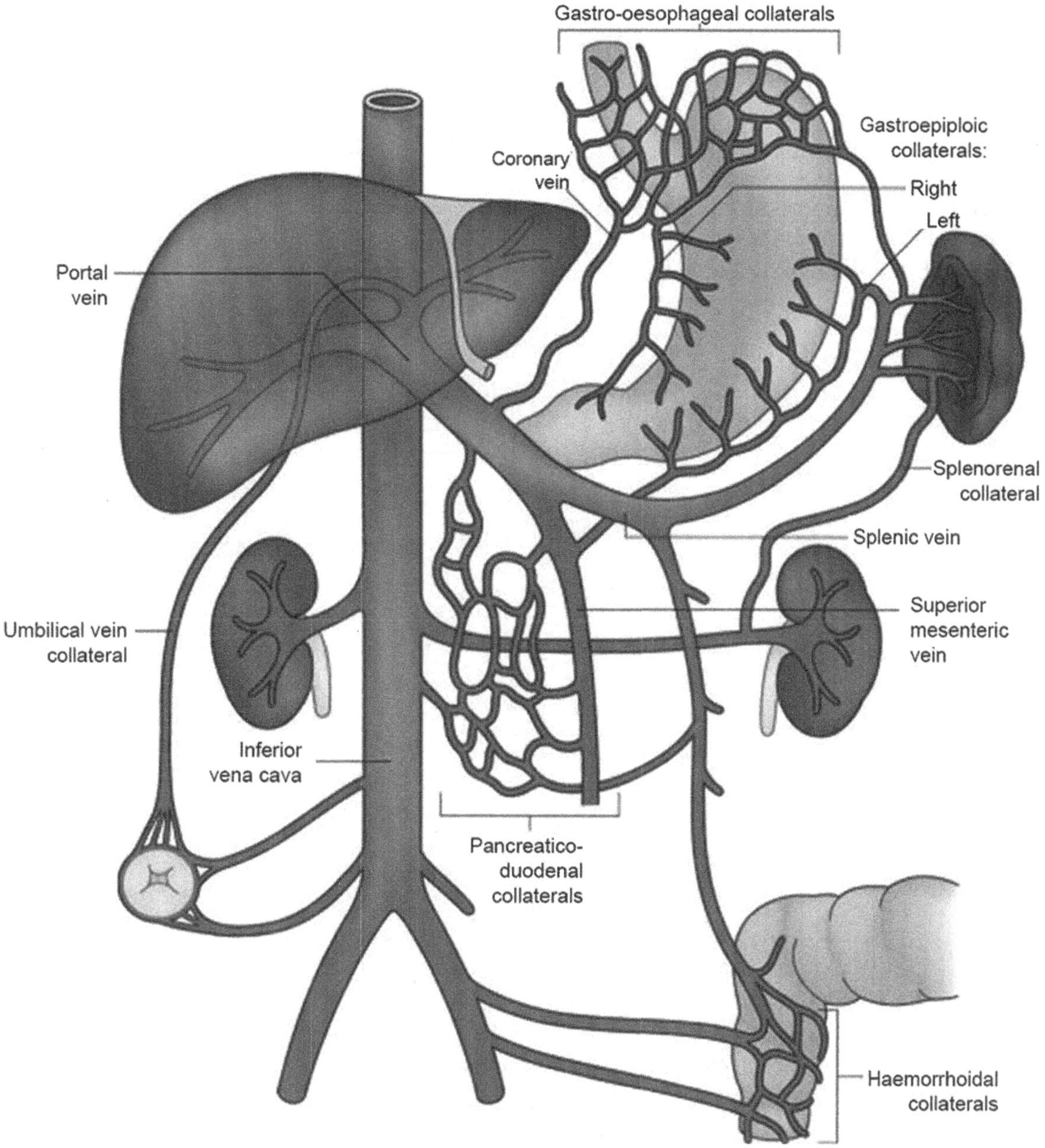

Fig. 40.3: Portal vein

Branches:

- ***Right branch:*** Is shorter and wider. Enters right lobe.
- ***Left branch:*** Is narrower and longer. Gives branches to left lobe and caudate and quadrate lobes. Receives paraumbilical vein and ligamentum teres and ligamentum venosum.

d. **Sites of portocaval anastomosis: (Fig. 40.4)**
   - Between the oesophageal branch of left gastric vein and oesophageal veins of azygous system.
   - Between the superior rectal branch of inferior mesenteric vein and inferior rectal veins draining into the internal iliac vein via internal pudendal artery.
   - Around the umbilicus between the paraumbilical vein and veins of anterior abdominal wall.
   - Between the portal tributaries in the mesentery and mesocolon and retroperitoneal veins communicating with the renal, lumbar and phrenic veins.
   - Between the portal branches in the liver and the veins of the diaphragm across the bare area of the liver.

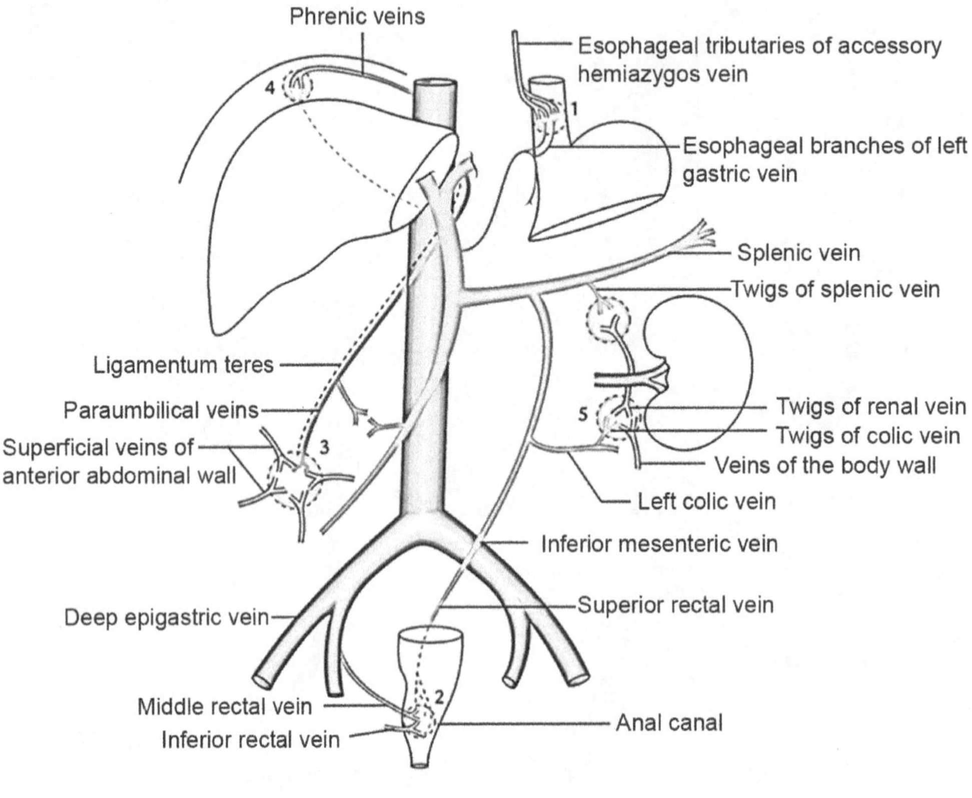

Fig. 40.4: Sites of portocaval anastomosis

41 CHAPTER URINARY BLADDER

1. **Describe the following features of urinary bladder:**
   a. **Location and shape**
   b. **External features and relations**

Ans. Urinary bladder is a hollow muscular viscus that acts as a reservoir of urine.

a. **Location:**
   - ***In adults:*** Empty bladder – in the pelvic cavity. Distended bladder – rises above the pubic symphysis in hypogastric region of abdominal cavity.
   - ***In infants:*** Abdominal cavity.

In adults as well as in infants, the urinary bladder is abdominal.

Shape: Empty – Tetrahedral, Distended – Ovoid.

b. **External features and relations:** Empty urinary bladder presents the following parts:
   - *An apex:*
     - Lies at the level of upper border of pubic symphysis.
     - Is connected to the umbilicus by median umbilical ligament (remnant of urachus).
   - *Base/Fundus/Posterior surface:*
     - Is triangular in shape.
     - In males, it is related to ampulla of vas deferens and seminal vesicle.
     - In females, it is related to anterior vaginal wall.
   - *Neck:*
     - Is the lowest and most fixed part.
     - Lies 3-4 cm behind the lower part of pubic symphysis.
     - In males, it is related to prostate gland and in females to pelvic fascia.
     - Is pierced by internal urethral meatus.
   - ***Borders:*** There are four borders:
     - Anterior.
     - Posterior.
     - Two lateral.
   - ***Surfaces:***
     - *Superior:* Is triangular in shape and is related to coils of ileum and pelvic colon.
     - *Two inferolateral surfaces:* Are related to pubic bone, retropubic fat and levator ani (Fig. 41.1a).

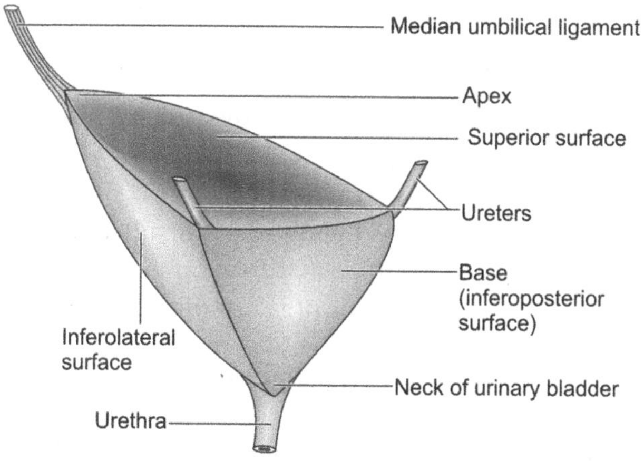

Fig. 41.1a: Surfaces and borders of urinary bladder

Posteroinferior surface is related to seminal vesicle, ampulla of vas deferens and ejaculatory duct (14.1b).

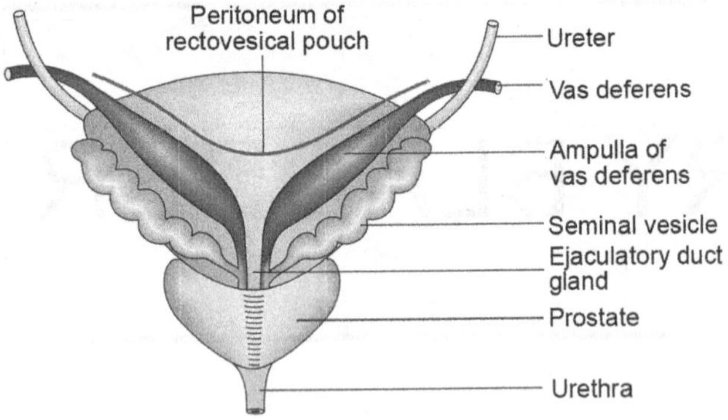

Fig. 41.1b: Relations of base of urinary bladder

2. **Describe briefly the trigone of bladder.**

Ans. Trigone of urinary bladder: (Fig. 41.2)

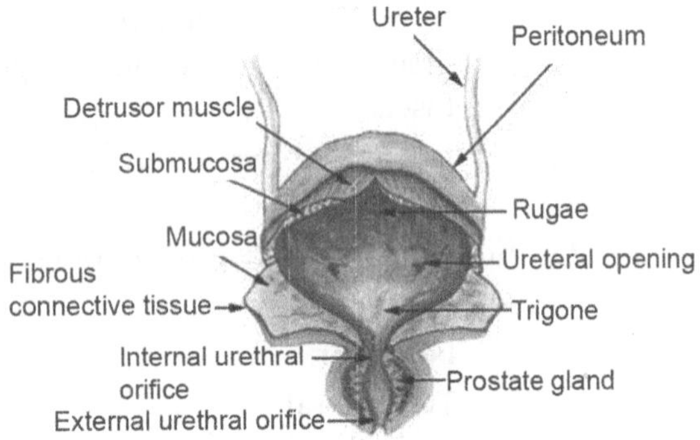

Fig. 41.2: Trigone of urinary bladder

- It is an equilateral triangular area on the inner surface of base of urinary bladder.
- ***Boundaries:***
  - *Base* – Is formed by interureteric ridge which extends between the two openings of the ureters.
  - *Apex* – Is formed by the internal urethral orifice.
  - *Sides* – Formed by uretero ureteric ridge.
- ***Characteristic features:***
  - Mucous membrane is firmly adherent to the musculature.
  - Absence of rugae (temporary folds of mucosa).
  - Submucosa is absent.

> **Uvula vesicae:** Is a rounded elevation just behind the urethral orifice which is formed by the median lobe of the prostate.
>
> In old aged man, the uvula vesicae may be enlarged due to enlargement of prostate and obstruct the outflow of urine through the internal urethral orifice.

3. **Enumerate:**
   a. **Supports of urinary bladder**
   b. **Arteries supplying urinary bladder**
   c. **Lymph nodes draining urinary bladder**
   d. **Relations**

Ans. a. **Supports of urinary bladder:**

- ***True ligaments:*** Are condensations of pelvic fascia.
  - *Pubovesical/puboprostatic ligaments:* From pubis to bladder.
  - *Lateral true ligaments:* From tendinous arch of levator ani muscle to inferolateral surface of bladder.
  - *Posterior true ligaments:* Base of bladder to pelvic wall along the internal iliac vessels.

> Neurovascular bundle for the urinary bladder passes along the posterior true ligaments. In males it includes the ductus deferens also.

- ***False ligaments:*** Are formed by peritoneal folds.
  - *Median umbilical ligament:* From the apex of bladder to the umbilicus (contains urachus – remnant of allantois).
  - *Lateral umbilical ligaments:* From bladder to the lateral pelvic walls.
  - *Posterior false ligaments/sacro-genital folds:* From base of bladder to sacrum.

b. **Arteries supplying urinary bladder:** Is supplied by branches of internal iliac artery.

- ***Superior vesical artery*** – Main artery.
- Obturator, inferior gluteal, uterine give small branches to the bladder.
- Inferior vesical artery – In males and vaginal artery in females also supply the bladder.

c. **Lymph nodes draining urinary bladder:**

- Chiefly internal iliac lymph nodes.
- External iliac lymph nodes.

d. **Relations:**

Surface of urinary bladder	*Males*	*Females*
Superior	Pelvic colon Coils of ileum	Body of the uterus Cervix
Inferolateral	Retropubic space (of Retzius) containing pubovesical and puboprostatic ligaments	Retropubic space (of Retzius) containing pubovesical and puboprostatic ligaments
Posterior/base	Rectum Ductus deferens Seminal vesical	Vagina

4. Describe briefly the nerve supply of urinary bladder.

Ans. Urinary bladder is supplied by autonomic nervous system.

a. **Parasympathetic innervations:**

- ***Efferent fibers:*** From S2-S4 spinal segments via pelvic splanchnic nerves/ nervi erigentes. They are concerned with emptying of the bladder.
  - Motor to the detrusor muscle.
  - Inhibitory to the sphincter urethrae.
- ***Afferent fibers:*** Convey the sensation of bladder distension.

> Parasympathetic innervaion is concerned with emptying of the bladder as it contracts the detrusor muscle and relaxes the sphincter urethrae.

b. **Sympathetic innervations:**

- ***Efferent fibers:*** From T11 – L2 spinal segments via hypogastric plexus.
  - Motor to sphincter urethrae muscle.
  - Inhibitory to detrusor muscle.
- ***Afferent fibers:*** Carry pain sensation.

> Sympathetic innervations is concerned with filling of the bladder as it relaxes the detrusor muscle and contracts the sphincter urethrae.

5. Describe neurogenic bladder.

Ans. Neurogenic bladder: Dysfunction of urinary bladder due to injury/disease of nervous system (CNS/PNS) involved in control of urination.

- ***Automatic reflex bladder:***
  - Is an UMN lesion due to spinal cord lesions above T12-L1.
  - The lesions may be due to trauma, infection, vascular infarction.
  - There is disruption of both the sensory and motor nerve tracts above sacral segments (S2, S3, S4).
  - The cortical or voluntary control is lost.
  - The spinal reflex arc takes over control of micturition, as a result the bladder fills and empties reflexly every one to four hours.
- ***Autonomous bladder:***
  - Occurs in LMN lesions, which involve disruption of the sacral spinal reflex arc at S2-S4.
  - In this case both voluntary and reflex control of micturition is lost.
  - The bladder capacity is greatly increased due to loss of tone of detrusor muscle.
  - The bladder overfills and overflows.

42 CHAPTER

PROSTATE

1. Describe prostate gland under the following headings:
   a. Location
   b. Measurements
   c. Gross features and relations
   d. Capsules
   e. Lobes

Ans. Prostate is a pyramidal shaped fibromuscular and glandular organ.

a. **Location:** It is located in the lower part of the pelvic cavity below the neck of the urinary bladder, behind the lower part of pubic symphysis, in front of the rectum and surrounds the prostatic part of urethra.

b. **Measurements:** ***Length*** – 3 cm, ***Breadth*** – 4 cm, ***Weight*** – 8 gm.

c. **Gross features and relations:** Prostate gland has:
   - ***An apex:*** Directed downwards between the medial margins of levator ani muscles. It rests on the superior fascia of urogenital diaphragm.
   - ***Base:*** Directed upwards. It surrounds the neck of the urinary bladder and is pierced by urethra near its anterior surface.
   - ***Four surfaces:***
     – *Anterior surface:* Is narrow and convex. Is separated from the pubic symphysis by extraperitoneal fat of retropubic space (cave of Retzius) containing:
       - Prostatic venous plexus.
       - Deep dorsal vein of penis.
       - Puboprostatic ligaments.
     – *Posterior surface:* Is broad, flat and triangular. It is separated from the ampulla of rectum by the rectovesical fascia (fascia of Denonvilliers).
       - It is divided by a horizontal groove into smaller upper part (median lobe) and larger lower part (further divided by median sulcus into two lateral lobes).
       - Ejaculatory ducts (formed by joining of ductus deferens and duct of seminal vesicle) pierce the horizontal sulcus near the median plane.

> Carcinoma of prostate rarely penetrates fascia of Denonvilliers, therefore ulceration into the rectum is unusual.

     – *Two inferolateral surfaces:* Are related to levator ani muscle.

d. **Capsules:** Prostate gland is surrounded by normally two capsules: (Fig. 42.1)

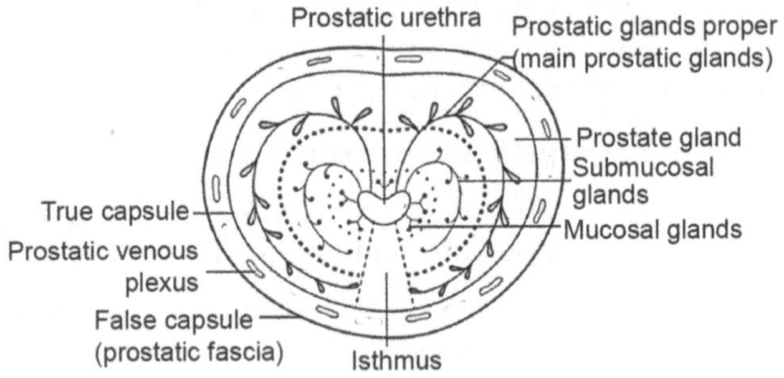

Fig. 42.1: Capsules of prostate gland and prostatic venous plexus

   - ***True capsule:*** Formed by condensation of the fibrous stroma of the gland.
   - ***False capsule:*** Formed by condensed extraperitoneal fascia.

> - Prostatic venous plexus lies between the true and false capsule.
> - **Pathological capsule:** In benign (adenomatous) hypertrophy of prostate, the normal peripheral part is compressed into a capsule surrounding the enlarged adenomatous mass. While performing

enucleation of the prostate, the plane between the adenomatous mass and the compressed normal peripheral tissue is entered, the tumor is enucleated and the condensed rim of prostatic tissue deep to true capsule is left behind. The prostatic venous plexus lying between the true and false capsule is thus undisturbed.

e. **Lobes:** Prostate gland is divided into five lobes: by prostatic urethra and ejaculatory ducts.
  - ***Anterior lobe:*** Lies anterior to urethra (formed by a small part called isthmus connecting the two lateral lobes). Is mainly formed of fibromuscular tissue. Adenoma rarely occurs.
  - ***Posterior lobe:*** Lies behind the urethra and the median lobe and below the ejaculatory ducts. Adenoma never occurs but primary carcinoma may begin here.
  - ***Median lobe:*** Lies behind the urethra and above the ejaculatory ducts.
  - ***Right and left lateral lobes:*** Lie on each side of the urethra. Contain glandular tissue and adenoma may arise in old age.

- Median lobe forms the uvula vesicae, an elevation in the lower part of the trigone of bladder behind the internal urethral meatus. It contains much glandular tissue and is the most common site of adenoma formation.
- Benign enlargement after the age of 60 years mostly involves median lobe, causing obstruction of the internal urethral meatus. This results in difficulty in passing the urine.

2. **Draw labeled diagram of the following:**
   a. **Lobes of prostate gland**
   b. **Structures inside the prostate gland**

Ans. a. **Lobes of prostate gland: (Fig. 42.2)**

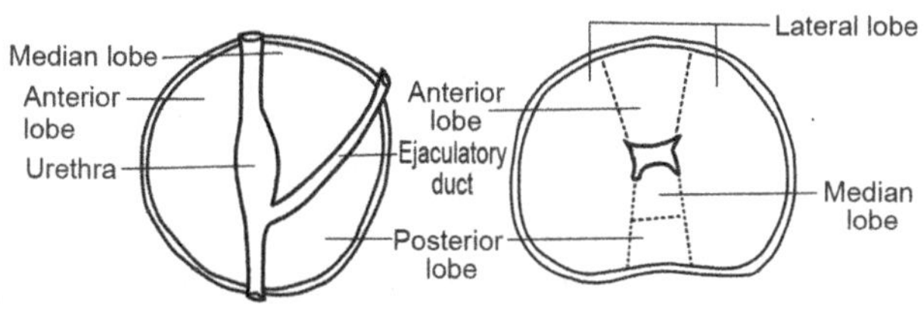

Fig. 42.2: Lobes of prostate gland

b. **Structures inside the prostate gland:**

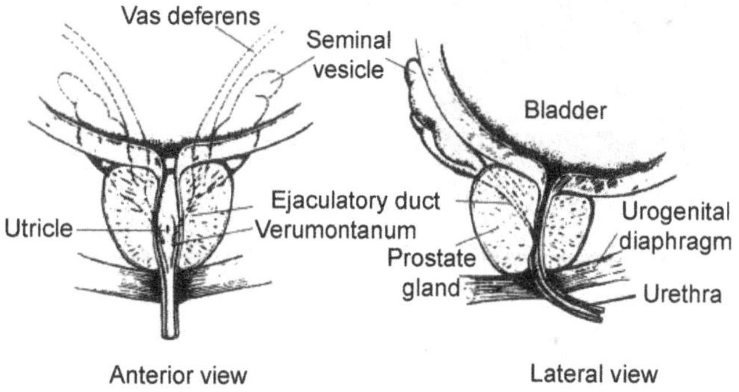

3. **Enumerate:**
   a. **Arteries supplying prostate**
   b. **Lymph nodes into which lymph from prostate drains**

Ans. a. **Arteries supplying prostate:** Are branches of internal iliac artery.
  - Inferior vesicle artery.
  - Internal pudendal artery.
  - Middle rectal artery.

b. **Lymph nodes into which lymph from prostate drains:**
  - Mainly into internal iliac lymph nodes.
  - Some lymphatics from posterior surface into sacral and external iliac lymph nodes.

4. **Describe briefly the venous drainage of prostate gland and its applied anatomy.**

Ans. The veins draining the prostate form prostatic venous plexus which is located between the true and the false capsule of the prostate gland. The prostatic venous plexus:
- Receives the deep dorsal vein of the penis.
- Communicates with the vesicular venous plexus and drains into the internal iliac vein on either side.
- Also communicates with the veins lying in front of the vertebral bodies and the vertebral venous plexus in the vertebral canal.

Applied Anatomy:

Carcinoma of prostate spreads to the pelvis and vertebrae due to the absence of valves in the veins connecting the prostatic venous plexus and the vertebral venous plexus.

43 CHAPTER

URETHRA

1. Describe in brief the extent and parts of male urethra.

Ans. Urethra is a fibrous tube that transports urine from the urinary bladder to the exterior.

a. **Extent:** From internal urethral meatus (neat neck of the bladder) to external urethral meatus.

b. **Length:** In males – 20 cm.

c. **Parts of male urethra:** Male urethra is divided into three parts:

- *Prostatic urethra:*
  - Lies within the prostate gland.
  - Extends from the internal urethral meatus (at the neck of urinary bladder) to the superior fascia of urogenital diaphragm.
  - Is 3 cm in length.
  - Is the widest and most dilatable art of the urethra.
  - Upper part is lined by transitional epithelium and lower part by stratified columnar/ pseudostratified columnar epithelium.
- *Membranous urethra:*
  - It lies in the deep perineal pouch between the superior and inferior fascia of urogenital diaphragm.
  - Is surrounded by sphincter urethrae muscle (voluntary sphincter).
  - Is 1.25 cm long.
  - Is the narrowest and least dilatable part of urethra.
  - Is lined by stratified columnar/ pseudostratified columnar epithelium.
- *Spongy or penile urethra:*
  - It lies in bulb of the penis (called bulbar urethra, lies in superficial perineal pouch) and the corpus spongiosum of penile body and glans penis.
  - Extends from the inferior fascia of urogenital diaphragm to external urethral meatus.
  - Is the longest part of the urethra – 15 cm in length.
  - *It has two dilatations:*
    - Intrabulbar fossa – in the bulb of penis.
    - Navicular fossa – in the glans penis.
  - *Shape of penile urethra in cross section:*
    - Bulbar urethra – trapezoid.
    - Urethra in penile body – transverse slit.
    - Urethra in glans penis (navicular fossa) – vertical slit.
  - Is lined by stratified columnar epithelium but the navicular fossa is lined by stratified squamous epithelium.
  - Urethral glands (glands of Littre) open along the whole of penile urethra in pit like recesses of mucosa called Lacunae. The lacuna in the roof of the navicular fossa is deep and called *lacuna magna.*

During urethral catheterization in males the following points should be kept in mind.

- External urethral meatus is the narrowest part of the urethra.
- The tip of the catheter may get caught in the lacuna magna present in the roof of the navicular fossa and result in perforation. Therefore, the catheter should be kept close to the floor of the navicular fossa.
- The membranous urethra is thin walled, narrow and least distensible part, therefore force applied during passage of catheter through this part may rupture it.

2. Where will urine accumulate in case of rupture of:

a. Membranous urethra

b. Bulbar urethra

Ans. a. In case of rupture of **membranous urethra** urine will accumulate in the deep perineal pouch.

b. In case of rupture of **bulbar urethra,** urine will accumulate in superficial perineal pouch, and may extravasate in scrotum, penis and lower part of anterior abdominal wall.

3. Describe the urethral sphincters.

Ans. Urethra is surrounded by two sphincters:

- **Internal urethral sphincter (sphincter vesicae):**
  - It surrounds the preprostatic part of urethra.
  - Is composed of smooth muscle fibers.
  - Is innervated by autonomic fibers.
  - Is involuntary.
- **External urethral sphincter (sphincter urethrae):**
  - The sphincter urethrae muscle surrounds the membranous part of urethra in the deep perineal pouch.
  - Is composed of striated muscle.
  - Is innervated by pudendal (somatic) nerve.
  - Is voluntary in nature.

4. Draw labeled diagram to show the parts of male urethra.

Ans. Parts of male urethra: (Fig. 43.1)

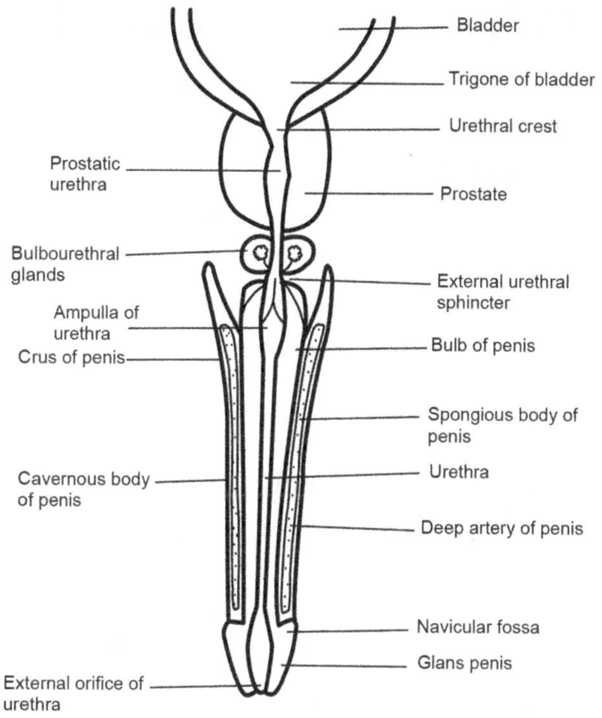

Fig. 43.1: Parts of male urethra

5. Describe briefly the female urethra.

Ans. Female urethra:

- Is 4 cm long.
- Extends from the internal urethral meatus (in the neck of urinary bladder) to external urethral meatus (in the vestibule of vagina).
- It is intimately related to the anterior wall of vagina.
- Is lined by transition epithelium in the uppermost part followed by stratified columnar/pseudostratified and near the external urethral meatus by stratified squamous epithelium.

Urinary tract infections are more common in females due to short urethra.

44 CHAPTER SCROTUM, TESTES & SPERMATIC CORD

1. **Enumerate:**
   a. **Coverings of spermatic cord**
   b. **Coverings of testis**
   c. **Layers of wall of scrotal sac**
   d. **Contents of spermatic cord**

Ans. a. **Coverings of spermatic cord:** See Table below.
   b. **Covering of testis:** See Table below.
   c. **Layers of wall of scrotal sac:** See Table below.
   d. **Contents of spermatic cord:**
   - Ductus deferens.
   - *Three arteries:* Testicular, artery of ductus deferens, cremasteric artery.
   - Pampiniform venous plexus.
   - Genital branch of genitofemoral nerve.
   - Lymphatics from testis and epididymis.
   - Autonomic nerves.
   - Fibrous remnant of processus vaginalis.

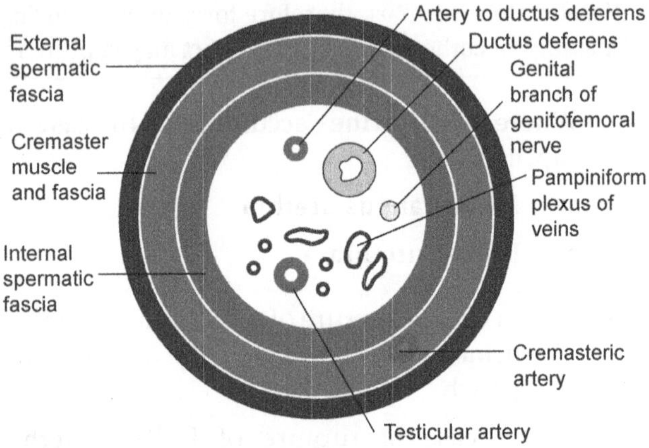

Fig. 44.1: Transverse section of spermatic cord

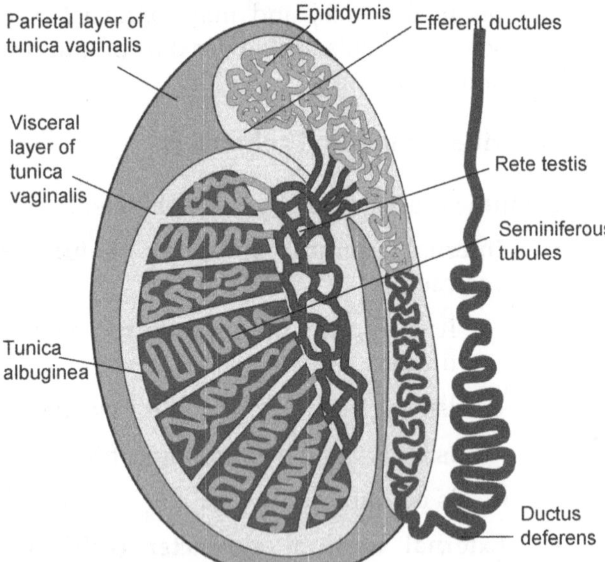

Fig. 44.2: Coronal section of testis and epididymis

2. **Draw labeled diagram of the following:**
   a. **Transverse section of spermatic cord**
   b. **Coronal section of testis and epididymis**

Ans. a. See Figure 44.1.
   b. See Figure 44.2.

Coverings of spermatic cord	*Layers of wall of scrotal sac*	*Coverings of testis*
Internal spermatic fascia (from fascia transversalis)	Skin	Tunica vasculosa (delicate connective tissue containing plexuses of blood vessels)
Cremaster muscle and fascia (derived from internal oblique muscle)	Dartos muscle (replaces fat in subcutaneous tissue)	Tunica albuginea (thick layer of fibrous tissue)
External spermatic fascia (derived from aponeurosis of external oblique muscle)	Membranous layer of superficial fascia (Colles' fascia)	Tunica vaginalis (Closed serous sac – the resistant lower end of processus vaginalis)
	All the layers covering spermatic cord	All the layers of wall of scrotal sac

3. **What is processus vaginalis and add a note on its applied anatomy?**

Ans. **Processus vaginalis** is a peritoneal pouch and precedes the testis in its descent through the vaginal canal to scrotum. Its proximal part gets obliterated and the distal part forms the tunical vaginalis around testis and epididymis.

Applied anatomy:

- Persistent patent processus vaginalis (more common on the right than the left) may result in congenital indirect inguinal hernia.
- The closed off tunica vaginalis may become distended with fluid to form *hydrocele.* Hydrocele can be classified into four types, i.e.:
  - Vaginal (confined to scrotum).
  - Infantile (up to deep inguinal ring.
  - Congenital (communicates with peritoneal cavity).
  - Encysted (Upper and lower parts are obliterated, fluid accumulates in the middle part).

4. **What is varicocele and why it is more common on left side?**

Ans. Dilatation of pampiniform plexus of veins is called varicocele. The incidence of varicocele is high on left side due to the following reasons:

- Obstruction of left testicular vein by the loaded sigmoid colon.
- Left testicular vein opens into the left renal vein at right angle.
- Left testicular vein is subjected to spasm due to adrenalin rich blood entering into left renal vein from the left adrenal vein.

5. **Describe briefly the chronology and factors responsible for the descent of testis.**

Ans. Testis develop in the lumbar region from the genital ridge and then descend into the scrotum.

- **The chronology of testicular descent is as follows:**
  - 3rd month (of fetal life) – reaches iliac fossa.
  - 4th to 7th month – at deep inguinal ring.
  - 7th month – transverses the inguinal canal.
  - 8th month – reaches superficial inguinal ring.
  - 9th month – enters scrotum.
- **Factors responsible for the descent of testes:**
  - *Hormonal factor:* Gonadotropins and androgens help in descent of testis.
  - Outgrowth followed by regression of gubernaculums testis (mesenchymal band extending from lower pole of testis to scrotum).
  - Intra-abdominal pressure.

- **Cryptorchidism (undescended testis):** Can be unilateral or bilateral. The descent could be arrested anywhere in its normal course of descent. It can be located in the iliac fossa, at deep inguinal ring, inguinal canal or at superficial inguinal canal. Undescended testis is incapable of spermatogenesis.
- **Ectopic testis:** If the testis completes the descent, but to an unusual position, i.e., other than scrotal sac. The testis may be located in the anterior abdominal wall, root of penis, perineum, femoral triangle in the upper thigh.

45 CHAPTER
UTERUS

1. Describe uterus under the following headings:

a. Location

b. Shape and size

c. Parts and external features

d. Uterine cavity

e. Relations

Ans. a. Location: Uterus is a fibromuscular organ located in the pelvis between urinary bladder in front and rectum behind.

b. Shape and size: Pear shaped, flattened anteroposteriorly. Size in adult nulliparous female:

- *Length* – 7.5 cm.
- *Width* – 5 cm.
- *Thickness* – 2.5 cm.

c.
- **Parts:** Uterus consists of the following three parts (Fig 45.1):
  - *Fundus:* Is the part above the openings of the uterine tubes (superolateral part of uterus where fallopian tube opens is called cornu).
  - *Body:* Upper 2/3rd of the organ below the fundus.
  - *Cervix:* Lower 1/3rd of the organ separated from the body by a constricted part (isthmus).
    - *Cervix is divided into two parts:*
      - Supravaginal part: Upper half.
      - Vaginal part: Lower half.
- **Surfaces and borders:**
  - Anteroinferior surface (vesical) surface.
  - Posterosuperior (intestinal) surface.
  - Right and left borders.

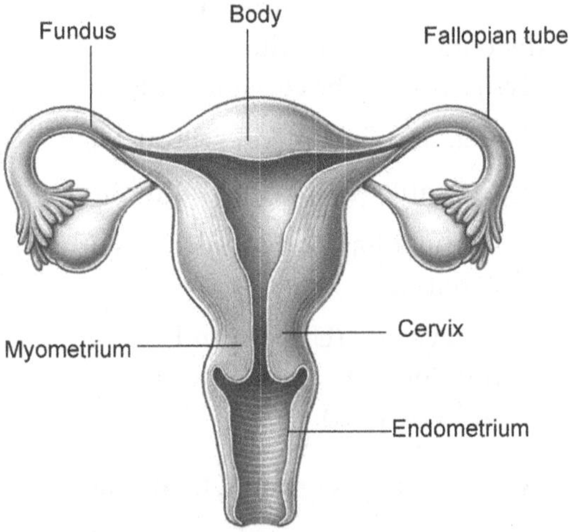

Fig. 45.1: Parts of uterus

d. Uterine cavity:

- Is triangular in shape in coronal section.
- In sagittal plane is merely a slit.
- The cavity communicates with the cervical canal via internal os.
- The cervical canal opens into vagina via external os.

e. Relations:

- ***Relations of the body:***
  - *Anteroinferior surface:*
    - Uterovesical pouch.
    - Superior surface of urinary bladder.
    - Loose of small intestine.
  - *Posterosuperior surface:*
    - Rectouterine pouch.
    - Sigmoid colon.
    - Rectum.

– *Attachments to lateral borders:*
  - Broad ligament (transverse fold of peritoneum extending from lateral border of uterus to the lateral pelvic wall).
  - Ligament of the ovary: Attached to uterus below and behind the uterine tube.
  - Round ligament of uterus: Attached below and in front of the uterine tube.

2. What is the normal position of uterus?

Ans. The normal uterus is anteverted and antiflexed.

- **Angle of antiversion:** The uterus is bent forwards at right angle to the vagina. This is called angle of antiversion (90°).
- **Angle of antiflexion:** The body of uterus is slightly bent forwards on the cervix and this angle is known as angle of antiflexion (120° – 170°).

> - Uterus is retroverted if the body of uterus is bent backwards. Retroversion redisposes to relapse of uterus.
> - If the uterine body is bent backwards on the cervix, it is said to be retroflexed, which may cause painful menstruation.

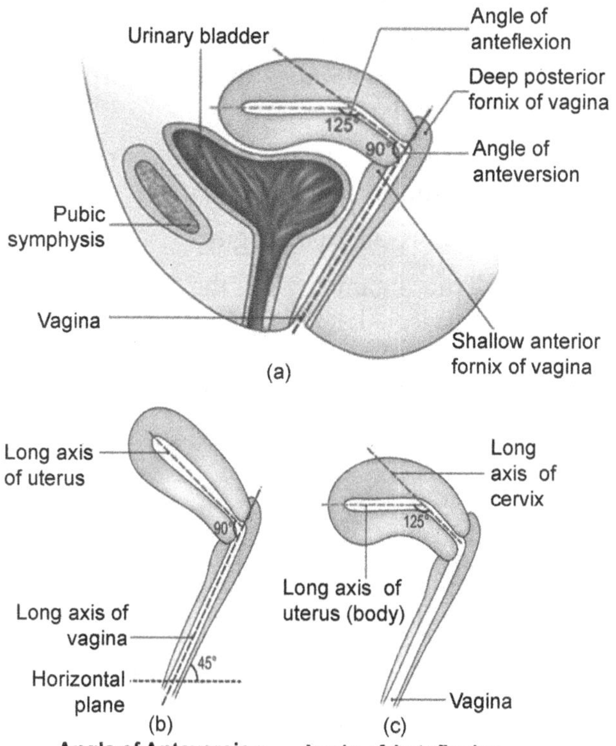

Fig. 45.2: Normal position of uterus

3. Enumerate:

a. Contents of broad ligament

b. Arteries supplying uterus

c. Lymh nodes draining uterus

d. True ligaments of uterus

e. False ligaments of uterus

Ans. a. Contents of broad ligament:

- Uterine tube.
- Round ligament of uterus.
- Ligament of ovary.
- Uterine artery.
- Ovarian vessels.
- Vestigial remnants of mesonephric duct epoophoron and paroophoron.
- Parametrium (connective tissue).

b. Arteries supplying uterus: (Fig. 45.3)

- Uterine artery (main supply).
- Ovarian artery.

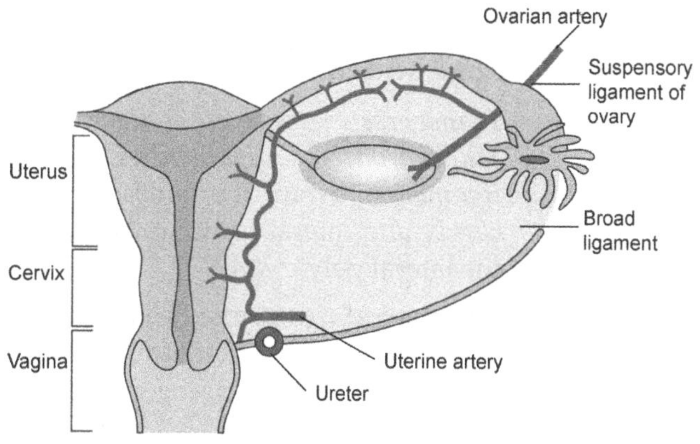

Fig. 45.3: Arterial supply of uterus

c. Lymh nodes draining uterus:

- *From the fundus and upper part of the body:*
  - Preaortic and lateral aortic lymph nodes (following ovarian vessels).
  - Superficial inguinal lymh nodes (along round ligament of uterus).
- *From the lower part of the body:*
  - External iliac lymph nodes.
- *From the cervix:*
  - *Upper part* – External iliac lymph nodes.

- *Lower part* – Internal iliac and obturator lymph nodes.
- *Posterior wall of cervix* – Sacral lymph nodes (Fig. 45.4).

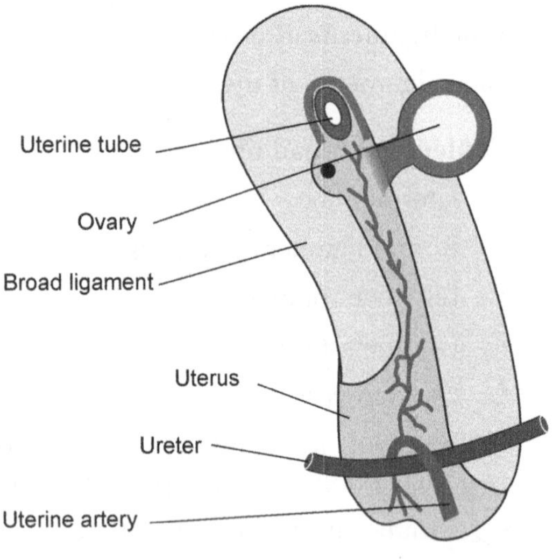

Fig. 45.4: Lymphatic drainage of uterus

Cancer of cervix is the most common type of cancer in women. It spreads widely due to widespread lymphatic drainage.

d. **True ligaments of uterus:**
   - ***Transverse cervical ligaments/ Mackenrodt's ligaments/Cardinal ligaments:*** From the sides of the cervix and lateral fornix of uterus to the lateral pelvic wall.
   - ***Uterosacral ligaments:*** From body of uterus and cervix to sacrum.
   - ***Pubocervical ligament:*** From cervix to the body of pubis.
   - ***Round ligament of uterus/ligamentum teres uteri:*** From anteroinferior part of the cornu of uterus to labia majora (Fig. 45.5).

e. **False ligaments of uterus:** Formed by peritoneal folds:
   - Broad ligaments.
   - Uterovesical fold.
   - Rectovesical fold.

4. **Enumerate the supports of uterus.**

Ans. The following factors support the uterus by maintaining the normal position of uterus:

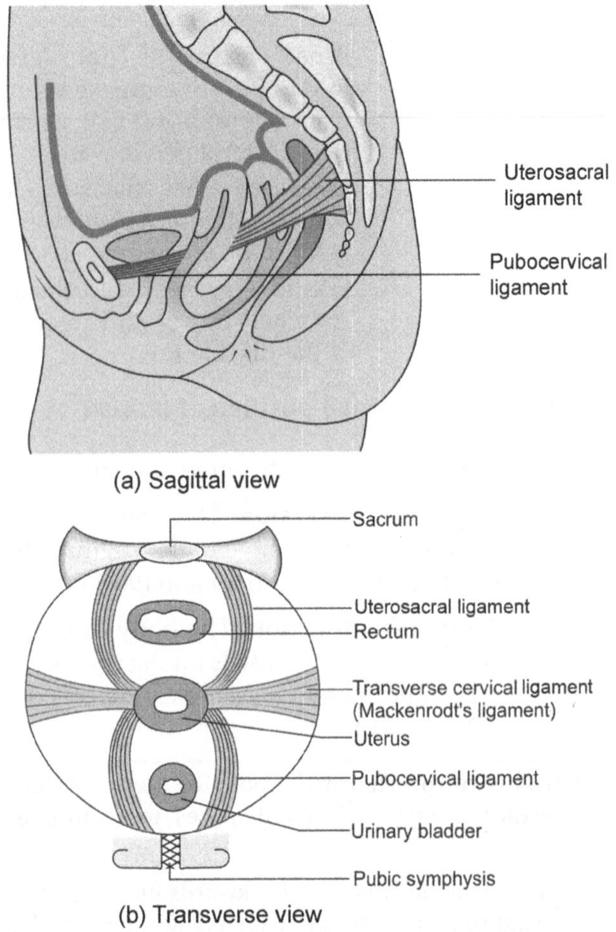

Fig. 45.5: True ligaments of uterus

- Pelvic diaphragm formed by levator ani muscles – cradles the uterus from below (Fig. 45.6).
- Perineal body provide support to uterus by supporting vagina.
- Urogenital diaphragm.
- True ligaments of the uterus – pubocervical, lateral cervical and uterosacral

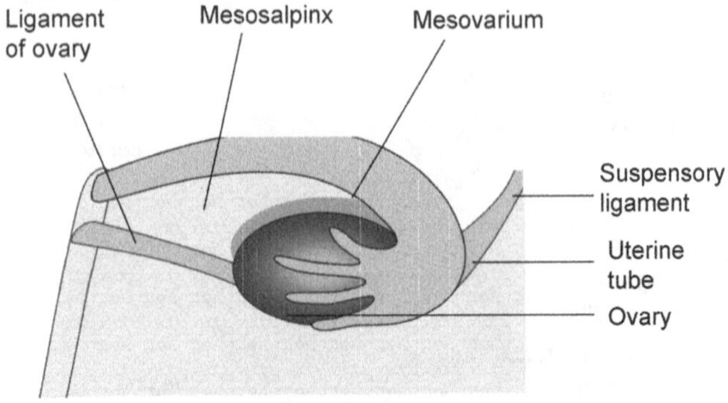

Fig. 45.6: Broad ligament

– the ligaments pass from cervix in three directions and fix it to the pelvic walls.

- Round ligament of uterus – forward pull of this ligament help in maintaining anteflexed and antiverted position of uterus.
- Surrounding organs.
- Intra-abdominal pressure.

Prolapse of uterus: When the uterus descends into the vagina. It results due to failure/rupture of various factors that support the uterus.

46 CHAPTER

UTERINE TUBE

1. **Enumerate:**
   a. **Parts of uterine tube (fallopian tube)**
   b. **Arteries supplying uterine tube**

Ans. a. **Parts of uterine tube:** Uterine tube is divided into four parts (from lateral to medial end): (Fig. 46.1)

- ***Infundibulum (1.25 cm):*** Is the most lateral part which opens into the peritoneal cavity. It is funnel shaped and has finger like processes called fimbriae surrounding its opening (ostium). The longest fimbria is attached to the medial surface of the ovary.
- ***Ampulla (5 cm):*** Is the widest and the longest part of uterine tube. It is the site of fertilization.
- ***Isthmus (2.5 cm):*** Is narrow and thick walled.
- ***Intramural/interstitial part (1.25 cm):*** Passes through the wall of the uterus and opens into the uterine cavity.

b. **Arteries supplying uterine tube:**

- Uterine artery supplies medial 2/3rd of the uterine tube.
- Ovarian artery supplies lateral 1/3rd of the uterine tube.

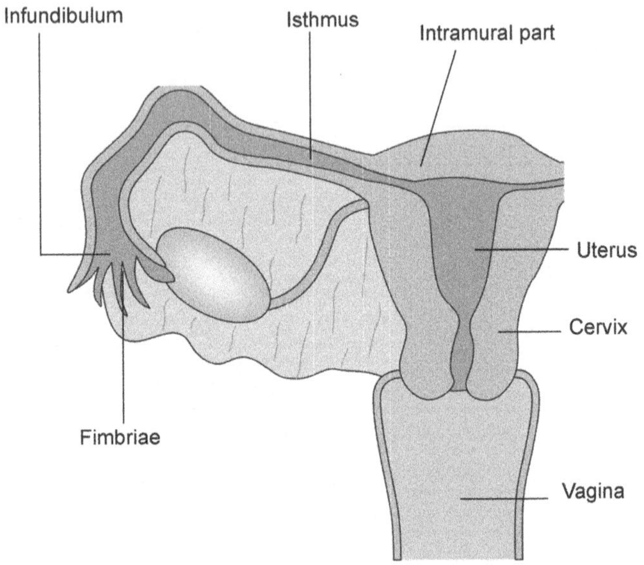

Fig. 46.1: Parts of uterine tube

- The exterior of genital tract in females communicates with the peritoneal cavity through the uterine tube. This is a potential pathway for spread of infection to the tube (salpingitis) and pelvic cavity (pelvic inflammatory disease).
- Ligation of uterine tube is one of the methods of birth control.

CHAPTER 47

OVARY

1. **Describe ovary under the following headings:**
   a. **Location**
   b. **Shape and size**
   c. **External features**
   d. **Arterial supply**
   e. **Nerve supply**

Ans. Ovaries are a pair of organs responsible for producing ovum (female gamete) and hormones.

a. **Location:** Ovary lies in the ovarian fossa on the lateral wall of the pelvis (with obturator nerve and vessels), between the ureter behind and the broad ligament in front (Fig. 47.1).

b. **Shape:** Almond shaped.

   Size: 3 cm long, 2 cm wide and 1 cm thick.

c. **External features:** Ovary has:
   - *Two surfaces:* Lateral and medial surfaces.
   - *Two poles:* Upper and lower poles.
   - *Two borders:* Anterior and posterior.

d. **Arterial supply:** Ovary is supplied by ovarian artery (branch of abdominal aorta).

e. **Nerve supply:** Sympathetic fibers from T10- T11 spinal segments.

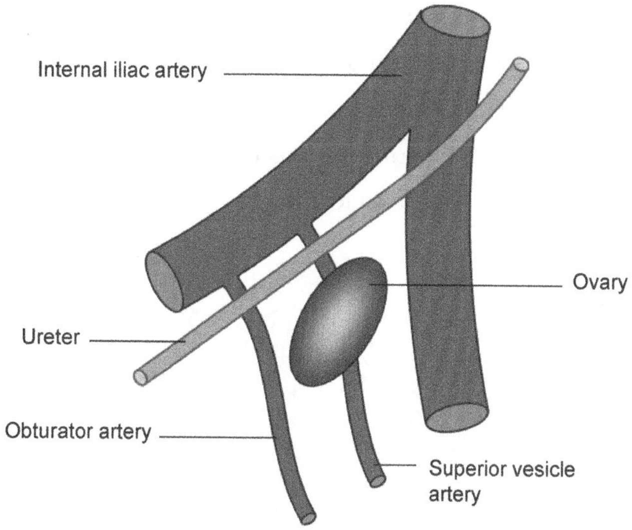

Fig. 47.1: Location of ovary

> Ovarian pain is referred to the umbilicus, lower abdominal and pubic region.

48 CHAPTER

PELVIC DIAPHRAGM, NERVES & VESSELS

1. **Enumerate:**
   a. **Muscles of true pelvis**
   b. **Branches of internal iliac artery**

Ans. a. Muscles of true pelvis: (Fig. 48.1)

- Obturator internus – Lateral wall.
- Levator ani – Floor.
- Coccygeus – Floor.
- Piriformis – Posterior wall.
- Muscles forming pelvic diaphragm.

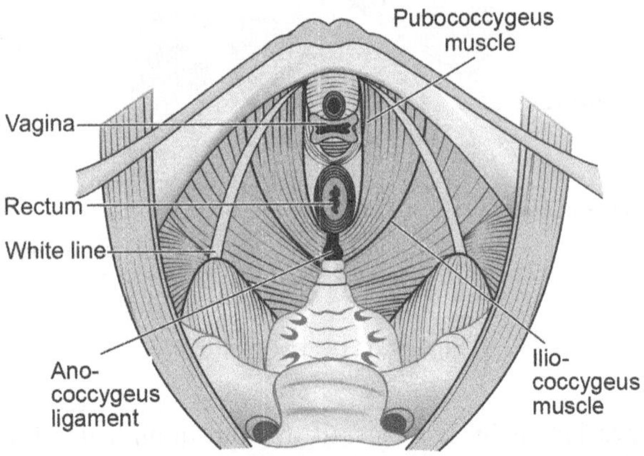

Fig. 48.1: Pelvic diaphragm

b. Branches of internal iliac artery: Internal iliac artery is one of the terminal branches of abdominal aorta. It divides into a larger anterior and a smaller posterior division (Fig. 48.2).

- *Branches of anterior division:*
  - *Parietal branches (3):*
    - Obturator artery – Leaves pelvis through obturator canal to reach thigh.
    - Inferior gluteal artery–Leaves pelvis by passing through greater sciatic foramen to reach gluteal region.
    - Internal pudendal artery–Leaves pelvis by passing through the greater sciatic foramen and enters perineum by passing through lesser sciatic foramen.
  - *Visceral branches (4):*
    - Superior vesical artery.
    - Inferior vesical artery (vaginal artery in females).
    - Uterine artery.
    - Middle rectal artery.
- *Branches of posterior division (3):*
  - Iliolumbar artery.
  - Lateral sacral arteries.
  - Superior gluteal artery.

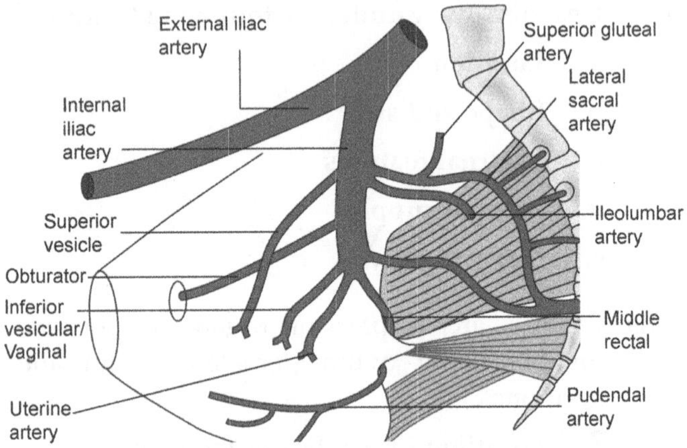

Fig. 48.2: Internal iliac artery branches

2. **Describe briefly pelvic diaphragm.**

Ans. Pelvic diaphragm forms the V-shaped floor of the true pelvis.

- It separates pelvis from the perineum.
- **Structures passing through it:** Urethra, anal canal and in females vagina.
- **Structures forming pelvic diaphragm:**
  - Pelvic fascia.
  - Levator ani muscle.
  - Coccygeus muscle.
- **Pelvic fascia:**
  - Covers the superior and inferior surfaces of the muscles forming pelvic diaphragm.
  - *Superior fascia:*
    - Is attached anteriorly to the posterior surface of body of pubis and superior ramus of pubis.
    - Is continuous laterally with obturator fascia.
    - Is continuous posteriorly with the fascia on the piriformis.
  - *Inferior fascia:*
    - Is continuous with obturator fascia laterally.
    - Medially blends with the fascia on sphincter ani externus.
  - *Levator ani:*
    - Is a broad flat muscle.
    - Takes origin from the inner aspect of pelvis along a line extending from the body of the pubis to the ischial spine.
    - Muscle fibers sweep downwards and backwards towards the median plane to unite with the muscle of the opposite side.
    - Is supplied by ventral rami of S3,S4 on the pelvic surface and pudendal nerve on the perineal surface.
    - It consists of two parts:
      - Pubococcygeus.
      - Iliococcygeus.
- **Pubococcygeus:** According to the attachment of fibers it is subdivided into three parts.
- **Levator prostate (in males)/Pubovaginalis (in females):**
  - *Origin:* Posterior surface of body of pubis.
  - Form a U-shaped sling around the prostate gland in males and vagina in females.
  - *Insertion:* Perineal body.
- **Puborectalis:**
  - *Origin:* Posterior surface of pubis.
  - Muscle fibers pass medially and downwards to join the fibers of the opposite side and form U-shaped sling around the anorectal junction.
  - Some fibers blend with the fibers of the deep part of the external anal sphincter to form the conjoint longitudinal coat of the anal canal.
- **Pubococcygeus proper:**
  - *Origin:* Posterior surface of body of pubis and anterior half of tendinous arch of obturator fascia.
  - *Insertion:* Anococcygeal ligament and coccyx.
- **Iliococcygeus:**
  - *Origin:* Posterior half or tendinous arch of obturator fascia and ischial spine.
  - *Insertion:* Anococcygeal ligament and side of coccyx.
- **Coccygeus (Ischiococcygeus):**
  - *Origin:* Ischial spine.
  - *Insertion:* Coccyx and fifth sacral vertebra.
  - Is supplied by perineal branch of S4.
- Sacrospinous ligament is regarded as degenerated tendon of coccygeus muscle.
- **Functions/actions of pelvic diaphragm:**
  - To support the pelvic viscera whenever there is rise in intra-abdominal pressure.
  - Assists in increasing intra-abdominal pressure during defecation, micturition and parturition.

- Puborectalis pulls the anorectal junction forward and maintain the rectal continence. The muscle relaxes during defecation.
- Puboprostatic part may help in expelling the urine during micturition.
- Muscles of the pelvic diaphragm guide the fetal head in anteroposterior direction during second stage of labor.

Pelvic diaphragm may be torn during difficult childbirth resulting in weakness of the muscles of pelvic diaphragm which in turn causes defective support of pelvic viscera. It may cause uterine prolapsed or prolapsed of the rectum or urinary incontinence.

3. **Draw labeled diagram of lumbosacral plexus.**

Ans. See Figure 48.3.

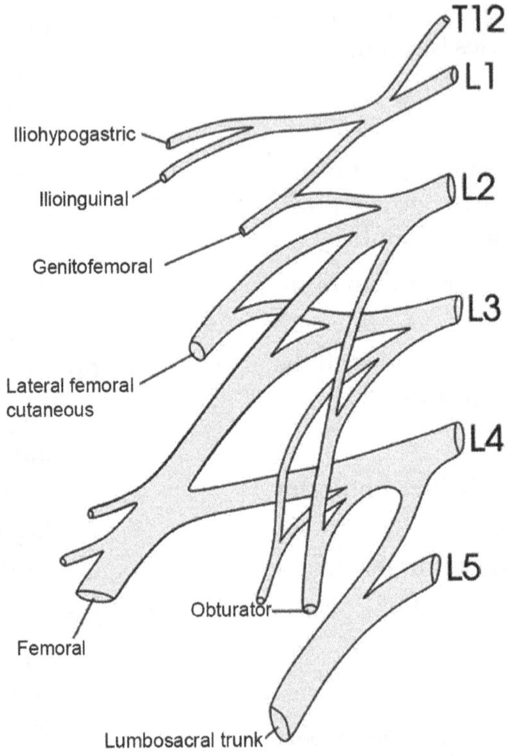

Fig. 48.3: Lumbosacral plexus

CHAPTER 49 PERINEUM

1. **Describe the boundaries and subdivisions of perineum.**

Ans. Perineum consists of structures that fill the inferior aperture of the pelvis.

- **Anteroposteriorly:** It extends from the inferior margin of pubic symphysis to the coccyx.
- **Laterally:** It is bounded by the inferior rami of pubis, rami and tuberosities of ischium and sacrotuberous ligaments.
- **Subdivisions:** Perineum is subdivided into two regions by an imaginary line passing through the ischial tuberosities:
  - Urogenital region anteriorly.
  - Anal triangle posteriorly (Fig. 49.1).

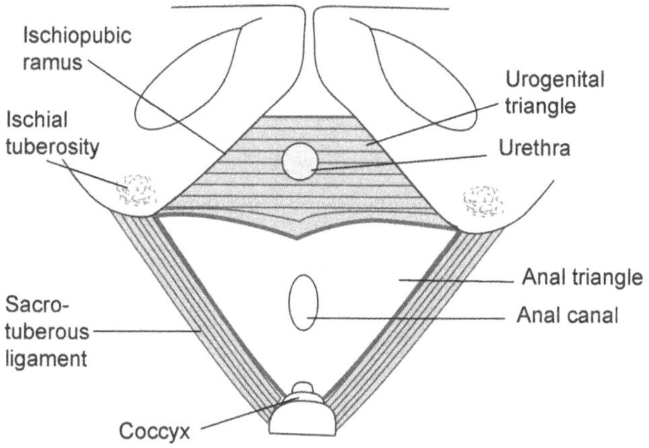

Fig. 49.1: Boundaries and subdivisions of perineum

2. **Enumerate:**
   a. **Fascial layers and spaces of urogenital region**
   b. **Contents of superficial perineal space/pouch**
   c. **Contents of deep perineal space/pouch**

Ans. a. Fascial layers and spaces of urogenital region: It has three layers of fascia separated by two spaces. The fascial layers consist of:

- ***Membranous layer of superficial fascia of perineum (Colles' fascia):*** Its attachments are as follows:
  - *Posteriorly:* To the posterior border of perineal membrane/inferior layer of urogenital diaphragm.
  - *Laterally:* To the ischial tuberosities, ischiopubic ramus.
  - *Anteriorly:* To the front of the bodies of pubis, pubic tubercle, Holden's line and is continuous with the membranous layer of superficial fascia of abdomen.
- ***Inferior fascia of urogenital diaphragm/perineal membrane:*** It is attached:
  - Laterally to the pubic arch.
  - Posteriorly fuses with the superior layer of urogenital diaphragm (above) and membranous layer of superficial fascia of perineum (below).
  - Anteriorly fuses with the superior layer of urogenital diaphragm.
  - Anteriorly it does not reach pubis but forms thickened transverse ligament of the perineum. The gap between the symphysis pubis and the transverse ligament gives passage to the dorsal vein of the penis.
  - It divides the urogenital region into superficial and deep perineal pouches.
- ***Superior fascia of urogenital diaphragm:*** Is attached:

- Laterally to the pubic arch.
- Anteriorly and posteriorly to the perineal membrane.

Spaces between the three fascial layers are:

- ***Superficial perineal space/pouch (is open anteriorly):***
  - Is between the membranous layer of superficial fascia (Colles' fascia) of perineum and perineal membrane.
  - Is closed laterally (the two layers are attached to the pubic arc and ischial tuberosities) and posteriorly (both the layers are fused).
  - Anteriorly the pouch is open and communicates with the space in the anterior abdominal wall between the membranous layer of superficial fascia (Scarpa's fascia) and external oblique muscle.

In case of injury to the bulbar urethra in the superficial perineal pouch *extravasation of urine* occurs in:

- Superficial perineal pouch and it may pass above and in front to scrotum, penis and lower part of anterior abdominal wall.

It cannot pass:

- Posteriorly due to attachment of Colles' fascia to the perineal membrane.
- Laterally due to the attachment of the fascia to the conjoint ischiopubic ramus.
- Into the thigh because of the attachment of the Scarpa's fascia to the fascia of thigh along the Holden's line (horizontal line below the inguinal ligament).

- ***Deep perineal pouch (Is closed on all the sides):***
  - Is between the superior and inferior (perineal membrane) fascia of urogenital diaphragm.
  - Both the fascial layers are attached laterally to the ischiopubic rami.
  - Anteriorly and posteriorly both the layers are fused.

b. Contents of superficial perineal space/pouch:

	Males	*Females*
Root of penis/ clitoris	Bulb of penis Two crura of penis	Two crura of clitoris Two bulbs of the vestibule
Muscles	Bulbospongiosus Two ischiocavernosus Two superficial transverse perinei	Two bulbospongiosus Two ischiocavernosus Two superficial transverse perinei
Nerves	Perineal branch of posterior cutaneous nerve of thigh Posterior scrotal nerves	Perineal branch of posterior cutaneous nerve of thigh Posterior labial nerves
Blood vessels	Posterior scrotal vessels	Posterior labial vessels
Other contents		Greater vestibular glands

- Superficial perineal pouch (a) Males (b) Females (Fig. 49.2).

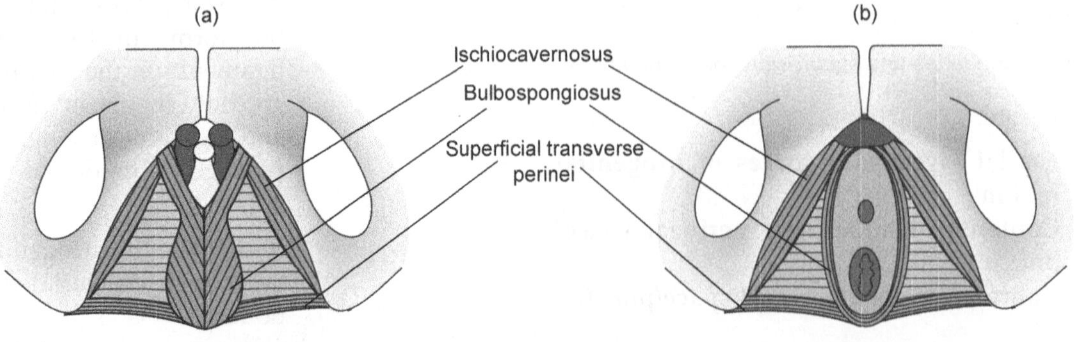

Fig. 49.2: Muscles of superficial perineal pouch in (a) Males (b) Females

c. **Contents of deep perineal space/pouch:**

	Males	*Females*
	Membranous part of urethra	Part of urethra Part of vagina
Muscles	Sphincter urethrae Two deep transverse perinei	Sphincter urethrae Two deep transverse perinei
Nerves	Nerve of the bulb of penis Pudendal nerve	Dorsal nerve of clitoris
Blood vessels	Artery of the bulb of penis Internal pudendal vessels	Internal pudendal vessels
Other contents	Two bulbourethral glands (Cowper's glands)	

- Deep perineal pouch (a) Males (b) Females (Fig. 49.3).

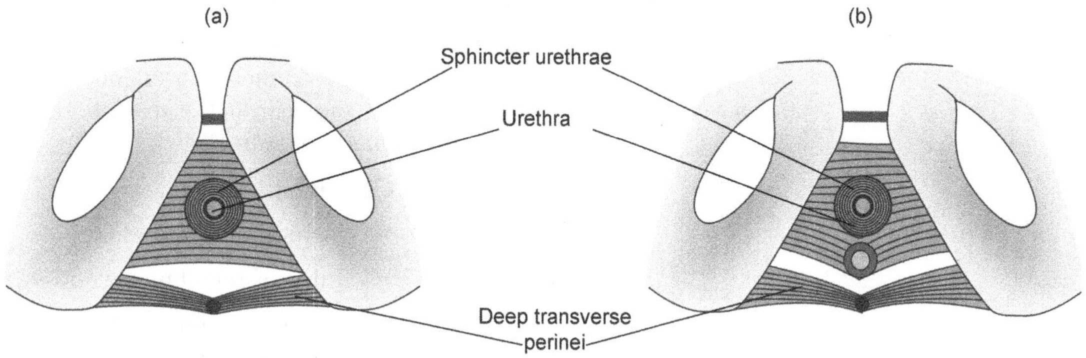

Fig. 49.3: Muscles of deep perineal pouch in (a) Males (b) Females

3. **Enumerate the branches of:**
   a. **Pudendal nerve**
   b. **Internal pudendal artery**

Ans. a. Branches of pudendal nerve (S2,S3,S4):

- *Inferior rectal nerve:* Supplies sphincter ani externus and skin around the anus.
- *Perineal nerve:* Divides into:
  - *Posterior scrotal/labial nerves (medial and lateral):* Supply skin of the posterior part of the scrotum/labium majus.
  - *Muscular branches* to the muscles of superficial and deep perineal pouches.
- *Dorsal nerve of the penis/clitoris:* Supplies penis/clitoris.

b. **Branches of internal pudendal artery:**

- *Inferior rectal artery.*
- *Perineal artery:* Gives following branches:
  - Transverse perineal branch.
  - Medial and lateral scrotal/labial arteries.
- *Deep artery of the penis/clitoris.*

4. **Draw labeled diagram of the following:**
   a. **Structures piercing perineal membrane in males**
   b. **Structures piercing perineal membrane in females**

Ans. a. See Figure 49.4a.

b. See Figure 49.4b.

5. **Describe ischiorectal fossa under the following headings:**
   a. **Location**
   b. **Boundaries**
   c. **Contents**
   d. **Applied anatomy**

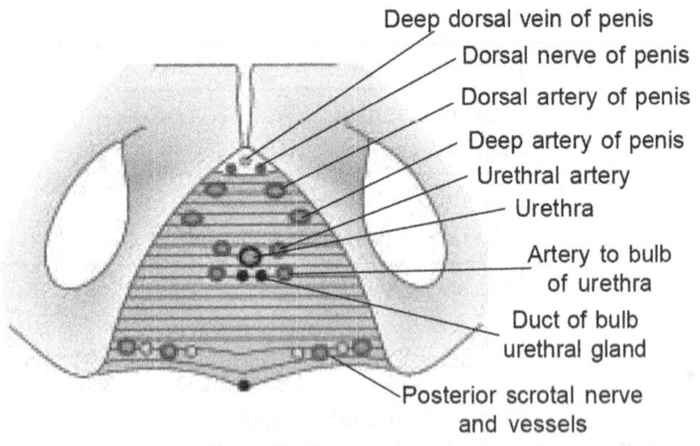

Fig. 49.4a: Structures piercing the perineal membrane (male)

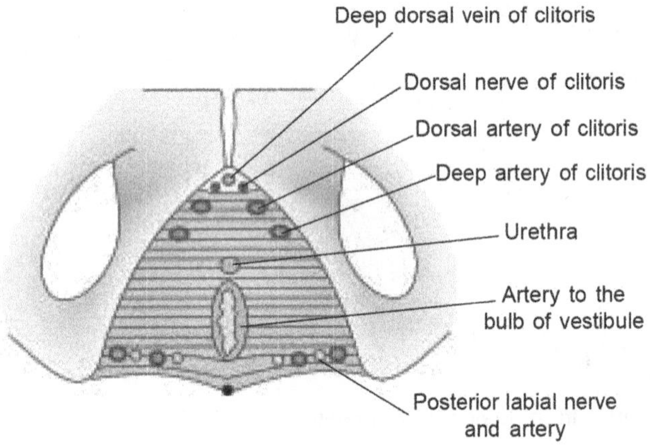

Fig. 49.4b: Structures piercing the perineal membrane (female)

Ans. a. Location: Ischiorectal fossae are located in the lateral part of the anal triangle on either side of the anal canal. They are pyramidal in shape with apex directed upwards and base downwards (Fig. 49.5).

b. Boundaries:

- *Anteriorly:* Posterior free border of urogenital diaphragm.

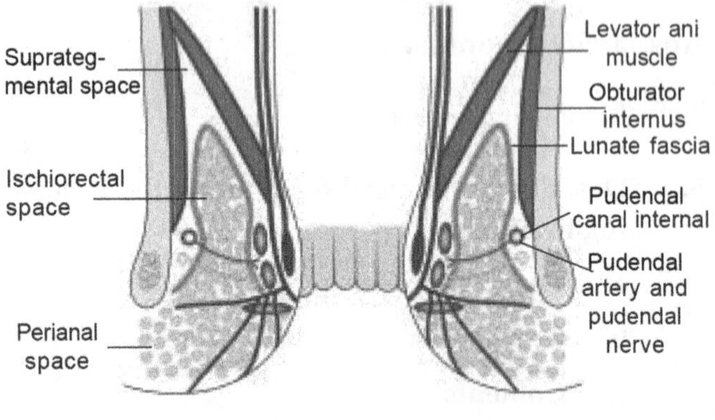

Fig. 49.5: Ischiorectal fossa

- *Posteriorly:* Lower border of gluteus maximus and sacrotuberous ligament.
- *Medially:* Levator ani above and sphincter ani externus below.
- *Laterally:* Obturator internus with obturator fascia above and ischial tuberosity below.
- *Apex:* Where the fascia lining the perineal surface of levator ani (inferior fascia of pelvic fascia) meets the obturator fascia.
- *Floor:* Perineal skin.

> - Posteriorly the two ischiorectal fossae communicate with each other behind the anal canal.
> - Herniation of pelvic viscera into the ischiorectal fossa may occur if there is a gap due to separation of levator ani muscle from the obturator fascia. The gap is called *hiatus of Schwalbe.*

c. Contents:

- Ischiorectal pad of fat.
- Inferior rectal nerve and vessels.
- Perineal branch of S4.
- Branches of posterior cutaneous nerve of thigh (S2,S3).

d. Applied anatomy:

- Ischiorectal abscess is common because the fat in the fossa is poorly vascularized and may be infected from the anal canal or infections in the perianal skin.
  - The abscess may burst on the skin forming a sinus.
  - It may open on the skin as well as in the anal canal forming fistula.
  - The abscess may spread to the other side behind the anal canal forming horseshoe-shaped abscess.
  - The abscess is painful due to compression of sensory nerves passing through the fossa.
- While draining the ischiorectal abscess, if inferior rectal nerve is cut, it may result in anal incontinence due to loss of action of sphincter ani externus which is supplied by inferior rectal nerve.

6. **What is lunate fascia and perianal fascia?**

Ans. The perianal fascia and lunate fascia divide the ischiorectal fossa into three compartments:

- **Lunate fascia:** The subcutaneous fat raises the deep fascia in the region of ischiorectal fossa to form a dome shaped lunate fascia.
- **Perianal fascia:** Is the lateral most septum from the lower end of the conjoint longitudinal tendon of anal canal.
- **Perianal space:** Between skin below and perianal fascia above.
- **Ischioanal space proper:** Between perianal fascia below and lunate fascia above.
- **Suprasegmental space:** Above the lunate fascia.

7. **Describe briefly pudendal canal.**

Ans. Pudendal canal is an elongated fascial canal located in the lateral wall of ischiorectal fossa (Fig. 49.6).

- Is present between the fascia lunata medially and obturator fascia laterally.
- It extends from the lesser sciatic foramen to the anterior end of the ischiorectal fossa.
- It contains:
  - **Pudendal nerve (S2, S3, S4):** Divides in the canal into its terminal branches:
    - Dorsal nerve of penis/clitoris.
    - Perineal nerve.
  - **Internal pudendal vessels.**
- Inferior rectal nerve and vessels (branches of pudendal nerve and internal pudendal vessels) pierce the fascia lunata to reach the anal canal.

> **Pudendal block:** The pudendal nerve can be blocked in the pudendal canal by injecting local anaesthetic agent via perineal route. The needle is inserted along the medial side of the ischial tuberosity and the anaesthetic solution is injected in the canal about 2.5 cm from the surface.

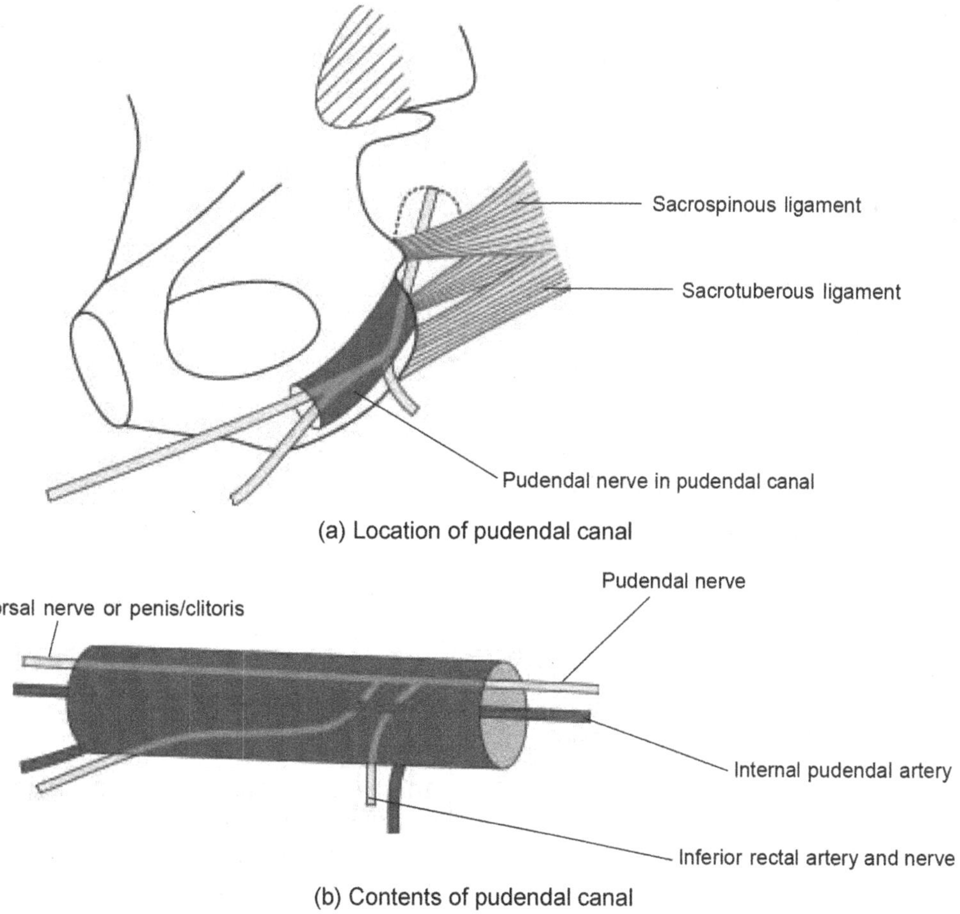

Fig. 49.6: Pudendal canal

50 CHAPTER ANAL CANAL

1. **Describe anal canal under the following headings:**
   a. **Location**
   b. **Relations**
   c. **Parts and internal features**

Ans. It is the terminal part of the large intestine. It extends from anorectal junction to the anal orifice.

a. **Location:** It is located in the anal triangle of the perineum below the pelvic diaphragm. It is 3-4 cm long and is directed downwards and backwards.

b. **Relations:**
   - ***Anteriorly:*** Perineal body which separates it from bulb of penis (in males) and vagina (in females).
   - ***Posteriorly:*** Anococcygeal raphe which separates it from tip of coccyx.
   - ***Laterally:*** Levator ani and ischiorectal fossa.

c. **Parts and internal features:** The interior of the anal canal is divided into 3 parts by pectinate line and Hilton's line (Fig. 50.1).
   - ***Upper part (1.5 cm):***
     - It extends from anorectal junction to pectinate line.
     - It is lined by columnar epithelium.
     - It is reddish in colour and shows following features:
       - *Anal columns/Columns of Morgagni:* These are 6-10 permanent vertical mucosal folds. Each fold contains terminal radicles of superior rectal vessels.
       - *Anal valves:* Are semilunar shaped transverse mucosal folds which connect the lower end of the anal columns. Free margins of the valves are directed upwards.
       - *Anal sinuses:* Are the spaces bounded below by the anal valves and on sides by the anal columns.
       - *Pectinate line:* The line of attachment of the valves is wavy and is called pectinate line. Pectinate line is called watershed line because it separates the two different parts of the anal canal in terms of development, nerve supply, blood supply and lymphatic drainage.

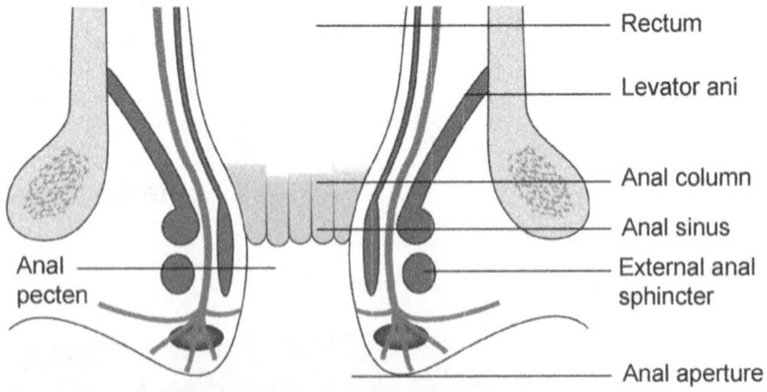

Fig. 50.1: Parts of anal canal

Anal fissure: The passage of hard stools may tear the anal valves thereby causing anal fissure. Being extremely painful fissure produces reflex spasm of the external anal sphincter.

Haemorrhoids/piles:

- Are dilatation of submucosal internal plexus of veins.
- The terminal radicles of superior rectal vessels are well developed in the left lateral (3 O'clock) position, right posterior (7 O'clock) position and right anterior (11 O'clock) position (when patient is examined in the lithotomy position) hence haemorrhoids (varicosity of veins in this region) are common at these three sites.
- Piles above the pectinate line (internal haemorrhoids) are painless, whereas below the pectinate line (external haemorrhoids).

- ***Intermediate area/area pecten (1.5 cm):***
  - Extends from pectinate line to Hilton's line.
  - Is lined by stratified squamous epithelium. Is bluish in colour due to the presence of venous plexus underneath.
  - *Hilton's line/White line:* Corresponds to the intersphincteric groove (lower end of internal sphincter muscle).
- ***Lower part (0.8 cm):***
  - Is below the Hilton's line.
  - Is lined by skin containing sweat and sebaceous glands.

2. **Write short notes on:**
   a. **Anal sphincters**
   b. **Blood supply of anal canal**

Ans. a. **Anal sphincters:** The musculature of anal canal forms two anal sphincters – internal and external anal sphincters.

- ***Sphincter ani internus:***
  - Is formed by thickened circular smooth muscle.
  - It surrounds the upper 3/4th of the anal canal, i.e., above the white line.
  - Is supplied by autonomic nerves and therefore involuntary in nature.
- ***Sphincter ani externus:***
  - Is formed by voluntary (skeletal) muscle.
  - Is supplied by somatic nerves (inferior rectal nerve).
  - It surround the entire length of the anal canal. Is divided into the following three parts:
    - *Deep part:* Surrounds the upper part of internal anal sphincter. Has no bony attachment.
    - *Superficial part:* Lies below the deep part and extends up to the intersphincteric groove. Is attached anteriorly to perineal body and posteriorly to coccyx.
    - *Subcutaneous part:* Encircles the lowest part of anal canal below the intersphincteric groove. Has no bony attachment.
- ***Longitudinal muscle of the anal canal:***
  - Separates the internal anal sphincter from the external anal sphincter.
  - Fuses with part of puborectalis muscle to form the conjoint longitudinal sheet.
  - It becomes progressively fibroelastic and breaks into number of fibrous strands which pass through the subcutaneous part of external anal sphincter and attach to the skin around the anus.

b. **Blood supply of anal canal:**

- ***Arterial supply of anal canal (Fig. 50.2):*** Anal canal is supplied by the following two arteries:
  - *Superior rectal artery:*
    - Is a branch of inferior mesenteric artery.
    - Its branches form submucosal plexus which extends as terminal radicals in the anal columns.

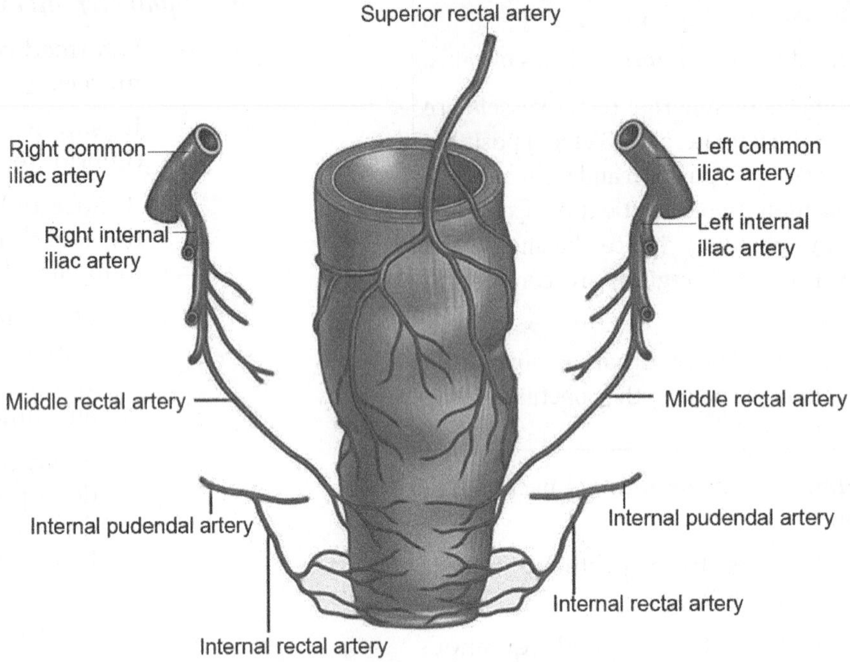

Fig. 50.2: Arterial supply of anal canal

- It supplies the mucosa of the anal canal above the pectinate line.

– *Inferior rectal artery:*
- Is a branch of internal pudendal artery.
- It supplies the mucosa of the anal canal below the pectinate line.

• ***Venous drainage of anal canal:***

– *Above the pectinate line:* Is drained by the internal venous plexus into the superior rectal vein which drains ultimately into the *portal circulation.*

– *Below the pectinate line:* Is drained by inferior rectal vein, a tributary of *systemic vein.*

> The internal venous plexus situated in the submucosa of the anal canal is tone of the site of porto-systemic anastomosis. In portal hypertension this anastomosis may dilate to form internal piles (haemorrhoids).

51

CHAPTER

LOWER LIMB–THIGH

1. **Enumerate:**
   - a. **Structures piercing cribriform fascia/ passing through saphenous opening**
   - b. **The compartments of thigh, their muscles and nerves supplying them**
   - c. **Branches of femoral artery**
   - d. **Branches of femoral nerve**
   - e. **Branches of profunda femoris artery**
   - f. **Muscles supplied by obturator nerve**

Ans. a. Structures piercing cribriform fascia/ passing through saphenous opening:

- Great saphenous vein.
- Superficial epigastric artery.
- Superficial external pudendal artery.
- Few lymph vessels connecting superficial and deep inguinal lymph nodes.

b. The compartments of thigh, their muscles and nerves supplying them: (Fig. 51.1)

> Nerve supplying muscles of anterior compartment of thigh–**Femoral.**
>
> Nerve supplying muscles of medial compartment of thigh–**Obturator.**

Contd.

Compartment	*Muscles*		*Action*	*Nerve supply*
	Quadriceps femoris	Rectus femoris	Flexion at hip joint Extension at knee joint	Femoral
		Vastus medialis	Extension at knee joint	
		Vastus intermedius		
		Vastus lateralis		
	Sartorius		Flexion and lateral rotation at hip joint Flexion at knee joint	Femoral
Medial/adductor	Adductor longus		Adduction of thigh	Obturator
	Adductor brevis			
	Adductor magnus		Adduction of thigh Extension at hip joint (Ischial part)	Obturator and tibial division of sciatic
	Pectineus		Flexion and adduction at hip joint	Obturator and femoral
	Gracilis		Adduction of thigh Flexion at knee joint Medial rotation of leg	Obturator
Posterior/flexor	Biceps femoris	Long head	Extension at hip joint Flexion at knee joint Lateral rotation of leg	Tibial division of sciatic
		Short head		Common peroneal division of sciatic
	Semitendinosus		Extension at hip joint Flexion at knee joint	Tibial division of sciatic
	Semimembranosus		Medial rotation of leg	

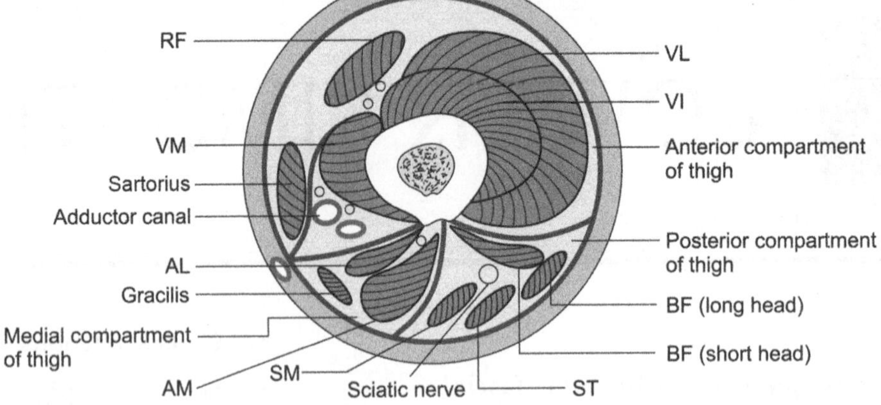

Fig. 51.1: T.S. of thigh showing the three compartments and their contents

Contd.

> Nerve supplying muscles of posterior compartment of thigh-**Sciatic.**
>
> **Composite muscles:** Muscles that have dual nerve supply:
> - ***Pectineus:*** Femoral and obturator nerve.
> - ***Adductor magnus:*** Obturator and tibial part of sciatic nerve.
> - ***Biceps femoris:*** Tibial and common peroneal divisions of sciatic nerve.

c. **Branches of femoral artery: (Fig. 51.2)**
- ***Superficial branches:***
  - Superficial epigastric.
  - Superficial circumflex iliac.
  - Superficial external pudendal.
- ***Deep branches:***
  - Deep external pudendal.
  - *Profunda femoris:*
    - Medial circumflex femoral.
    - Lateral circumflex femoral.
  - Muscular branches.
  - Descending genicular.

> Pulsations of femoral artery can be felt in the femoral triangle just below the midinguinal point against the head of femur.

d. **Branches of femoral nerve (Fig. 51.3a and Fig. 51.3b): Root value:** L2, L3, L4 (dorsal divisions).
- Femoral nerve divides into anterior and posterior divisions.
- ***Branches of anterior division:***

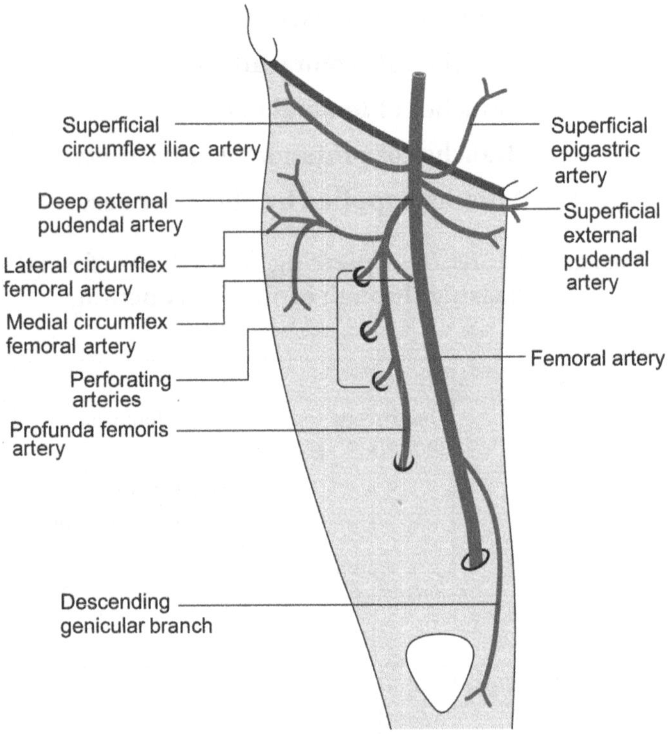

Fig. 51.2: Branches of femoral artery

  - *Muscular branches to:*
    - Pectineus.
    - Sartorius.
  - *Cutaneous branches:*
    - Medial cutaneous.
    - Intermediate cutaneous.
- ***Branches of posterior division:***
  - *Muscular branches to:*
    - Quadriceps femoris.

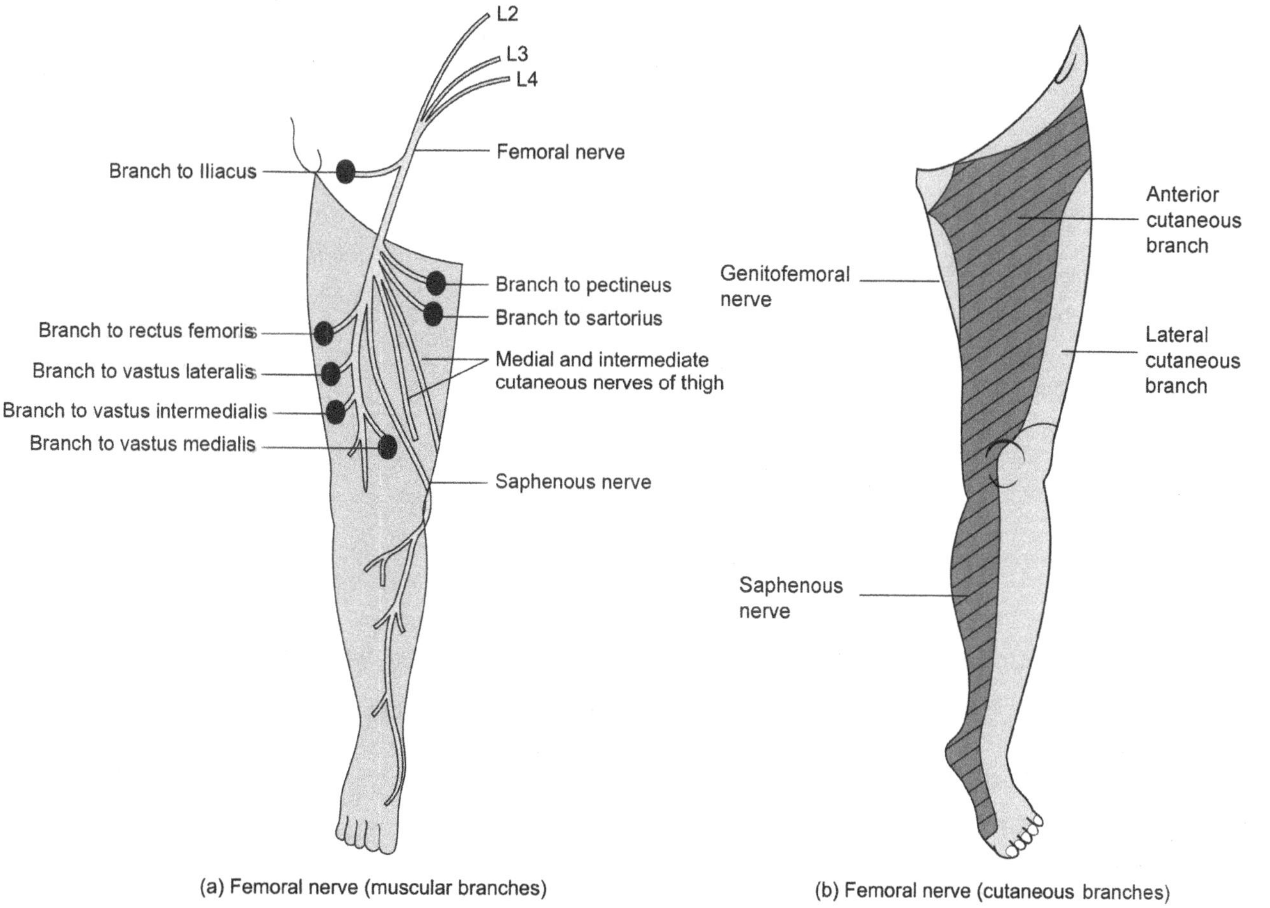

Fig. 51.3: Branches of femoral nerve

- Sartorius.

– *Cutaneous branches:*

- Saphenous nerve (longest cutaneous nerve of the body).

– *Articular branches:*

- Hip joint via nerve to rectus femoris.
- Knee joint via branches to vasti.

Effects of injury to femoral nerve:

Motor loss: Paralysis of quadriceps femoris and sartorius.

Sensory loss: Loss of sensations on the anterior and medial aspect of thigh, medial aspect of leg, medial aspect of foot till the head of 1st metatarsal.

e. **Branches of profunda femoris artery:**

- Medial circumflex artery.
- Lateral circumflex artery.
- Muscular branches.
- Three perforating arteries.

It ends by piercing adductor magnus as fourth perforating artery.

f. **Muscles supplied by obturator nerve (Fig. 51.4a and Fig. 51.4b):** Root value: L2,3,4 (ventral divisions).

- Is the nerve of the adductor compartment of thigh.
- Divides into anterior and posterior divisions.
- ***Muscles supplied by anterior division:***
  - Adductor longus.
  - Adductor brevis.
  - Gracilis.
  - Pectineus.
- ***Muscles supplied by posterior divisions:***

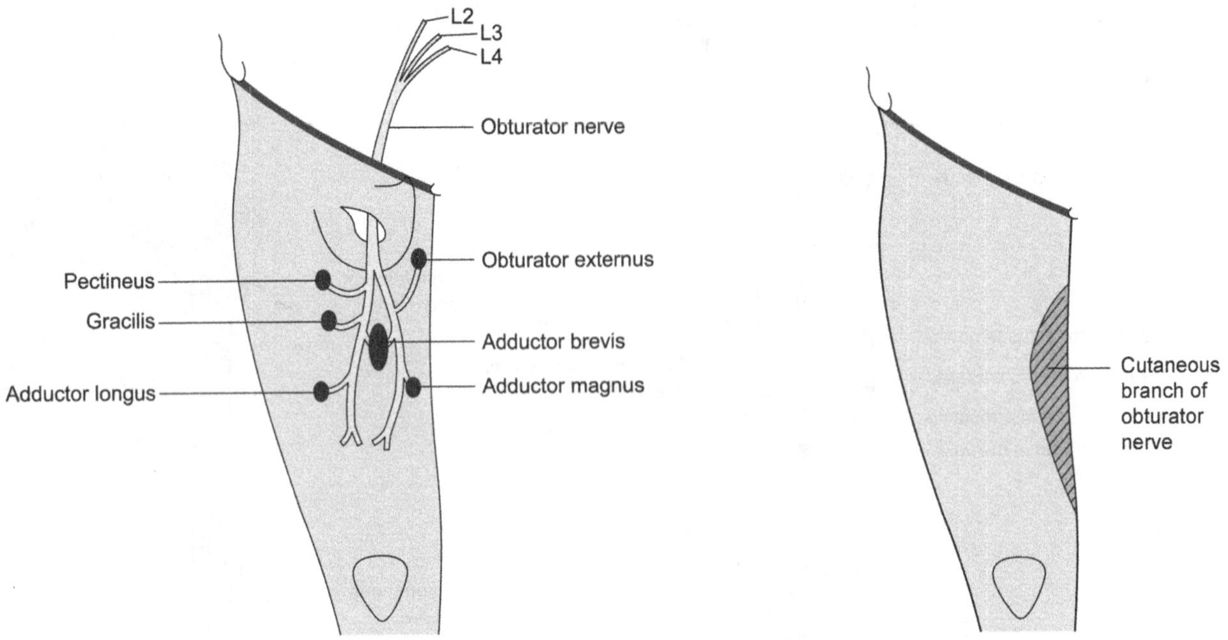

(a) Obturator nerve (muscular branches)

(b) Cutaneous innervation of obturator nerve

Fig. 51.4: Muscular and cutaneous innervation of obturator nerve

- Adductor brevis.
- Adductor magnus.
- Obturator externus.

2. **Describe briefly:**
   - a. **Femoral triangle**
   - b. **Femoral sheath, canal and hernia**
   - c. **Adductor canal**
   - d. **Hamstring muscles**
   - e. **Iliotibial tract**

Ans. a. **Femoral triangle:** It is a triangular intermuscular space on the front of upper 1/3rd of thigh.

Its boundaries are: (Fig. 51.5a)

- ***Lateral:*** Medial border of sartorius.
- ***Medial:*** Medial border of adductor longus.
- ***Apex:*** Where sartorius overlaps adductor longus.
- ***Base:*** Inguinal ligament.
- ***Roof:*** Is formed by:
  - Skin.
  - Superficial fascia with superficial blood vessels and superficial inguinal lymph nodes.
  - Deep fascia (fascia lata).
- ***Floor is formed by the following muscles (lateral to medial): (Fig. 51.5b)***
  - Iliacus.
  - Psoas major.
  - Pectineus.
  - Adductor longus.
- ***Contents: (Fig. 51.5c)***
  - *Arteries:* Femoral artery and its branches:
    - Superficial branches: Superficial epigastric, superficial circumflex iliac, superficial external pudendal.
    - Deep external pudendal.
    - Profunda femoris and its branches: Lateral and medial circumflex femoral.
  - *Veins:* Femoral vein and its tributaries.
  - *Nerves:*

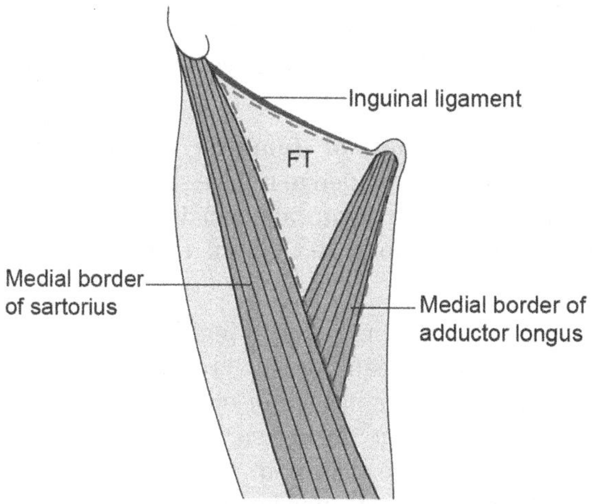

Fig. 51.5a: Boundaries of femoral triangle

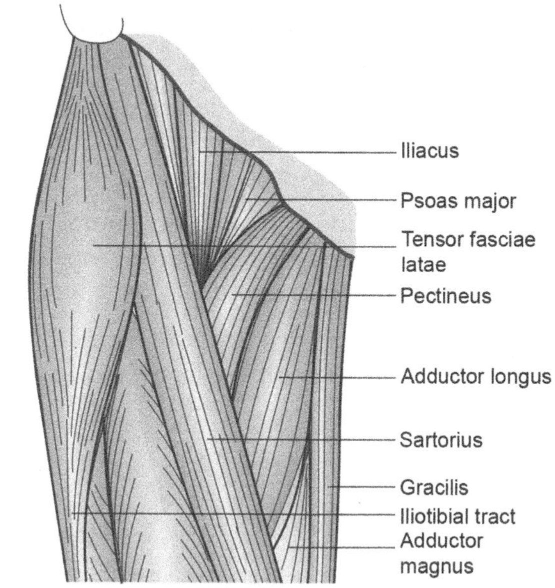

Fig. 51.5b: Muscles forming floor of femoral triangle

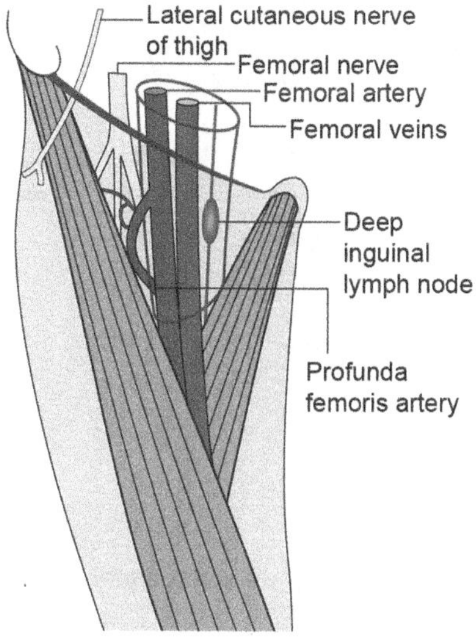

Fig. 51.5c: Contents of femoral triangle

- Femoral nerve and its branches.
- Lateral cutaneous nerve of thigh.
- Femoral branch of genito-femoral nerve.

– Deep inguinal lymph nodes.

– Fibrofatty tissue.

b. **Femoral sheath (Fig. 51.6a and Fig. 51.6b):**

- Is a funnel shaped fascial sheath that surrounds the upper part of femoral vessels and also encloses femoral canal.
- It is formed:
  - Anteriorly by fascia transversalis.
  - Posteriorly by fascia iliaca.

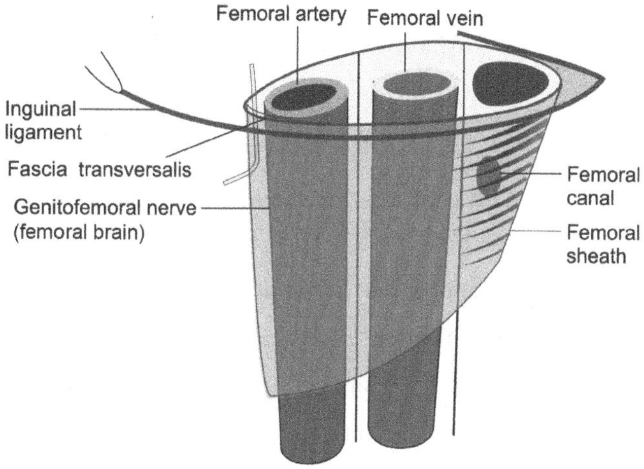

Fig. 51.6a: Femoral sheath and its contents

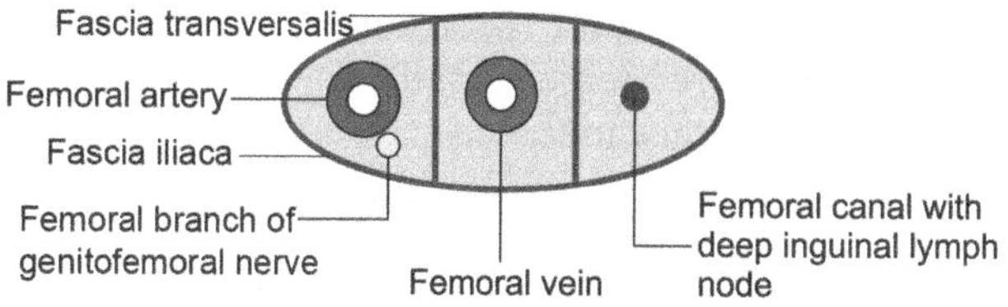

Fig. 51.6b: T.S. of right femoral sheath showing its three compartments and their contents

- Is divided into three compartments:
  - *Medial compartment:* Is called femoral canal is filled with areolar tissue and contain a lymph node (Gland of Cloquect) which drains glans penis/clitoris.

- *Intermediate compartment:* Femoral vein passes through it.
- *Lateral compartment:* Allows the passage of femoral artery and femoral branch of genitofemoral nerve.

> Femoral nerve lies outside the femoral sheath, lateral to the femoral artery.

- Is the funnel shaped medial compartment of the femoral sheath.
- Is 1.2 cm long.
- Contains some areolar tissue and a lymph node of deep inguinal group.
- Its upper end opens towards abdominal cavity and is bounded by femoral ring.
- Boundaries of femoral ring are:
  - *Lateral* – Femoral vein.
  - *Medial* – Lacunar ligament.
  - *Anterior* – Inguinal ligament.
  - *Posterior* – Pectineal line of pubic bone.
- Femoral ring is closed by a plug of fat called femoral septum.

> **Femoral canal is wider in females because:**
> - Bony pelvis is wider.
> - Femoral vessels are smaller in diameter.
>
> Therefore, *femoral hernia is more common in females.*

Femoral hernia:

- Is abnormal protrusion of abdominal content (e.g., small intestine) through femoral canal.
- Lies inferior and lateral to the pubic tubercle.
- The herniated structure enters the canal through the femoral ring, then bulge anteriorly through the saphenous opening and bends superolaterally towards the inguinal ligament.
- Strangulation of a femoral hernia may occur due to the sharp, stiff boundaries of the femoral ring.

> Femoral hernia lies inferior and lateral to pubic tubercle whereas inguinal hernia lies above and medial to pubic tubercle.
>
> **Surgical reduction of femoral hernia:** Lacunar ligament has to be divided to relieve strangulation. Care has to be taken to ligate abnormal obturator artery which may run along the lateral margin of lacunar ligament.
>
> Abnormal obturator artery (enlargement of the anastomosis between pubic branches of inferior epigastric and pubic branch of obturator artery) is in danger of being cut during surgery (femoral hernia reduction) as it lies close to the medial border of femoral ring (along lacunar ligament). This may cause severe bleeding.

c. **Adductor canal/Subsartorial canal/Hunter's canal: (Fig. 51.7a and Fig. 51.7b)**

- Is a narrow intermuscular canal located in the middle 1/3rd of the medial aspect of thigh.
- Extends from apex of femoral triangle to the osseoaponeurotic opening in adductor magnus.
- Allows the passage of femoral vessels from femoral triangle to popliteal fossa.

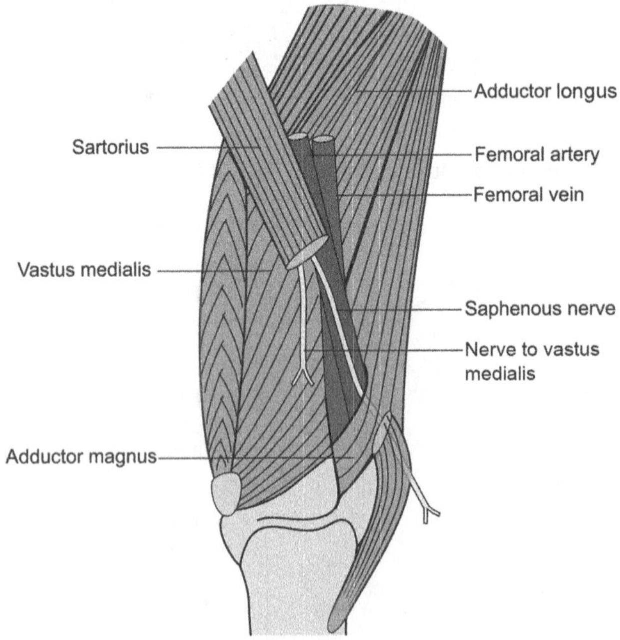

Fig. 51.7a: Location of adductor canal and its contents

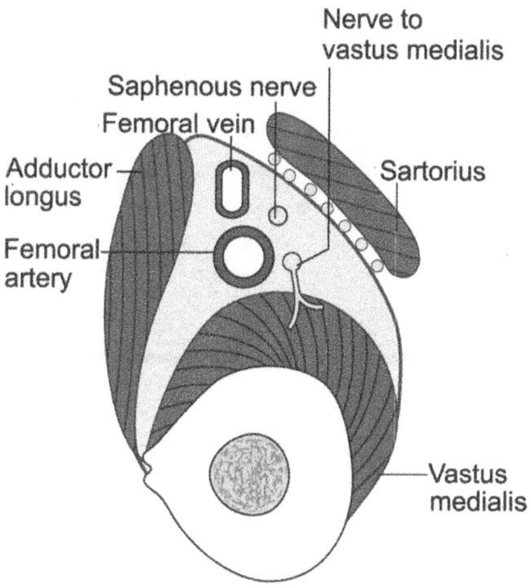

Fig. 51.7b: T.S. of adductor canal

- ***Its boundaries are:***
  - *Anterolateral:* Vastus medialis.
  - *Anteromedial (roof):* Fibrous covered by sartorius.
  - *Posterior:*
    - Adductor longus (in upper part).
    - Adductor magnus (in lower part).
- ***Contents:***
  - Femoral artery.
  - Femoral vein.
  - Saphenous nerve.
  - Nerve to vastus medialis.
  - Branches of obturator nerve.
  - Descending genicular branch of femoral artery.
- All the contents enter the canal through the apex of femoral triangle but femoral vessels leave it through the opening in adductor hiatus (lower end), saphenous nerve by piercing the roof and the nerve to vastus medialis by entering vastus medials (anterolateral wall).
- ***Applied:*** Femoral artery can be ligated in the adductor canal to treat popliteal aneurysm. Following ligation of femoral artery, blood can reach popliteal artery through the anastomotic channels around the knee. This was first described in the 18th century by John Hunter.

d. **Hamstring muscles:**

- Are the muscles of the posterior/flexor compartment of thigh.
- Include:
  - Semimembranosus.
  - Semitendinosus.
  - Long head of biceps femoris.
  - Ischial part of adductor magnus.
- Take origin from ischial tuberosity.
- Are inserted on one of the bones of leg.
- Are supplied by tibial division of sciatic nerve (all the branches arise from the medial side of the sciatic nerve).
- Act as extensors of hip joint and flexor of knee joint.

> Short head of biceps femoris takes origin from lateral lip of linea aspera and is supplied by common peroneal part of sciatic nerve.

e. **Iliotibial tract:**

- Is thickened fascia lata along the lateral surface of thigh.
- Is about 2.5 cm width.
- Receives insertion of two muscles, i.e., tensor fascia latae and superficial 3/4th of gluteus maximus.
- Above it splits to enclose tensor fascia latae; superficial layer is attached to the iliac crest and the deep layer is attached to capsule of hip joint.
- Inferiorly it is attached to flattened triangular area on anterior surface of lateral condyle of tibia.
- It maintains the knee in extended position.

52 CHAPTER GLUTEAL REGION

1. **Enumerate:**
   a. **Muscles of gluteal region and their nerve supply**
   b. **Structures passing through the greater sciatic notch**
   c. **Structures passing through the lesser sciatic notch**
   d. **Muscles inserted into iliotibial tract**
   e. **Arteries participating in trochanteric anastomosis**
   f. **Arteries participating in cruciate anastomosis**

Ans. a. **Muscles of gluteal region and their nrerve supply:** See the following Table.

b. **Structures passing through the greater sciatic foramen: (Fig. 52.1)**
   - *Piriformis muscle.*
   - *Structures passing above the piriformis:*
     - Superior gluteal nerve.
     - Superior gluteal vessels.
   - *Structures passing below the piriformis:*
     - Inferior gluteal nerve.
     - Inferior gluteal vessels.
     - Sciatic nerve.
     - Posterior cutaneous nerve of the thigh.
     - Nerve to obturator internus.
     - Nerve to quadratus femoris.
     - Internal pudendal vessels.
     - Pudendal nerve.

> Intramuscular injections in the gluteal region are given in its upper and outer quadrant to avoid injury to sciatic nerve.

c. **Structures passing through the lesser sciatic foramen: (Fig. 52.1)**
   - Tendon of obturator internus.
   - Nerve to obturator internus.
   - Internal pudendal vessels.
   - Pudendal nerve.

d. **Muscles inserted into iliotibial tract:**
   - Gluteus maximus.
   - Tensor fasciae latae.

	Name	*Nerve supply*
Gluteal muscles	Gluteus maximus	Inferior gluteal nerve (L5,S1,S2)
	Gluteus medius	Superior gluteal nerve (L4,L5,S1)
	Gluteus minimus	Superior gluteal nerve (L4,L5,S1)
Lateral rotators of thigh	Piriformis	Ventral ramii of S1,S2
	Obturator internus	Nerve to obturator internus (L5,S1,S2)
	Superior gamellus	Nerve to obturator internus (L5,S1,S2)
	Inferior gamellus	Nerve to Quadratus femoris (L4,L5,S1)
	Quadratus femoris	Nerve to Quadratus femoris (L4,L5,S1)
	Obturator externus	Obturator nerve (L2,L3,L4)
	Tensor fasciae latae	Superior gluteal nerve (L4,L5,S1)

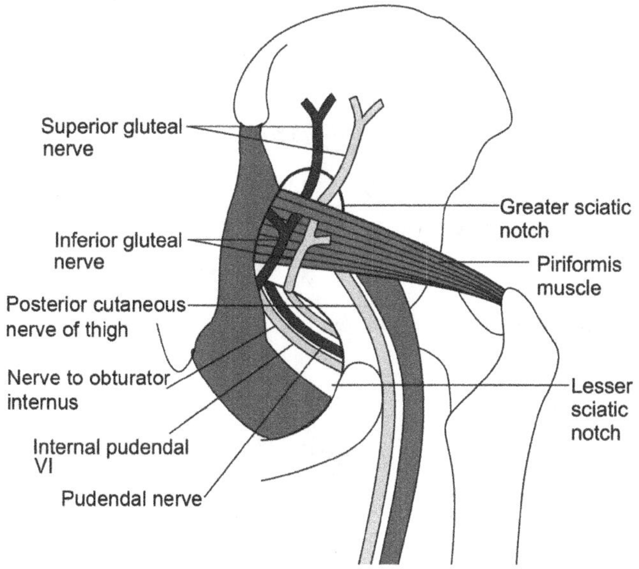

Fig. 52.1: Structures passing through greater and lesser sciatic foramina

e. **Arteries participating in trochanteric anastomosis (in the trochanteric fossa): (Fig. 52.2)**

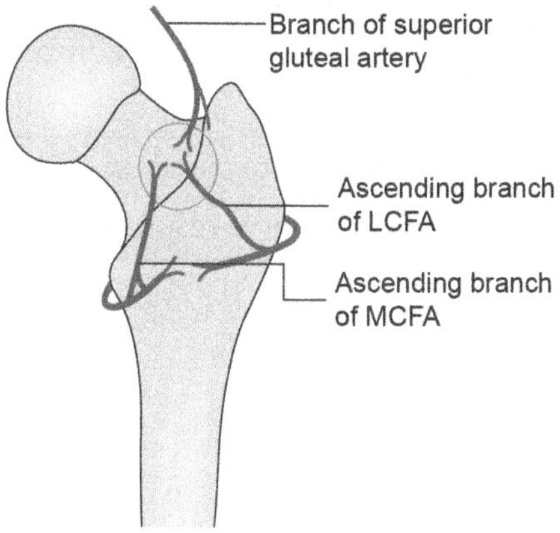

Fig. 52.2: Trochanteris anastomosis

- Descending branch of superior gluteal.
- Ascending branch of lateral circumflex femoral.
- Ascending branch of medial circumflex femoral.
- A branch from inferior gluteal artery.

f. **Arteries participating in cruciate anastomosis (at the root of the greater trochanter): (Fig. 52.3)**

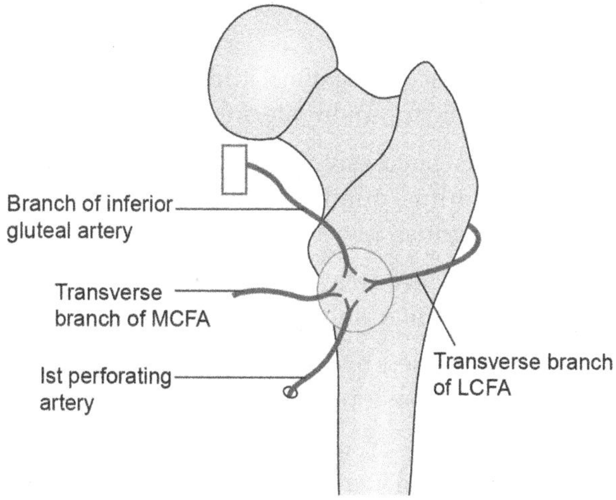

Fig. 52.3: Cruciate anastomosis

- Transverse branch of medial circumflex femoral.
- Transverse branch of lateral circumflex femoral.
- Descending branch of inferior gluteal.
- Ascending branch of first perforating.

2. **Write in a tabulated form the origin, insertion and actions of gluteal muscles.**

Ans. Gluteal muscles:

Muscle	*Origin*	*Insertion*	*Action/s*
Gluteus maximus	Gluteal surface of ilium behind the posterior gluteal line Dorsal surface of sacrum and ilium Sacrotuberous ligament	Superficial 3/4th into iliotibial tract Deep 1/4th into gluteal tuberosity	Powerful extensor of hip joint (in getting up from sitting position, running, jumping)
Gluteus medius	Gluteal surface of ilium between anterior and posterior gluteal lines	Lateral surface of greater trochanter	Abductors of hip joint Medial rotators of hip joint
Gluteus minimus	Gluteal surface of ilium between anterior and inferior gluteal lines	Anterior surface of greater trochanter	Prevents sagging of pelvis on the unsupported side

Trendelenburg's sign: If gluteus medius and minimus of one side are paralysed (due to injury to superior gluteal nerve) then if the patient is asked to stand on the paralysed side of foot, the pelvis sinks on the unsupported side (opposite side - foot is off the ground). The affected person walks with a lurching gait. This is known as *Trendelenburg's sign.*

3. Describe briefly sciatic nerve.

Ans. Sciatic nerve: (Fig. 52.4)

- Arises from the ventral ramii of L4-S3 spinal nerves.
- Leaves the pelvis through the greater sciatic foramen inferior to the piriformis.
- Lies successively on ischium, obturator internus, quadratus femoris and adductor magnus.
- Lies midway between the greater trochanter and ischial tuberosity.
- Is crossed by long head of biceps femoris in the posterior compartment of thigh.
- Usually divides into tibial and common peroneal nerves at the superior angle of popliteal fossa.
- Has no branches in the gluteal region.

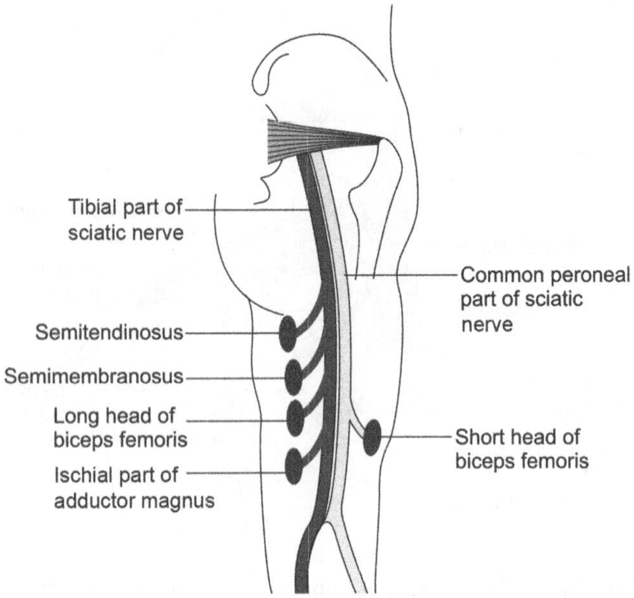

Fig. 52.4: Sciatic nerve

- Supplies all the hamstring muscles (semitendinosus, semimembranosus, biceps femoris and ischial part of adductor magnus) in the posterior compartment of thigh.

- Sciatic nerve injury leads to *foot drop.*
- Compression of sciatic nerve results in *'sleeping foot'.*

53 CHAPTER POPLITEAL FOSSA

1. Describe popliteal fossa under the following headings:

a. Boundaries

b. Contents

Ans. Popliteal fossa is a diamond shaped fossa on the back of the knee (Fig. 53.1).

a. **Boundaries:**

- *Roof:*
  - Is formed by skin, superficial fascia and deep fascia (popliteal fascia).
  - Is pierced by posterior cutaneous nerve of thigh and small saphenous vein.
- *Floor:*
  - Is formed by popliteal surface of femur, capsule of knee joint and fascia over popliteus muscle (from above downwards).
- *Side boundaries:*
  - *Superolateral:* Biceps femoris.
  - *Superomedial:* Semitendinosus and semimembranosus.
  - *Inferolateral:* Lateral head of gastrocnemius and plantaris.
  - *Inferomedial:* Medial head of gastrocnemius.

b. **Contents:**

- Popliteal artery and its branches.
- Popliteal vein and its tributaries.
- Tibial nerve and its branches.
- Common peroneal nerve.
- Popliteal group of lymph nodes.

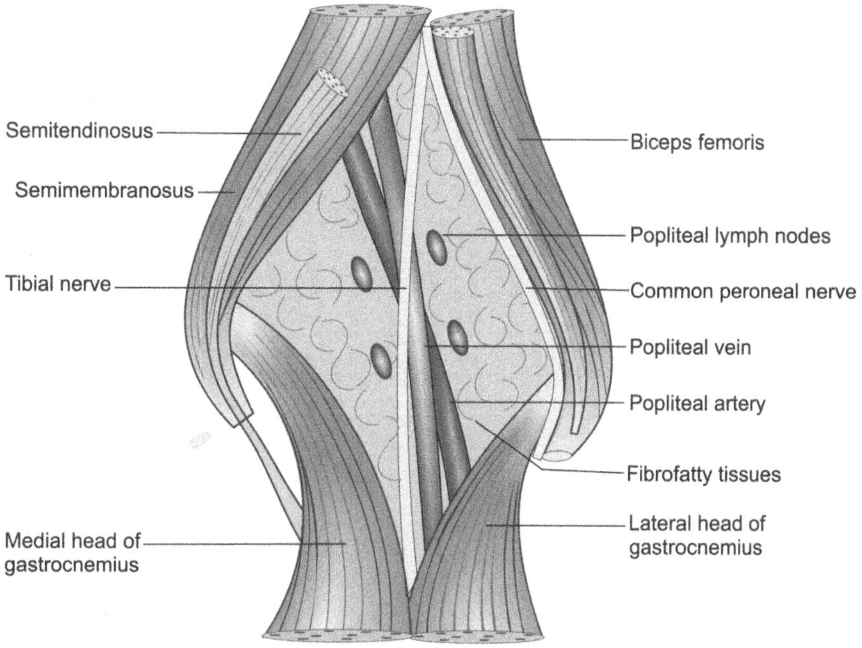

Fig. 53.1: Right popliteal fossa (boundaries and contents)

2. **Enumerate:**

   a. **Branches of tibial nerve in the popliteal fossa**

   b. **Branches of popliteal artery**

   c. **Areas of lower limb draining into popliteal lymph nodes**

Ans. a. **Branches of tibial nerve in the popliteal fossa:**

- *Muscular branches to:*
  - Gastrocnemius.
  - Soleus.
  - Plantaris.
  - Popliteus.
- *Cutaneous branch:* Sural nerve (supplies skin of the lower part of the calf).

b. **Branches of popliteal artery:**

- *Terminal branches:*
  - Anterior and posterior tibial arteries.
- *Other branches:*
  - Superior medial and lateral genicular arteries.
  - Middle genicular artery.
  - Muscular branches.

Genicular arteries form anastomosis around knee joint.

c. **Areas of lower limb draining into popliteal lymph nodes:**

- *Cutaneous lymphatics from the:*
  - Little toe.
  - Lateral margin of foot.
  - Lateral side of back of leg.

Efferents from popliteal lymph nodes drain into deep inguinal lymph nodes.

54 CHAPTER LEG

1. **Draw labeled diagram showing various compartments of leg and their contents.**

Ans. Compartments of leg and their contents: (Fig. 54.1)

2. **Enumerate:**

   a. **Muscles of the anterior/extensor compartment of leg and their nerve supply**

   b. **Muscles of the lateral/peroneal compartment of leg and their nerve supply**

   c. **Muscles of the posterior/flexor compartment of leg and their nerve supply**

   d. **Structures passing deep to superior extensor retinaculum from medial to lateral side**

   e. **Structures passing deep to flexor retinaculum from medial to lateral side**

   f. **Muscles inserted on the upper part of the medial surface of tibia and their nerve supply**

   g. **Muscles responsible for dorsiflexion of foot**

   h. **Muscles responsible for plantar flexion of foot**

   i. **Muscles responsible for inversion of foot**

   j. **Muscles responsible for eversion of foot**

Ans. a. **Muscles of the anterior/extensor compartment of leg and their nerve supply:**

- Tibialis anterior.
- Extensor hallucis longus.
- Extensor digitorum longus.
- Peroneus tertius.

* All the muscles of the anterior compartment of leg are supplied by *deep peroneal nerve.*

b. **Muscles of the lateral/peroneal compartment of leg and their nerve supply:**

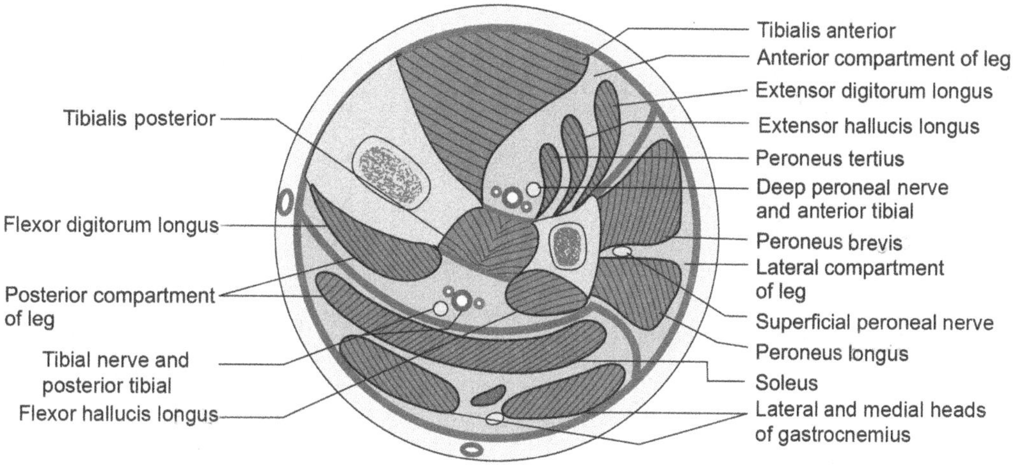

Fig. 54.1: T.S. of right leg showing the three compartments and their contents

- Peroneus longus.
- Peroneus brevis.

* All the muscles of the lateral compartment of leg are supplied by *superficial peroneal nerve.*

c. **Muscles of the posterior/flexor compartment of leg and their nerve supply:** Muscles of this compartment are divided into three groups: superficial, middle and deep group.

- ***Muscles of superficial group:***
  - Gastrocnemius.
  - Soleus.
  - Plantaris.
- ***Muscles of middle group:***
  - Flexor digitorum longus.
  - Flexor hallucis longus.
- ***Muscles of deep group:***
  - Tibialis posterior.
  - Popliteus.

* All the muscles of the posterior compartment of leg are supplied by *tibial nerve.*

d. **Structures passing deep to superior extensor retinaculum from medial to lateral side: (Fig. 54.2)**

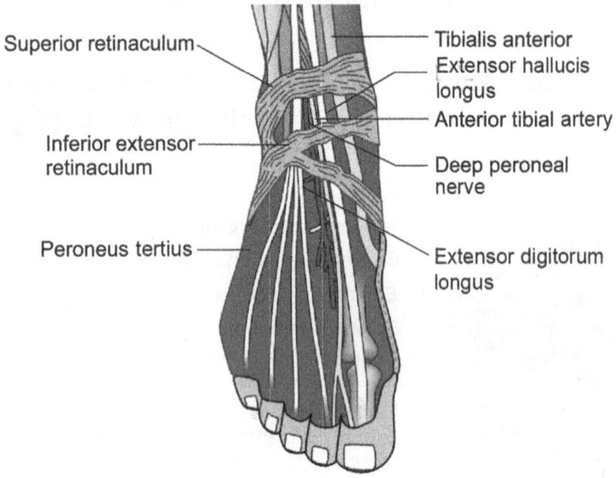

Fig. 54.2: Structure passing deep to superior extensor retinaculum

- Tibialis anterior.
- Extensor hallucis longus.
- Anterior tibial vessels.
- Deep peroneal nerve.
- Extensor digitorum longus.
- Peroneus tertius.

e. **Structures passing deep to flexor retinaculum from medial to lateral side: (Fig. 54.3)**

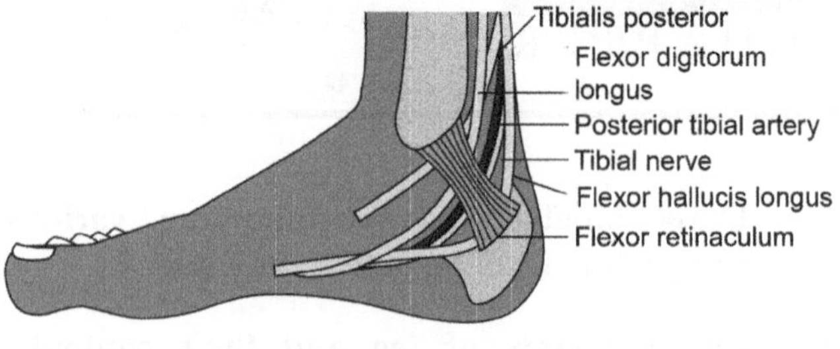

Fig. 54.3: Structure passing deep to flexor retinaculum

- Gastrocnemius.
- Soleus.
- Plantaris.
- Flexor digitorum longus.
- Flexor hallucis longus.
- Tibialis posterior.

f. **Muscles inserted on the upper part of the medial surface of tibia and their nerve supply:**

- Sartorius – supplied by femoral nerve.
- Gracilis – supplied by obturator nerve.
- Semitendinosus – supplied by tibial part of sciatic nerve.

g. **Muscles responsible for dorsiflexion of foot:**

- Tibialis anterior.
- Extensor hallucis longus.
- Extensor digitorum longus.
- Peroneus tertius.

h. **Muscles responsible for plantar flexion of foot:**

- Tibialis posterior.
- Extensor digitorum longus.
- Posterior tibial vessels.
- Tibial nerve.
- Extensor hallucis longus.

i. **Muscles responsible for inversion of foot:**

- Tibialis anterior.
- Tibialis posterior.

j. **Muscles responsible for eversion of foot:**
- Peroneus longus.
- Peroneus brevis.
- Peroneus tertius.

3. **Write in a tabulated form the origin, insertion and action of tibialis anterior, tibialis posterior, peroneus longus, gastrocnemius, soleus and popliteus.**

Ans. See the following Table.

4. **What is the triceps surae?**

Ans. The triceps surae comprises the gastrocnemius (two heads) and the underlying soleus. It is inserted via tendocalcaneus on the posterior surface of calcaneum. It is the chief plantar flexor of the foot.

Anterior tibial compartment syndrome: Occurs following excessive exertion of the muscles of anterior compartment of leg. Muscles within the tight compartment swell resulting in compression of anterior tibial artery and its branches, leading to ischemia and pain. The boundaries of anterior compartment of leg are:
- Anterior – Deep fascia.
- Posterior – Interosseous membrane.
- Lateral – Anterior intermuscular septum and fibula.
- Medial – Lateral surface of tibia.

Intermittant Claudication (derived from word Claudicare (Latin) means 'to limp'): Occurs due to ischemia of the muscles of lower limb chiefly the calf muscles. Is seen in occlusive peripheral arterial diseases particularly involving popliteal artery and its branches. The pain usually causes the person to limp. Pain is typically felt while walking and subsides with rest.

Foot drop: Foot is plantar flexed, dorsiflexors of foot are paralysed. Is caused due to injury to sciatic or common peroneal or deep peroneal nerve.

Muscle	*Origin*	*Insertion*	*Action*
Tibialis anterior	Upper 2/3rd of lateral surface of tibia and adjoining part of interosseous membrane.	Medial side of base of 1st metatarsal. Adjoining surface of medial cuneiform.	Inversion of foot. Maintains medial longitudinal arch of foot.
Tibialis posterior	*Posterior surface of:* • Tibia (below the soleal line). • Fibula (medial to medial crest). • Interosseous membrane.	Chiefly on *tuberosity of navicular* bone. All tarsals except talus. Bases of 2nd, 3rd and 4th metatarsals.	Invertor of foot. Plantar fexion of foot. Maintains medial longitudinal and transverse arches of foot.
Peroneus longus	Upper 2/3rd of lateral surface of fibula.	Lateral side of base of 1st metatarsal. Adjoining surface of medial cuneiform.	Eversion of foot. Maintains lateral longitudinal arch of foot.
Gastrocnemius	*Lateral head*: Lateral condyle of femur. *Medial head*: Popliteal surface of femur and adjoining aspect of medial condyle of femur.	Posterior surface of calcaneus via tendocalcaneus.	Plantar flexion at ankle joint. Flexion at knee joint.
Soleus	Upper 1/4th of the posterior surface of shaft of fibula. Soleal line and middle 1/3rd of the medial border of tibia. Tendinous arch between tibia and fibula.	Posterior surface of calcaneus via tendocalcaneus.	Plantar flexion at ankle joint.
Popliteus	Popliteal groove on the lateral condyle of femur.	Triangular area above the soleal line on the posterior surface of tibia.	Unlocks the knee joint by laterally rotating femur (foot on the ground) or medially rotating the tibia (foot off the ground) in the beginning of flexion of knee joint.

CHAPTER 55

FOOT

1. Draw labeled diagram showing cutaneous innervations of foot.

Ans. Cutaneous innervations of dorsum of foot (Fig. 55.1a) and sole of foot (Fig. 55.1b):

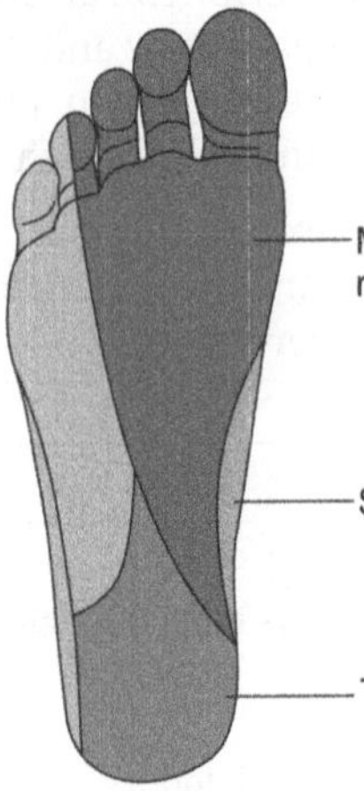

Fig. 55.1a: Cutaneous innervations of dorsum of foot

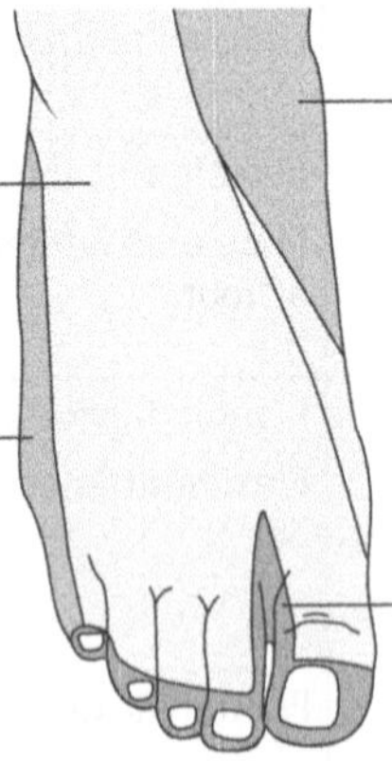

Fig. 55.1b: Cutaneous innervations of sole of foot

2. Enumerate:

a. **Muscles of 1st muscular layer of sole**

b. **Muscles of 2nd muscular layer of sole**

c. **Muscles of 3rd muscular layer of sole**

d. **Muscles of 4th muscular layer of sole**

e. **Branches of dorsalis pedis artery**

f. **Branches of medial plantar nerve**

g. **Branches of lateral plantar nerve**

Ans. a. **Muscles of 1st muscular layer of sole (two abductors and a flexor):**

- Abductor hallucis.
- Flexor digitorum brevis.
- Abductor digiti minimi.

b. **Muscles of 2nd muscular layer of sole (two tendons of longus muscles of toes and two associated muscles):**

- Tendon of flexor digitorum longus.
- Tendon of flexor hallucis longus.
- Flexor digitorum accessories.
- Four lumbricals.

c. **Muscles of 3rd muscular layer of sole (two flexors, one adductor):**

- Flexor hallucis brevis.
- Flexor digiti minimi brevis.
- Adductor hallucis.

d. **Muscles of 4th muscular layer of sole (all interossei):**

- 3 plantar interossei.
- 4 dorsal interossei.

e. **Branches of dorsalis pedis artery:**

- Medial tarsal artery.
- Lateral tarsal artery.
- Arcuate artery (gives 2nd-4th dorsal metatarsal arteries).
- First dorsal metatarsal artery.

> Pulsations of dorsalis pedis artery can be felt between the tendon of extensor hallucis and tendon of extensor digitorum longus.

f. **Branches of medial plantar nerve (similar to median nerve in palm):**
- ***Muscular branches (4 muscles):***
  - Abductor hallucis.
  - Flexor hallucis brevis.
  - Flexor digitorum brevis.
  - 1st lumbrical.
- ***Cutaneous branches (one proper digital and three common digital branches) innervate:***
  - Skin of medial part of sole.
  - Skin of plantar surface of medial 3½ toes.
  - Dorsum of terminal phalanx including nail bed of medial 3½ toes.

g. **Branches of lateral plantar nerve (similar to ulnar nerve in palm):**
- ***Muscular branches (All the intrinsic muscles of sole except the 4 muscles supplied by medial plantar nerve):***
  - Abductor digiti minimi.
  - Flexor digiti minimi.
  - Flexor digitorum accessories.
  - Adductor hallucis.
  - All palmar interossei.
  - All dorsal interossei.

2. **Describe arches of foot under the following headings:**
   a. **Functions of arches**
   b. **Classification (Types)**
   c. **Bony components**
   d. **Factors maintaining arches of foot**

Ans. a. **Functions of arches:**
- Distribution of body weight to the weight bearing points.
- Act as shock absorber (e.g., during jumping).
- Concavity of the arches protect underlying vessels and nerves.
- Help in walking on uneven surfaces.

b. **Classification:**
- ***Two longitudinal arches:***
  - Medial longitudinal arch.
  - Lateral longitudinal arch.
- ***Two transverse arches:***
  - Posterior (incomplete) transverse arch.
  - Anterior (complete) transverse arch.

c. **Bony components:**
- ***Medial longitudinal arch (medial half of calcaneum, talus, navicular, three cuneiforms and three metatarsals): (Fig. 55.2a)***

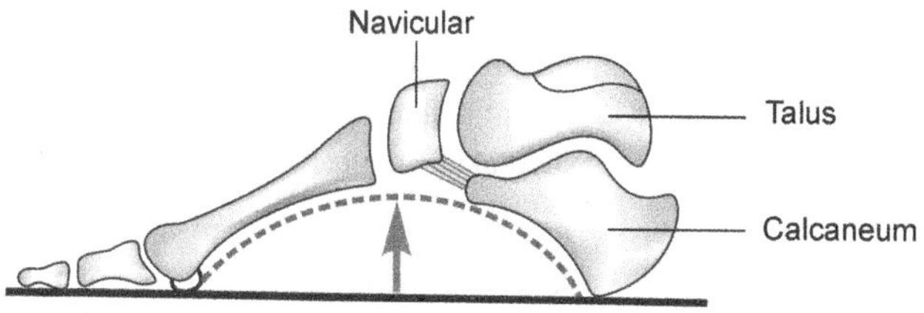

Fig. 55.2a: Medial longitudinal arch

  - *Posterior pillar:* Medial tubercle of calcaneum.
  - *Anterior pillar:* Heads of medial three metatarsals.
  - *Keystone:* Talus.
- ***Lateral longitudinal arch (lateral half of calcaneum, cuboid and lateral two metatarsals): (Fig. 55.2b)***

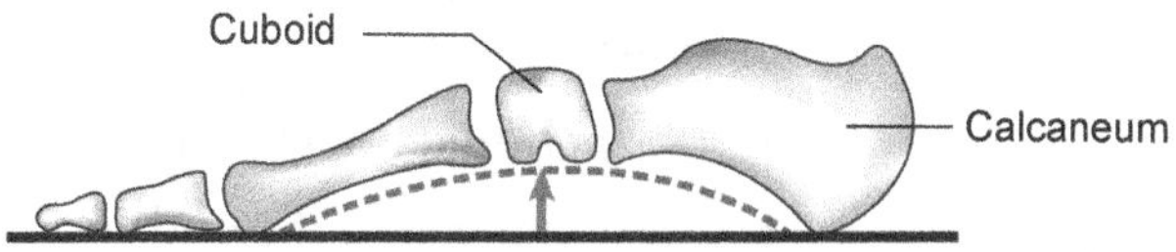

Fig. 55.2b: Lateral longitudinal arch

  - *Posterior pillar:* Lateral tubercle of calcaneum.
  - *Anterior pillar:* Heads of lateral two metatarsals.
  - *Summit:* At calcaneo – cuboid joint.
- ***Posterior transverse arch (is incomplete as its medial end does not touch the ground during standing position):*** Consists of:

Factors maintaining arches	*Medial longitudinal arch*	*Lateral longitudinal arch*	*Transverse arches*
Shapes of bones	Wedge shaped cuneiforms with narrow edge directed to the plantar surface Sustentaculum tali supports the head of talus	–	Wedge shaped cuneiforms and bases of middle three metacarpals with narrow edge directed to the plantar surface
Intersegmental ties	Ligaments: • Plantar calcaneonavicular • Interosseous talocalcanean • Dorsal ligaments connecting bony components	Ligaments: • Long plantar ligament • Short plantar ligament	• Deep transverse ligaments • Transverse and oblique heads of adductor hallucis
Slings	Tibialis anterior Tibialis posterior Deltoid ligament	Peroneus longus Peroneus brevis	Medially: Tibialis anterior Laterally: Peroneus tertius Peroneus brevis
Tie beams	Medial part of plantar aponeurosis Abductor hallucis Flexor hallucis brevis Flexor hallucis longus Medial half of flexor digitorum brevis	Lateral part of plantar aponeurosis Abductor digiti minimi Flexor digiti minimi Lateral half of flexor digitorum brevis	Tendons of: Peroneus longus Tibialis posterior

  - Bases of metatarsals, cuboid and cuneiforms.
- ***Anterior transverse arch (is complete as its medial and lateral end touch the ground during standing position):*** Consists of:
  - Heads of metatarsals.

d. **Factors maintaining arches of foot: (See above Table) (Fig. 55.3a and Fig. 55.3b)**
- Shapes of bones.
- Intersegmental ties (connecting adjacent bones).
- Slings (suspending arch from above).
- Tie beams (connecting the ends of the arches).

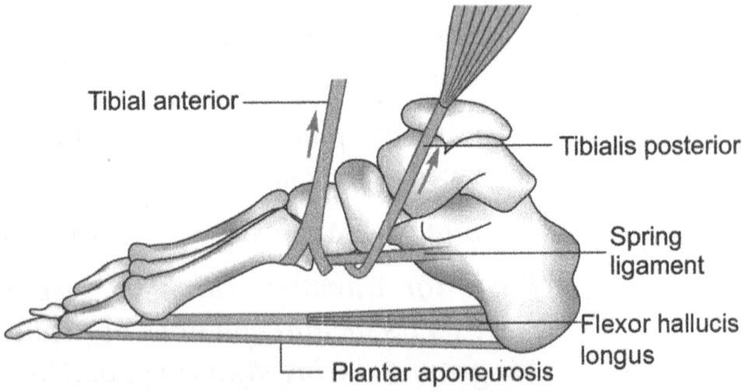

Fig. 55.3a: Factors maintaining medial longitudinal arch

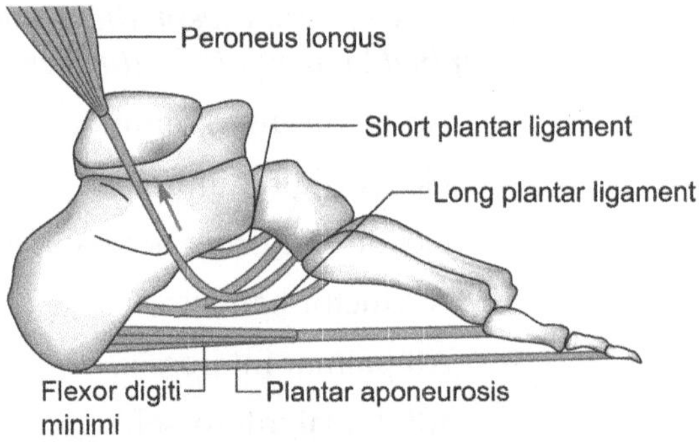

Fig. 55.3b: Factors maintaining lateral longitudinal arch

Flat foot (pes planus): Collapse of arches (especially medial longitudinal) of foot. Leads to compression of nerves and vessels in the sole of foot.

Pes cavus: Arches (mainly medial longitudinal) of foot are exaggerated.

Talipes equinovarus (club foot):
- Is a congenital deformity.
- Foot is plantar flexed, inverted and adducted.
- The four primary types are:
  - Talipes equinus – Foot is plantar flexed, toes touching the ground.
  - Talipes calcaneus – Foot is dorsiflexed, heel touching the ground.
  - Talipes varus – Foot is inverted and adducted.
  - Talipes equinus – Foot is everted and abducted.

56 CHAPTER

VENOUS AND LYMPHATIC DRAINAGE AND CUTANEOUS INNERVATIONS OF LOWER LIMB

1. **Describe the venous drainage of lower limb under the following headings:**
   a. **Superficial and deep veins**
   b. **Factors that help in venous return**
   c. **Varicose veins of lower limb**

Ans. a. **Superficial and deep veins:** The veins of the lower extremity are subdivided into two sets: *superficial* and *deep*. The two set of veins are connected by perforating veins. Both sets of veins are provided with valves, which are more numerous in the deep than in the superficial set.

- *Superficial veins:* The two important superficial veins are:
  - Great saphenous vein.
  - Small saphenous vein.
- *Great saphenous vein: (Fig. 56.1)*
  - Is the longest vein of the body.
  - Begins at the medial side of the dorsal venous arch of the foot.
  - Ascends in front of medial malleolus, crosses the medial surface of lower third of tibia and ascend along the medial border of tibia to reach the posteromedial aspect of knee (about one hand-breadth posterior to patella).
  - Then ascends along the medial side of thigh to reach the saphenous opening.
  - Passes through the saphenous opening, pierces cribriform fascia and femoral sheath to drain into femoral vein.
  - *Tributaries:*
    - Posterior arch vein, anterior leg veins, anterolateral and posteromedial veins of thigh; and
    - Three vein before it pierces cribriform fascia: Superficial epigastric, superficial circumflex iliac and superficial external pudendal veins.

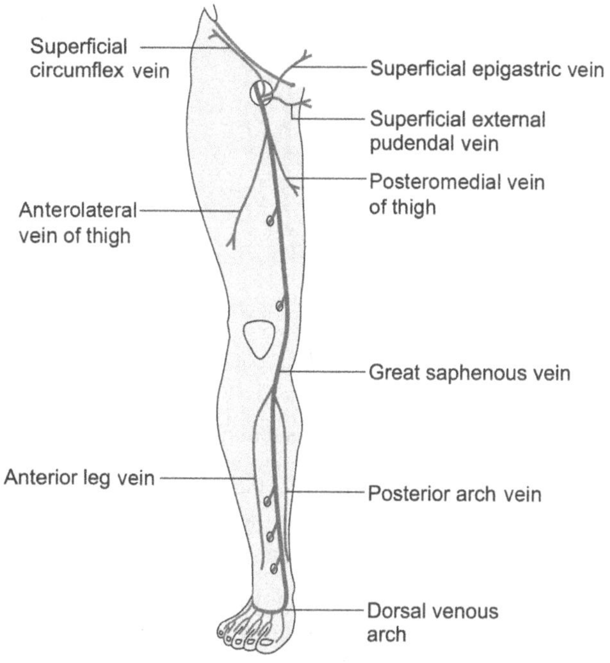

Fig. 56.1: Great saphenous vein

- Is accompanied by saphenous nerve in the leg and foot.
- Is connected to deep veins via perforating veins.

> Great saphenous vein can be used for venipuncture and coronary bypass. Care should be taken to reverse the vein so that its valves do not obstruct blood flow in the graft.

- *Small saphenous vein: (Fig. 56.2)*
  - Begins at the lateral side of the dorsal venous arch.

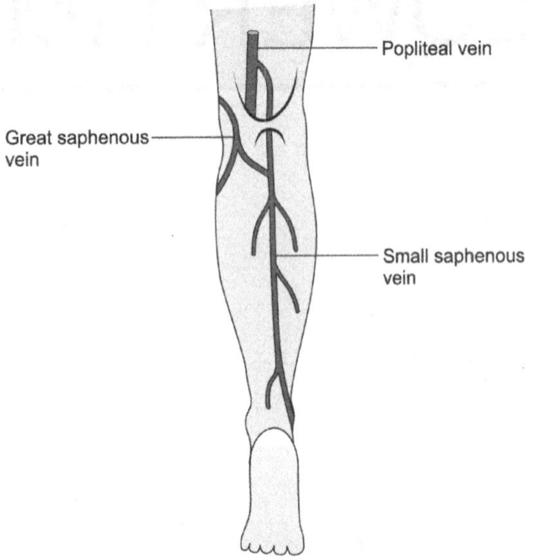

Fig. 56.2: Small saphenous vein

  - Ascend behind the lateral malleolus and then along the posterior aspect of leg.
  - Pierces popliteal fascia to open into the popliteal vein.
  - Drains lateral side of the foot and leg.
  - Is accompanied by sural nerve.
- *Deep veins:* Accompany the major arteries viz. anterior tibial, posterior tibial, popliteal and femoral.

b. **Factors that help in venous return:**
- Contraction of muscles (especially calf muscle).
- Presence of valves prevents back-flow.
- Pulsations of arteries.
- -ve intrathoracic pressure.

> **Soleus is known as peripheral heart:** The muscle is pierced by perforating veins draining blood from superficial veins to the deep veins (presence of valves allow blow to flow from superficial to deep veins). Soleus contains rich plexus of valveless veins (venous sinuses), the contraction of the muscle within the tight sleeve of fascia pushes the blood upwards along the deep veins.

c. **Varicose veins of lower limb:**
- The superficial veins of lower limb often become dilated and tortuous (varicose).
- The causes of varicosity are:
  - Incompetency of valves of perforating or superficial veins.
  - Persistent increase of intra-abdominal pressure (e.g., abdominal tumors, pregnancy).
  - Thrombosis of deep veins.

2. **Draw labeled schematic diagram showing lymph nodes of lower limb and the areas drained by them.**

Ans. Lymph nodes and lymphatic drainage of lower limb: (Fig. 56.3)

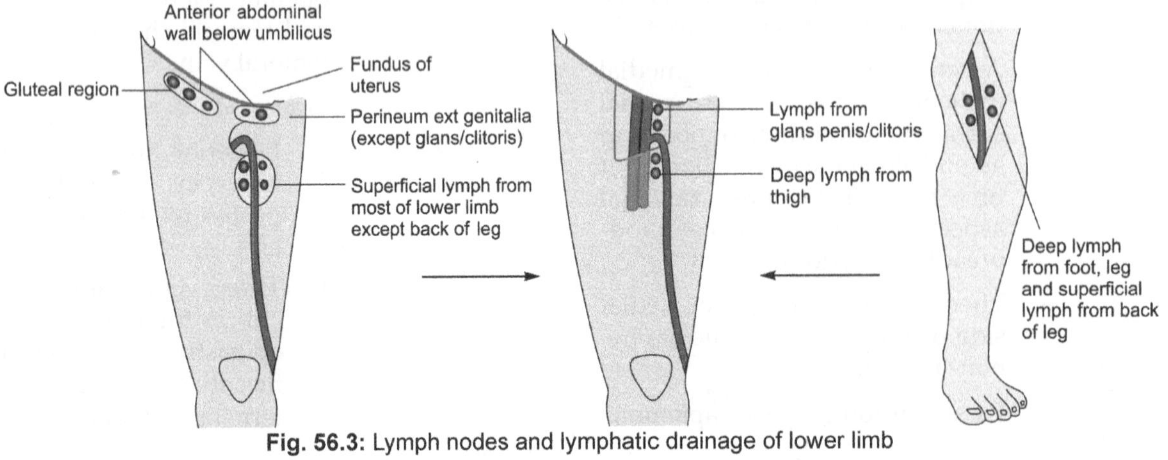

Fig. 56.3: Lymph nodes and lymphatic drainage of lower limb

3. **Draw labeled diagram showing cutaneous innervations of lower limb.**

Ans. Cutaneous innervations and dermatomes of lower limb: (Fig. 56.4a,b and Fig. 56.5)

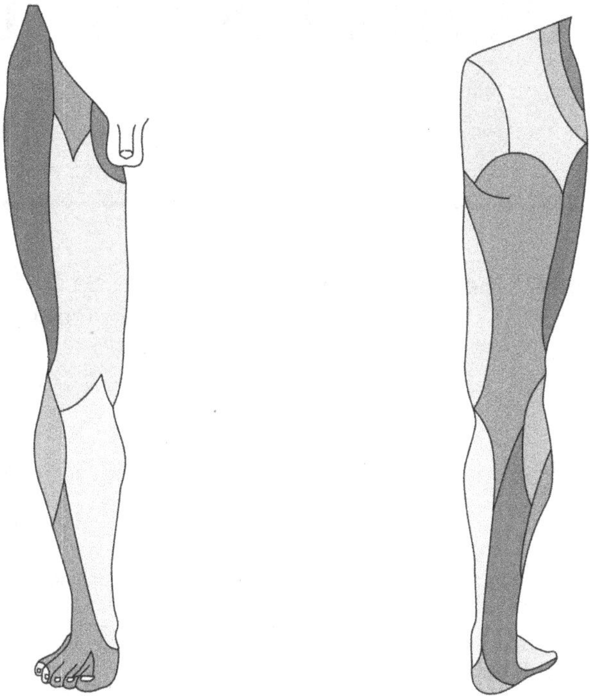

(a) Anterior aspect (b) Posterior aspect

Fig. 56.4: Cutaneous innervations of lower limb

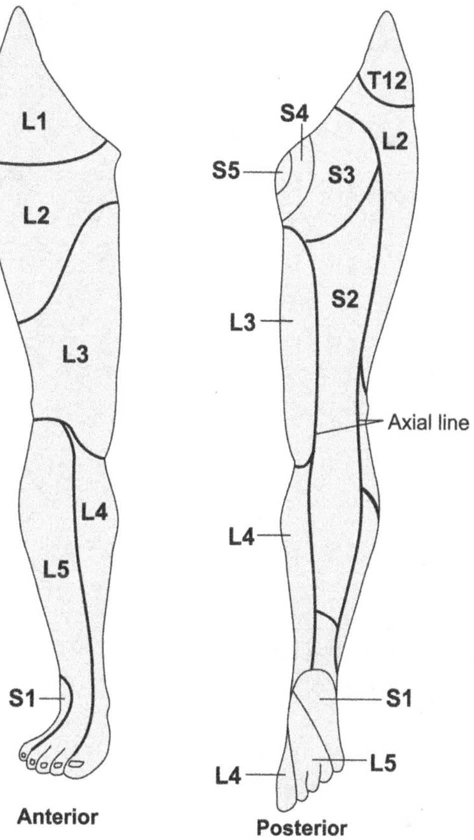

Fig. 56.5: Dermatomes of lower limb

57 CHAPTER

JOINTS OF LOWER LIMB

1. Describe hip joint under the following headings:

a. Type

b. Articular surfaces

c. Capsule and ligaments

d. Relations

e. Movements

f. Blood and nerve supply

Ans. a. **Type:** It is a multiaxial ball and socket synovial joint.

b. **Articular surfaces:** It is formed by the articulation of head of femur (ball) with the acetabulum (socket) of hip bone (Fig. 57.1).

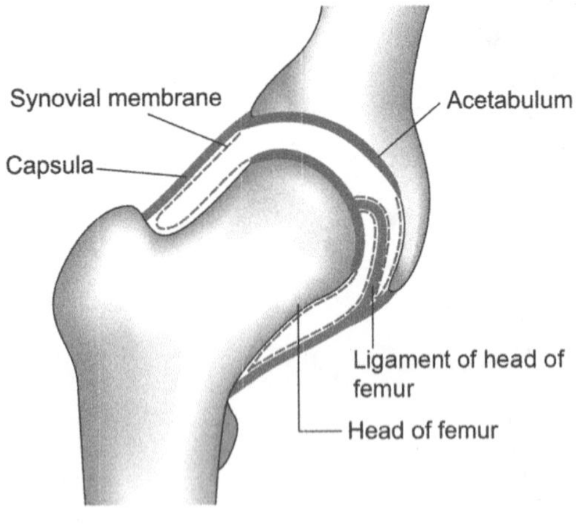

Fig. 57.1: Hip joint

Acetabulum labrum: Fibrocartilaginous rim attached to acetabulum that deepens the articular socket.

c. **Capsule:**

- Is attached proximally to the margins of the acetabulum and to the transverse acetabular ligament.
- Is attached distally to the neck of the femur as follows:
  - Anteriorly to the intertrochanteric line.
  - Posteriorly 1cm medial to inter-trochanteric crest.

Ligaments: (Fig. 57.2)

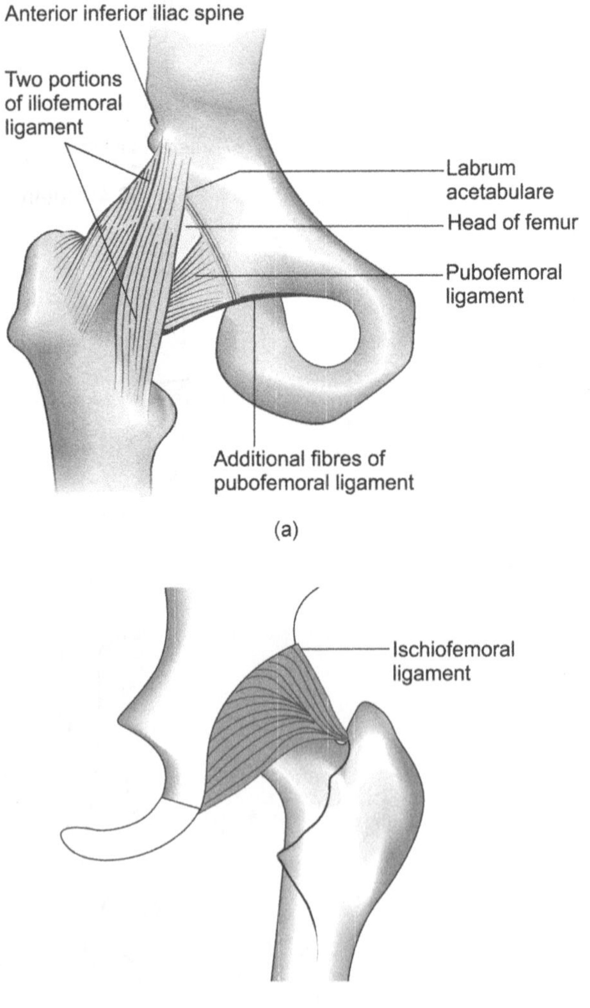

Fig. 57.2: Ligaments of hip joint

- ***Ileofemoral ligament:*** Is inverted Y-shaped ligament that extends from the anterior inferior iliac spine to the intertrochanteric line. It reinforces capsule anteriorly and resists/prevents hyperextension.
- ***Pubofemoral ligament:*** Is a triangular ligament with base above and apex below. It reinforces capsule inferiorly. Extends from iliopubic eminence and obturator crest to lower part of neck of femur. It prevents hyperabduction.
- ***Ischiofemoral ligament:*** It reinforces the capsule posteriorly, extends from ischium posteroinferior to acetabulum to intertrochanteric crest near the base of the greater trochanter.
- ***Ligament of head of femur (Ligamentus teres or Round ligament):*** Is a triangular ligament with its apex attached to the fovea of head of femur and base is attached to the transverse acetabular ligament.
- ***Transverse acetabular ligament:*** Bridge the acetabular notch.

d. **Relations: (Fig. 57.3)**

- ***Anteriorly:*** Iliopsoas and pectineus separate femoral nerve and vessels from the hip joint.
- ***Posteriorly:*** Lateral rotators of hip joint and sciatic nerve.
- ***Superiorly:*** Gluteus medius, minimus and piriformis.
- ***Inferiorly:*** Obturator externus.

e. **Movements:**

- ***Flexion:*** Iliopsoas, Rectus femoris, Sartorius.
- ***Extension:*** Gluteus maximus, Hamstring muscles.
- ***Abduction:*** Gluteus medius, Gluteus minimus.
- ***Adduction:*** Adductor longus, Adductor fibres of the adductor magnus, Adductor brevis.
- ***Lateral rotation:*** Piriformis, Obturator internus and externus, Quadratus femoris, Superior and inferior Gamelli.
- ***Medial rotation:*** Anterior fibres of gluteus medius, Gluteus minimus, Tensor fascia lata.

f. **Nerve supply:** Femoral, obturator, sciatic nerve and nerve to obturator externus.

Blood supply: Medial and lateral circumflex femoral, superior and inferior gluteal, obturator artery.

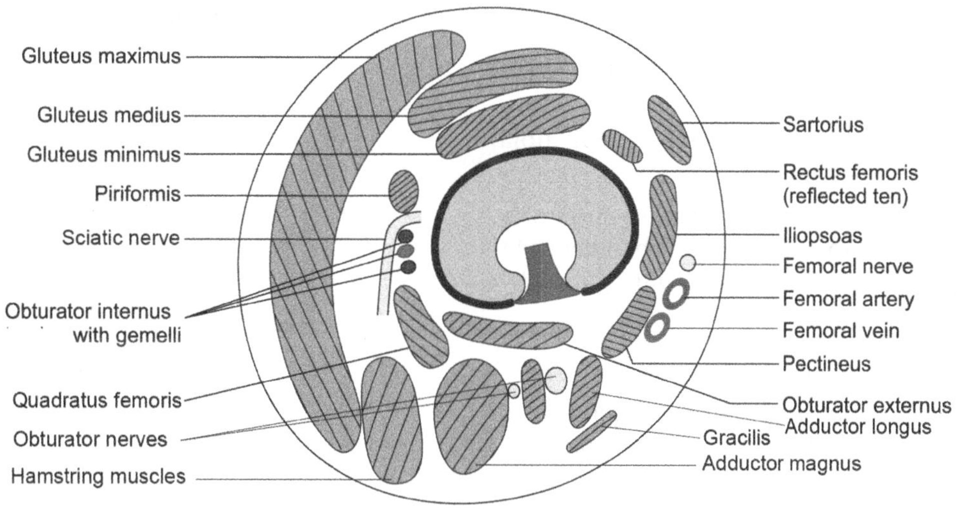

Fig. 57.3: Relations of hip joint

Dislocation of hip joint:

- ***Congenital dislocation:*** Upper margin of acetabulum is developmentally deficient therefore, the head of femur slips into gluteal region. Affected limb is shorter in length, patients has lurching gait with positive Trendelenburg's sign.
- ***Acquired posterior dislocation:*** May occur during automobile accident and is also called dashboard dislocation. It results in shortening and medial rotation of lower limb. Sciatic nerve may get injured.

Fracture of neck of femur: Can damage the blood vessels supplying femoral head resulting in non-union and avascular necrosis of head of femur. Generally the more proximal the fracture, the greater are the chances of interrupting the vascular supply. Usually seen in elderly woman, especially those who suffer from osteoporosis.

2. **Describe knee joint under the following headings:**
   a. **Type**
   b. **Articular surfaces**
   c. **Capsule and ligaments**
   d. **Movements**
   e. **Bursae around the knee joint**
   f. **Blood and nerve supply**

Ans. **Knee joint** is the largest joint. It is compound (more than two bones articulate) and complex (joint cavity is divided into two compartments – menicofemoral and meniscotibial) joint (Fig. 57.4).

a. **Type:** Is a condylar (modified hinge) synovial joint.

b. **Articular surfaces:** Femoral and tibial condyles, patella.

c. **Capsule:** Is thin and incomplete anteriorly. Is attached to femoral and tibial condyles and to the patella and patellar ligament.

Ligaments:

- ***Extracapsular ligaments:***
  - *Ligamentum patellae:* Extends from apex of patella to tibial tuberosity.
  - *Tibial collateral ligament:* Has superficial and deep parts. Both the parts are attached to medial epicondyle of femur above. Superficial part is attached to medial condyle and upper part of medial border of tibia. Deep part blends with fibrous capsule and is attached to medial meniscus.

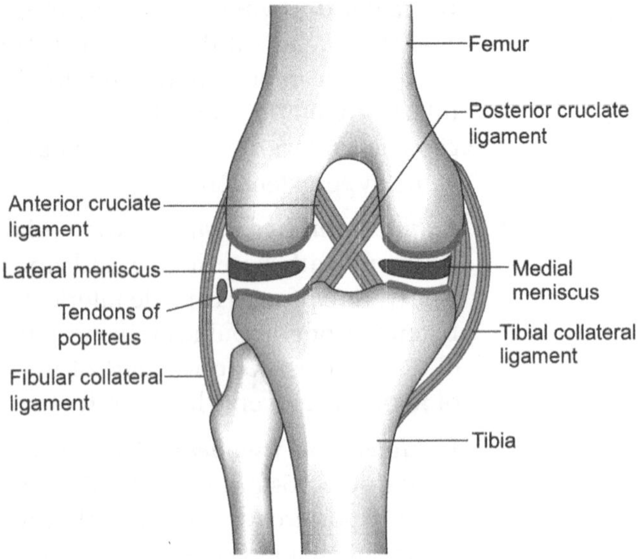

Fig. 57.4: Knee joint

  - *Fibular collateral ligament:* Extends as a fibrous cord from lateral epicondyle of femur to the head of the fibula.
  - *Oblique popliteal ligament:* Extends from medial condyle of tibia to lateral part of intercondylar line of femur.
- ***Intracapsular ligaments:*** Are intracapsular but extrasynovial:
  - *Anterior cruciate ligament:*
    - Is attached below to the anterior part of the intercondylar area of tibia.
    - Passes upward, backward and laterally.
    - Is attached above to the medial surface of the lateral condyle of femur.
    - Is taut during extension and prevents hyperextension of knee joint.
  - *Posterior cruciate ligament:*
    - Is attached below to the posterior part of the intercondylar area of tibia.

- Passes upward, forwards and medially.
- Is attached above to the lateral surface of the medial condyle of femur.
- Is taut during flexion and prevents hyperflexion of knee joint.

– *Medial and lateral menisci:*
  - Act as shock absorber and lubricates the articular surfaces by distributing synovial fluid.
  - Medial meniscus is 'C' shaped and lateral is circular.
  - Medial meniscus is attached to tibial collateral ligament and the lateral is attached to popliteus which separates it from fibular collateral ligament.

Medial meniscus is more prone to injury than lateral as its movement is restricted due to its attachment to tibial collateral ligament whereas medial fibers of popliteus attached to lateral meniscus pull it backwards and prevent it from being trapped between the articular surfaces.

d. **Movements:**

- ***Extension:*** Quadriceps femoris and tensor fascia lata.
- ***Flexion:*** Semimembranosus, semitendinosus, biceps femoris, sartorius, gracilis, popliteus.
- ***Medial rotation:*** Semitendinosus, semimembranosus, sartorius, gracilis, popliteus.
- ***Lateral rotation:*** Biceps femoris.

Locking of knee joint: The lateral femoral condyle is smaller than the medial femoral condyle. As the knee is extended the smaller condyle moves through its arc before the medial condyle which continues to move further posteriorly. This movement results in a medial rotation of the femur. Therefore, at the end of extension there is slight medial rotation, so that all the ligaments are taught and the joint is in close packed position called 'locking of knee joint'.

Contd.

Contd.

Unlocking of knee joint: In the beginning of flexion of knee joint, there is either lateral rotation of femur (foot on the ground) or medial rotation of tibia (foot off the ground) to unlock the knee joint from its tight packed position. This is done by popliteus muscle which is, therefore, also known as key muscle of the knee joint.

e. **Bursae around the knee joint: (Fig. 57.5)**

- ***Suprapatellar bursa:*** Lies deep to the quadriceps femoris and communicates with the knee joint cavity.

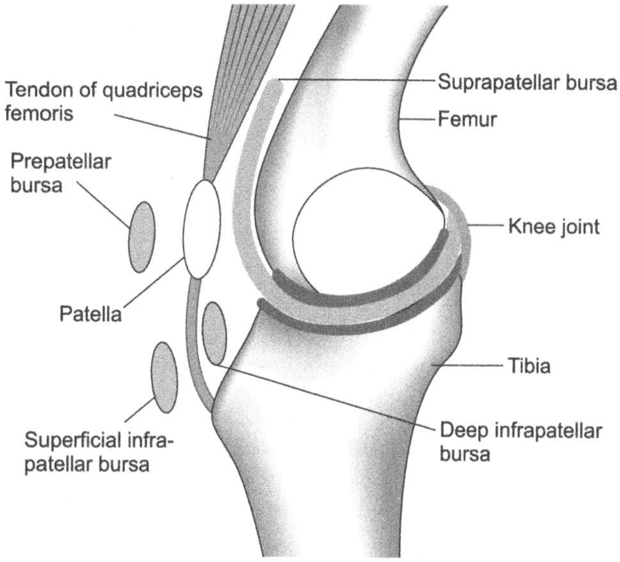

Fig. 57.5: Bursae around knee joint

- ***Subcutaneous prepatellar bursa:*** Lies superficial to lower part of patella and upper half of ligamentum patellae.
- ***Subcutaneous infrapatellar bursa:*** Between the skin and lower half of ligamentum patellae.
- ***Deep infrapatellar bursa:*** Deep to the ligamentum patellae.

Housemaid's knee: Inflammation of subcutaneous prepatellar bursa.

Clergyman's knee: Inflammation of subcutaneous infrapatellar bursa.

f. **Blood and nerve supply:**

- ***Blood supply:*** By anastomosis around the knee joint which is formed by:
  – 5 genicular branches of popliteal artery.

- Descending genicular branch of femoral artery.
- Descending branch of lateral circumflex femoral artery.
- Anterior and posterior recurrent branches of anterior tibial artery.
- Circumflex fibular branch of posterior tibial artery.

• *Nerve supply:* Femoral, obturator, tibial and common peroneal nerve.

> Femoral and obturator nerves supply both hip and knee joints, therefore, pain in one joint is referred to other.

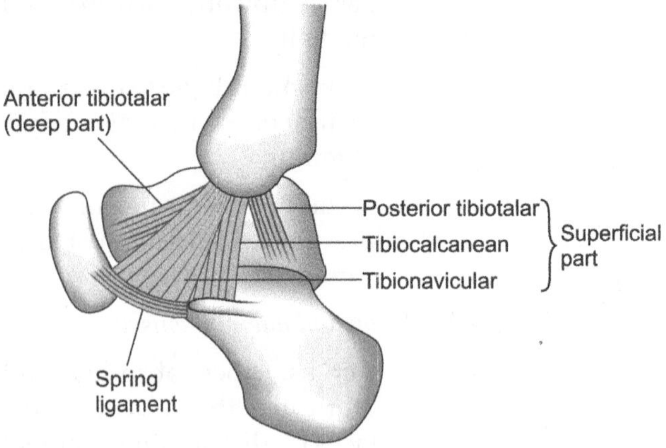

Fig. 57.6b: Ankle joint (Medial ligament – Deltoid ligament)

3. **Describe briefly:**
   a. **Ankle joint**
   b. **Intertarsal joints**

Ans. a. Ankle joint: (Fig. 57.6a)

- *Type:* Hinge synovial joint.
- ***Articular surfaces:*** Distal ends of tibia and fibula superiorly and trochlea of talus inferiorly.
- ***Articular capsule:*** Is thin anteriorly and posteriorly to allow movements. It is reinforced medullary by deltoid ligament and laterally by lateral ligament.
- ***Ligaments:***
  - *Medial (deltoid) ligament: (Fig. 57.6b)*
    - Is strong triangular ligament on the medial side of ankle.
    - Extends from medial malleolus to navicular, talus and calcaneus.
    - Is divided into superficial and deep parts.
    - Superficial part is further subdivided into three parts viz. tibionavicular, tibiocalcanean, posterior tibiotalar.
    - Deep part comprises anterior tibiotalar.
    - Prevents overeversion of foot and helps maintain the medial longitudinal arch.
  - *Lateral ligaments: (Fig. 57.6c)*

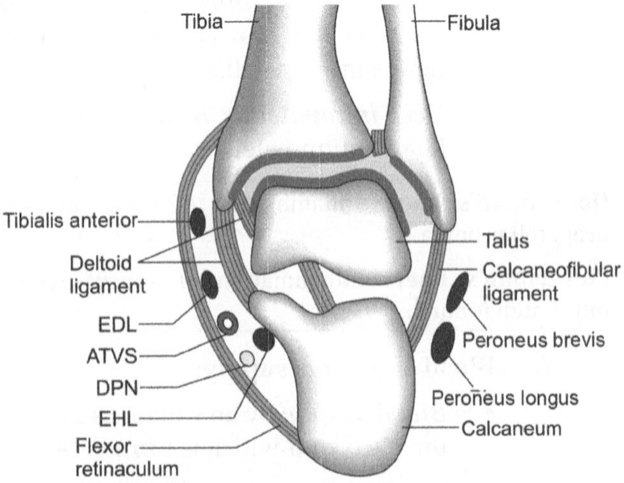

Fig. 57.6a: Ankle joint (Articular surfaces and relations)

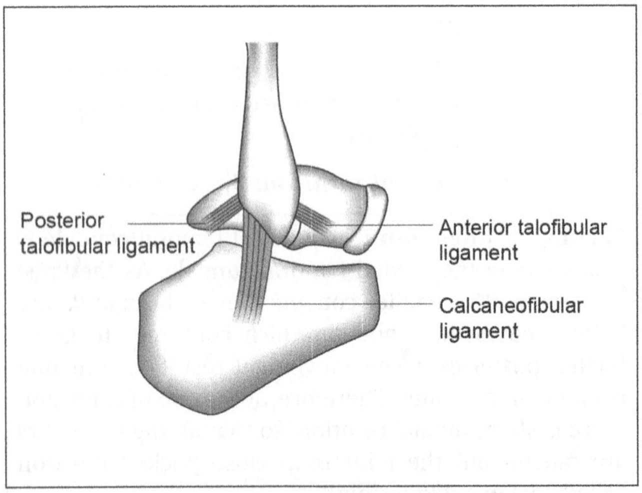

Fig. 57.6c: Ankle joint (Lateral ligaments)

- Extends from lateral malleolus to calcaneum and talus.
- Is divided into 3 parts: Anterior talofibular, posterior talofibular and calcaneofibular.

- ***Movements:***
  - *Dorsiflexion:*
    - The angle between the leg and foot decreases.
    - Is the close-packed position (stable position) of ankle joint.
    - Muscles responsible: Tibialis anterior, extensor hallucis longus, extensor digitorum longus and peroneus tertius.
  - *Plantar flexion:*
    - The angle between the leg and foot increases.
    - Is the loose-packed position (unstable position) of ankle joint.
    - Muscles responsible: Gastrocnemius, soleus, tibialis posterior, flexor hallucis longus, flexor digitorum longus.

> **Ankle sprains:** Occur due to the injury to medial/lateral ligaments due to excessive eversion/inversion respectively.
>
> **Pott's fracture:** Occurs when the foot is everted forcibly when caught in a hole. It may result in:
> - Torn deltoid ligament.
> - Oblique fracture of lower end of fibula.
> - Fracture of medial malleolus.
> - Fracture of l posterior margin of lower end of tibia.

b. **Intertarsal joints:** Are classified as:
- Subtalar joint.
- Talocalcaneonavicular joint.
- Calcaneocuboid joint.
- Transverse talar joint.
- ***Subtalar joint: (Fig. 57.7)***
  - *Type:* Plane synovial joint.
  - *Articular surfaces:* Inferior surface of talus and superior surface of calcaneum.
  - *Ligaments:* Lateral and medial talocalcanean, interosseous talocalcanean, cervical.
- ***Talocalcaneonavicular joint: (Fig. 57.7)***
  - *Type:* Ball and socket type of synovial joint.
  - *Articular surfaces:* Head of talus fits into socket formed by calcaneum, navicular and spring ligament.
  - *Ligaments:* Plantar calcaneonavicular ligament (spring ligament), calcaneonavicular part of bifurcate ligament.

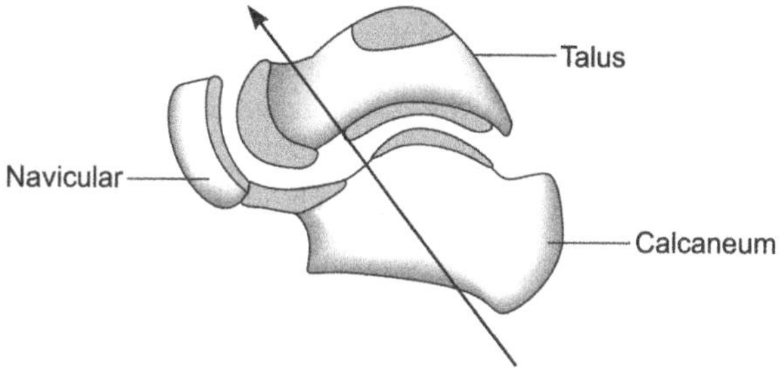

Fig. 57.7: Subtalar and talocalcaneonavicular joint (arrow indicates the axis along which inversion and eversion takes place)

- ***Calcaneocuboid joint: (Fig. 57.8)***
  - *Type:* Saddle type of synovial joint.

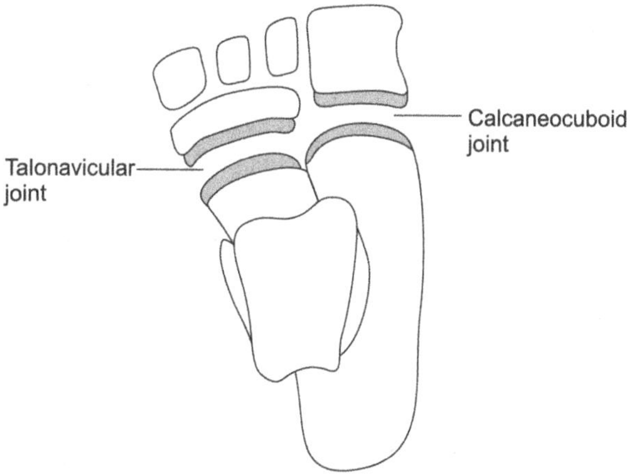

Fig. 57.8: Transverse tarsal joint (calcaneocuboid and talonavicular joints)

- *Articular surfaces:* Reciprocally concavoconvex surfaces of calcaneum and cuboid.
- *Ligaments:* Calcaneocuboid part of bifurcate ligament, long and short plantar ligaments.

• ***Transverse talar joint: (Fig. 57.8)***
  - Collective term used for talonavicular part of talocalcaneonavicular joint and calcaneocuboid joint.

• ***Movements occurring at intertarsal joints:***
  - *Inversion:*
    - Medial border of foot is raised so that sole faces medially.
    - Muscles responsible: Tibialis anterior, tibialis posterior, flexor hallucis longus and flexor digitorum longus.
  - *Eversion:*
    - Lateral border of foot is raised so that sole faces laterally.
    - Muscles responsible: Peroneus longus, peroneus brevis and peroneus tertius.
  - *Axis of movement:* Passes obliquely from the back of calcaneum through the sinus tarsi to the neck of the talus.

4. Classify the joint of lower limb.

Ans. See the following Table:

Joint	*Type*
Hip joint	Ball and socket type of synovial joint
Knee joint	Modified hinge type of synovial joint
Superior tibiofibular Intermediate tibiofibular Inferior tibiofibular	Plane type of synovial joint Syndesmosis Syndesmosis
Ankle joint	Hinge type of synovial joint
Intertarsal joints: Subtalar Talocalcaneonavicular Calcaneocuboid	 Plane type of synovial joint Ball and socket type of synovial joint Saddle type of synovial joint
Tarsometatarsal joints	Plane type of synovial joint
Metatarsophalangeal joints	Ellipsoid type of synovial joint
Interphalangeal joints	Hinge type of synovial joint

58 CHAPTER HEAD AND NECK – SCALP

1. Define scalp and write its extent.

Ans. a. Definition: Scalp is the soft tissue that covers the vault of the skull.

b. Extent:

- ***Anteriorly:*** Supraorbital margin.
- ***Laterally:*** Superior temporal lines.
- ***Posteriorly:*** External occipital protuberance and superior nuchal lines.

2. Enumerate:

a. Layers of scalp

b. Arteries supplying scalp

c. Sensory nerves of scalp

Ans. a. Layers of scalp: The scalp consists of five layers. Superficial three layers are intimately bound together and move as one unit. The five layers from superficial to deep are:

- S – Skin.
- C – Connective tissue (superficial fascia).
- A – Aponeurosis (epicranial aponeurosis).
- L – Loose areolar tissue.
- P – Pericranium.

> **Dangerous layer of scalp:** Subaponeurotic loose areolar connective tissue layer is known as dangerous layer of scalp because the blood and pus tend to collect in this layer and the infection from this layer may travel readily along the emissary veins into the intracranial venous sinuses.

b. Arteries supplying scalp: Scalp has a rich blood supply from branches of internal and external carotid arteries. There is anastomosis between the branches of internal and external carotid arteries. There are five arteries on each side, three in front of the auricle and two behind the auricle. The arteries are:

- ***In front of the auricle:***
  - Supratrochlear, Supraorbital } Branches of internal carotid artery
  - Superficial temporal – branch of external carotid artery.
- ***Behind the auricle:***
  - Posterior auricular, Occipital } Branches of external carotid artery

> - Scalp wounds bleed profusely but heal quickly due to rich blood supply of scalp.
> - Scalp wounds bleed profusely also due to the following reason:
>
>   The main arteries and veins supplying scalp lie in the dense connective tissue deep to the skin. The walls of the blood vessels are adherent to the fibrous network, therefore when the blood vessels are torn they are unable to retract, resulting in profuse bleeding.

c. Sensory nerves of scalp:

In front of the auricle	*Behind the auricle*
Supratrochlear (from ophthalmic division of trigeminal nerve)	Great auricular (from ventral rami of C2, C3 spinal nerves)
Supraorbital (from ophthalmic division of trigeminal nerve)	Lesser occipital (from ventral ramus of C2 spinal nerve)
Zygomaticotemporal (from maxillary division of trigeminal nerve)	Greater occipital (from dorsal ramus of C2 spinal nerve)
Auriculotemporal (from mandibular division of trigeminal nerve)	Third occipital (from dorsal ramus of C3 spinal nerve)

3. **Draw labeled diagram of the following:**
   a. **Layers of scalp**
   b. **Arterial supply of scalp**
   c. **Nerve supply of scalp**

Ans.

a. **Layers of scalp (Fig. 58.1).**
b. **Arterial supply of scalp (Fig. 58.2).**
c. **Nerve supply of scalp (Fig. 58.3).**

4. **Describe occipitofrontalis muscle under the following headings:**
   a. **Origin and insertion**
   b. **Nerve supply**
   c. **Action**

Ans. Occipitofrontalis muscle: It consists of a pair of occipital bellies (posteriorly) and a pair of frontal bellies (anteriorly). Both the parts are inserted into the intervening galea aponeurotica or epicranial aponeurosis (See Table on the next page).

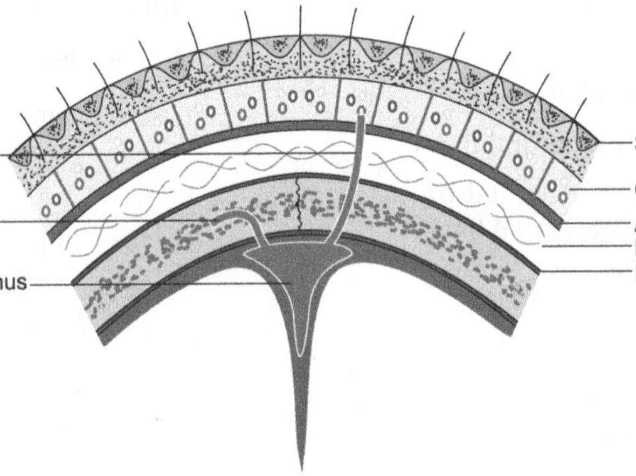

Fig. 58.1: Layers of scalp

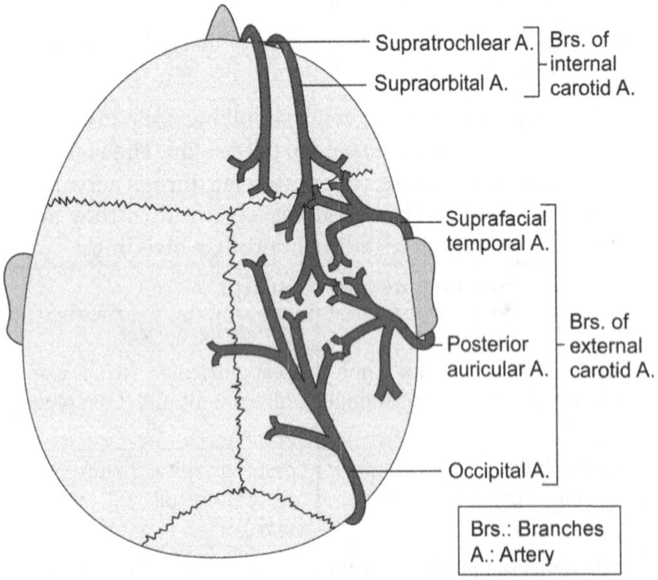

Fig. 58.2: Arterial supply of scalp

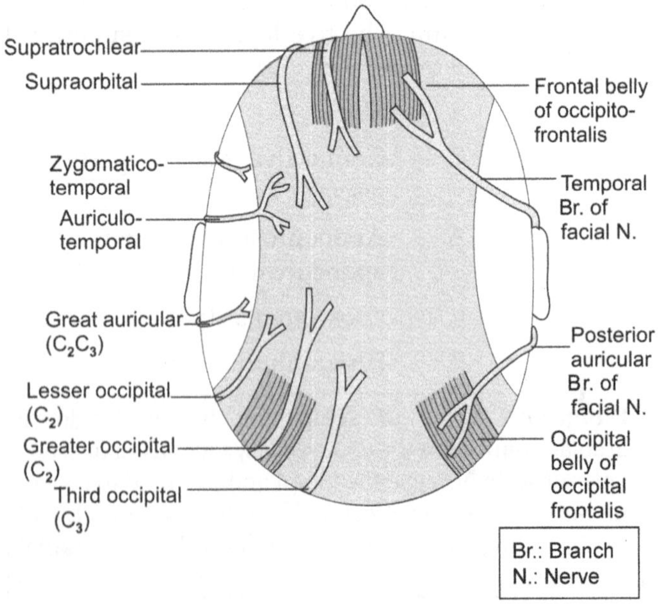

Fig. 58.3: Nerve supply of scalp

	Origin	*Insertion*	*Nerve supply*	*Action*
Occipital bellies	Lateral 2/3rd of superior nuchal lines of occipital bone	Into epicranial aponeurosis	Posterior auricular branch of facial nerve	Alternate contraction of occipitalis and frontalis move the scalp backward and forward
Frontal bellies	Skin and subcutaneous tissue over the eyebrows and root of nose	Into epicranial aponeurosis	Temporal branch of facial nerve	Frontal bellies raise the eyebrows as in surprise

5. **Give anatomical basis of:**
   a. **Deep wounds of scalp tend to gape**
   b. **A blow on head may lead to 'Black eye'**

Ans. a. **Deep wounds of scalp tend to gape:** Epicranial aponeurosis is under tension from the tone of occipitofrontalis muscle and therefore if aponeurosis is cut, the wound tend to gape.

b. **A blow on head may lead to collection of blood in the 4th layer (loose areolar tissue) of scalp:** The blood from this layer may gravitate into the eyelids resulting in 'black eye' because the frontalis muscle has no bony attachment. The blood cannot pass laterally or anteriorly due to the attachment of epicranial aponeurosis and occipitalis muscle to the superficial temporal lines and superior nuchal lines respectively.

CHAPTER 59 FACE

1. **What is the extent of face?**

Ans. Extent of face:

- *Superiorly:* Hairline.
- *Inferiorly:* Chin and base of the mandible.
- *Laterally:* Auricle.

2. **What are the characteristic features of skin of face?**

Ans. Characteristic features of skin of face:

- Is highly vascular and elastic.
- Contains large number of sweat and sebaceous glands (is common site for acne).
- Is lax except on nose where it is attached to the underlying cartilages (laxity of the skin facilitates rapid spread of edema).
- Provides insertion to the muscles of facial expression.

Deep fascia is absent in face except over the parotid gland and masseter muscle (parotidomasseteric).

3. **Enumerate the muscles of face (facial expression) and write their action.**

Ans. Muscles of facial expression are arranged around three orifices palpebral fissure, nostrils and mouth.

	Muscle		*Expression*
Muscle around palpebral fissure	Orbicularis oculi	Orbital part	Closes eyelids tightly (winking, protection from light)
		Palpebral part	Closes eyelids gently (blinking or sleep)
		Lacrimal part	Dilates lacrimal sac and helps and aids in drainage of lacrimal fluid
	Corrugator supercilii		Produce vertical lines in the forehead
	Levator palpebrae superioris		Elevate the upper eyelid
Muscles around nose	Procerus		Produces transverse wrinkles over the bridge of the nose
	Compressor naris		Compresses the nasal aperture
	Dilator naris		Draws the ala downwards and laterally, thus assists in widening the nasal aperture
	Depressor septi		Widens the nasal aperture
Muscles around mouth	Muscles attached to upper lip	Labial part of levator labii superioris	Elevates upper lip
		Levator labii superioris	Elevates and everts upper lip
		Zygomaticus minor	Elevates upper lip
	Muscles converging at angle of mouth	Levator anguli oris	Raises the angle of mouth
		Zygomaticus major	Pulls the angle of mouth upwards and laterally
		Depressor anguli oris	Draws the angle of mouth downwards and laterally
		Risorius	Pulls the angle of mouth laterally

Contd.

Contd.

	Muscle attached to lower lip	Depressor labii inferioris	Draws the lower lip downwards
		Platysma	Draws down the lower lip and angle of mouth
		Mentalis	Protrudes or everts the lower lip (although it is not attached to lower lip)
	Orbicularis oris		Closes the mouth

4. Name the muscles responsible for various facial expressions.

Ans. See the following Table.

Facial expression	*Muscle*
Frowning	Corrugator supercilii and procerus
Surprise	Frontalis
Laughing	Zygomaticus major
Grinning	Risorius
Grief	Depressor anguli oris
Anger	Dilator naris and depressor septi
Doubt	Mentalis

> Muscles of facial expression are derived from the 2nd pharyngeal arc and are therefore supplied by facial nerve.

5. Write short notes on:

a. **Buccinator**

b. **Facial artery**

c. **Bell's palsy**

Ans. a. Buccinator: It is quadrilateral shaped muscle of cheek occupying the interval between maxilla and mandible.

- ***Structures piercing buccinators muscle:***
  - Parotid duct.
  - Buccal branch of mandibular nerve.
- ***Paralysis of buccinators muscle:*** Paralysis of buccinators muscle (in facial palsy – injury to facial nerve), food tens to accumulate in the vestibule of mouth (Fig. 59.1).

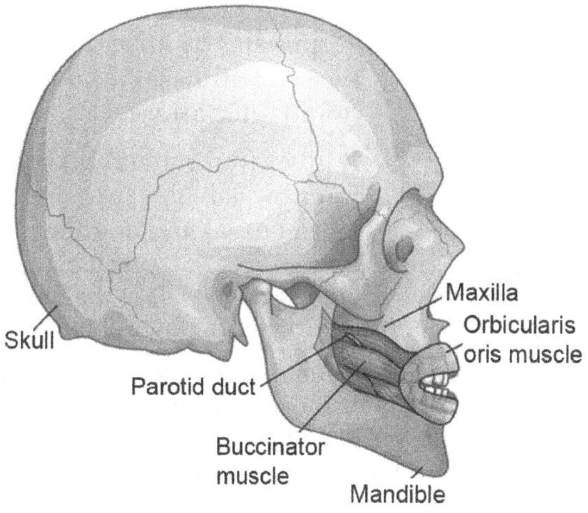

Fig. 59.1: Buccinators muscle

b. Facial artery:

- Is the anterior branch of external carotid artery.
- It arises in the carotid triangle.
- Its course is divided into two parts – Cervical and facial.

	Origin	*Insertion*	*Action*	*Nerve supply*
Buccinator	Upper fibers–Outer surface of maxilla opposite molar teeth	Upper lip	Compresses the cheek against teeth and gums	Buccal branch of facial nerve
	Middle fibers–Pterygomandibular raphe	Fibers decussate at angle of mouth and upper fibers pass to lower lip, lower fibers to upper lip	This preventing accumulation of food in the vestibule of mouth	
	Lower fibers – Outer surface of mandible opposite molar teeth	Lower lip	Helps in whistling, blowing	

- *Cervical part:*
  - Is intimately related to submandibular gland.
  - Gives four branches – Ascending palatine, tonsillar, glandular and submental.
- *Facial part:*
  - Enters face by crossing base of mandible at the anteroinferior angle of the masseter.
  - It then runs upwards and forwards towards angle of mouth (1.25 cm lateral to angle of mouth).
  - Then ascends by the side of the nose up to the medial angle of the eye.
  - Terminates by anastomosing with the dorsal nasal branch of the ophthalmic artery.
  - It gives four named branches viz. inferior labial, superior labial, lateral nasal and angular.

> - Facial artery pulsations can be felt at the base of the mandible at the anteroinferior angle of masseter.
> - Facial artery is tortuous throughout its course. The cervical part is tortuous to adapt to the movement of pharynx during deglutition and facial part is tortuous to adapt to the movements of mandible, lips and cheek.

c. **Bell's palsy:** A lesion of facial nerve usually at stylomastoid foramen results in ipsilateral paralysis of facial muscles. The symptoms include:

- Asymmetrical face.
- Loss of horizontal wrinkles on forehead.
- Inability to close eye.
- Loss of corneal reflex.
- Absence of nasolabial fold.
- Inability to show teeth.
- Drooling of saliva from corner of mouth.
- When the person tries to smile the angle of mouth of the normal side moves upwards and laterally.

6. **Draw labeled diagram of the following:**
   a. **Sensory innervations of face**
   b. **Muscles of face and their nerve supply**
   c. **Arteries supplying face**
   d. **Veins draining face**
   e. **Lymphatic drainage of face**
   f. **Components of lacrimal apparatus**

Ans. a. **Sensory innervations of face (Fig. 59.2):** Skin of face is supplied by the three subdivisions of trigeminal nerve. A small part over the angle of mandible is supplied by great auricular nerve (Ventral rami of C2,C3).

- *Branches of ophthalmic nerve:* Supply skin of forehead, upper eyelid, dorsum of nose including tip and scalp as far as vertex.

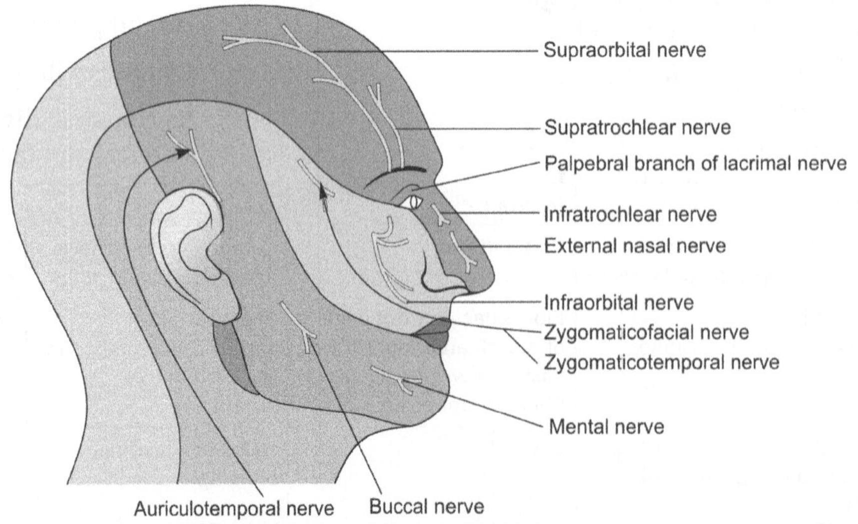

Fig. 59.2: Sensory innervations of face

- Supratrochlear.
- Supraorbital.
- Infratrochlear.
- Palpebral branch of lacrimal.
- External nasal.

• ***Branches of maxillary nerve:*** Supply lower eyelid, side of nose upper lip and upper part of cheek and anterior part of temporal region.

- Infraorbital.
- Zygomaticofacial.
- Zygomaticotemporal.

• ***Branches of mandibular nerve:*** Supply lower lip lower part of cheek and posterior part of temporal region.

- Mental.
- Buccal.
- Auriculotemporal.

b. Muscles of face and their nerve supply (Fig. 59.3).

c. Arteries supplying face (Fig. 59.4).

d. Veins draining face (Fig. 59.5).

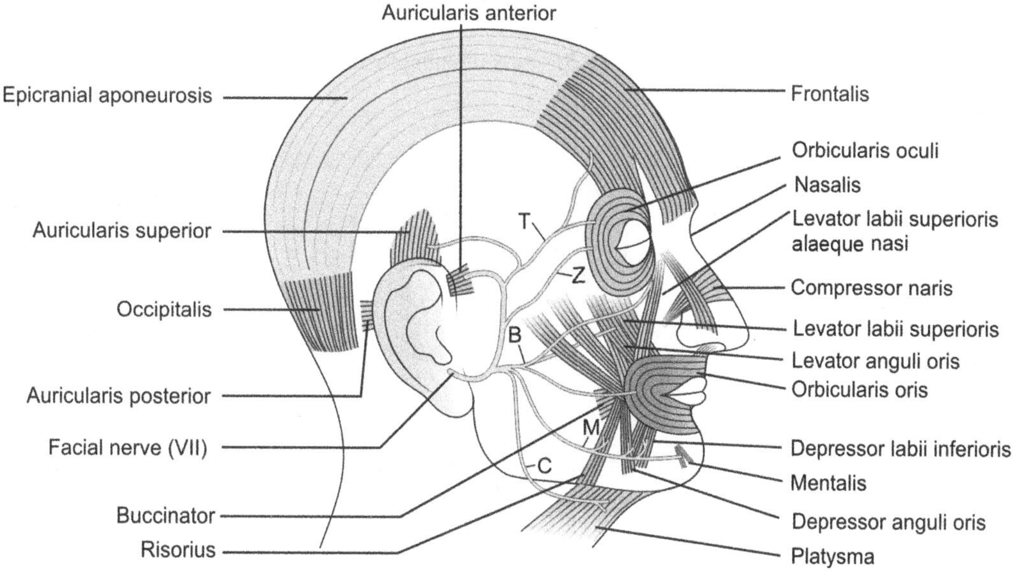

Branches of facial nerve: T-Temporal, Z-Zygomatic, B-Buccal, M-Marginal mandibular, C-Cervical

Fig. 59.3: Muscles of face and their nerve supply

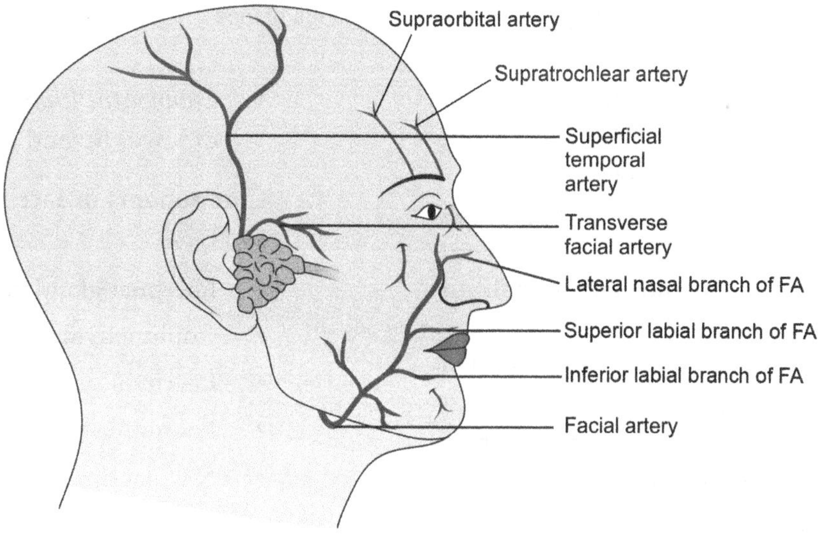

Fig. 59.4: Arteries supplying face

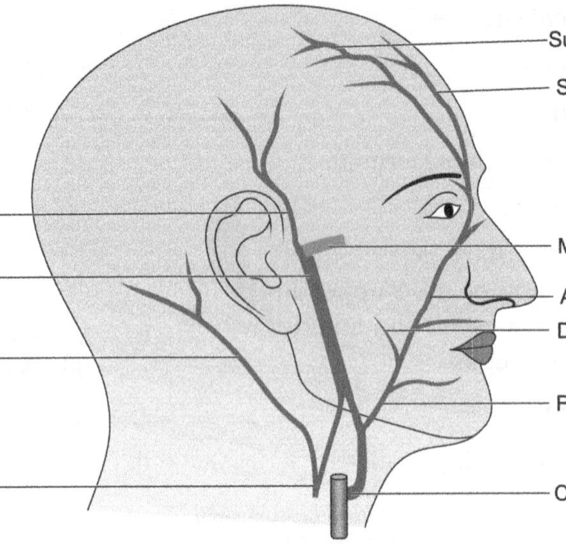

Fig. 59.5: Veins draining face

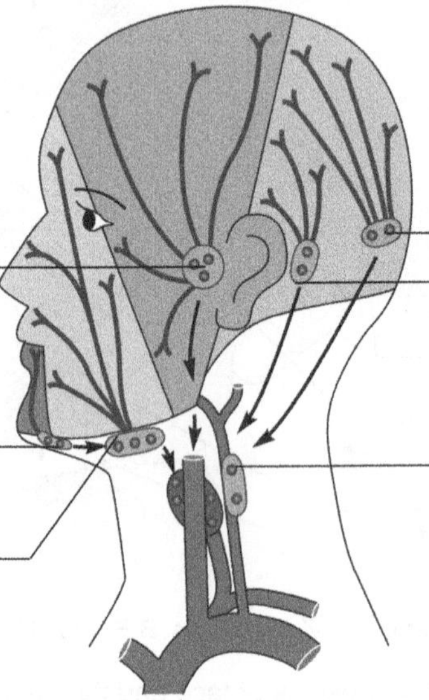

Fig. 59.6: Lymphatic drainage of face

e. **Lymphatic drainage of face (Fig. 59.6):** Lymphatics from face drain into following three groups of lymph nodes:
   - ***Preauricular/superficial parotid lymph nodes:*** Lateral part of forehead, lateral half of eyelids and lateral half of cheek.
   - ***Submandibular lymph nodes:*** Medial part of forehead, medial half of eyelids, nose, upper lip, lateral part of lower lip and medial part of cheek.
   - ***Submental lymph nodes:*** Central part of lower lip and chin.

f. **Components of lacrimal apparatus: (Fig. 59.7)**
   - Lacrimal gland and ducts.
   - Conjunctival sac.
   - Lacrimal puncta and canaliculi.
   - Lacrimal sac.
   - Nasolacrimal duct.

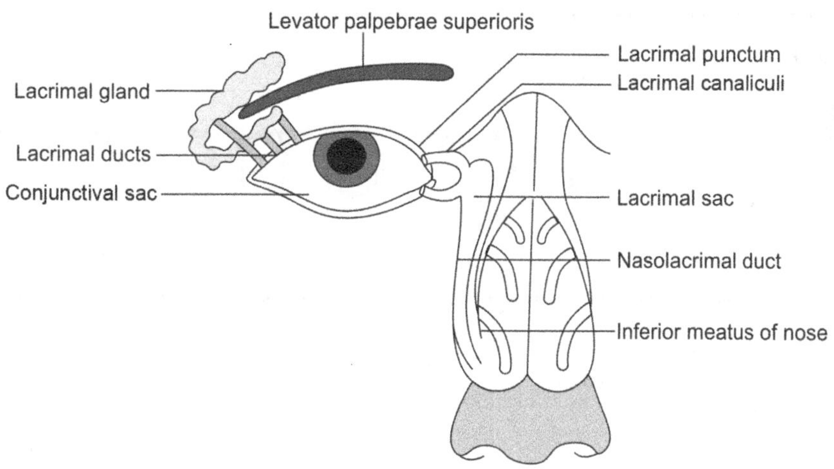

Fig. 59.7: Components of lacrimal apparatus

7. **Give anatomical basis of dangerous area of face.**

Ans. The dangerous area of face includes the upper lip, lower part of nose and adjoining cheek. The infection from a boil on the dangerous area of face may spread from facial vein to cavernous sinus along the following route:

Facial vein → Deep facial vein → Pterygoid plexuses of veins → emissary veins → cavernous sinus.

* Facial vein and its communicating veins do not possess valves, therefore blood can flow in both directions.

8. **Trace secretomotor fibers of lacrimal gland.**

Ans. Secretomotor fibers to lacrimal gland:

Preganglionic fibers originate in lacrimatory nucleus in pons

↓

Pass in nervus intermedius of facial nerve

↓

Pass in greater petrosal nerve → nerve of pterygoid canal

↓

Relay in pterygopalatine ganglion

↓

Postganglionic fibers are carried in zygomatic branch of maxillary nerve and then in zygomaticotemporal nerve

↓

Finally the postganglionic secretomotor fibers join lacrimal nerve to reach lacrimal gland

60 CHAPTER PAROTID GLAND

1. What is the extent of parotid region?

Ans. Parotid Region: Boundaries:

- ***Anteriorly:*** Posterior border of ramus of mandible with masseter and medial pterygoid attached to it.
- ***Posteriorly:*** Mastoid process and sternocleidomastoid muscle.
- ***Superiorly:*** External acoustic meatus and posterior part of temporomandibular joint.
- ***Inferiorly:*** Extends slightly below the posterior belly of digastric and stylohyoid muscle (into carotid triangle).
- ***Medially:*** Styloid process and muscles attached to it.

2. Describe parotid gland under the following headings:

a. External features and relations of parotid gland

b. Capsules of parotid gland

Ans. a. External features and relations of parotid gland:

- Is the largest of the salivary glands.
- Is purely serous in nature.
- Is irregular in shape (roughly 3 sided inverted pyramidal) and weighs approx. 25 gm. It has:
  - ***An apex:***
    - Directed below.
    - Overlaps posterior belly of digastric muscle and reaches carotid triangle.
    - Structures emerging through apex are:
      - Cervical branch of facial nerve.
      - Anterior and posterior divisions of retromandibular vein.
  - ***Base:***
    - Is concave and directed upwards.
    - Is related to external acoustic meatus and posterior part of temporomandibular joint.
    - Structures emerging through base are (anterior to posterior):
      - Temporal branch of facial nerve.
      - Superficial temporal vessels.
      - Auriculotemporal nerve.

Three surfaces–superficial, anteromedial and posteromedial.

- *Superficial (lateral) surface:* Is covered from superficial to deep by:
  - Skin.
  - Superficial fascia containing:
    - Anterior branch of great auricular nerve.
    - Pre auricular (superficial parotid) lymph nodes.
    - Platysma muscle fibers.
  - Superficial lamella of parotid fascia.
  - Deep parotid lymph nodes.
- *Anteromedial surface:*
  - Is grooved by posterior border of ramus of mandible.
  - Masseter.
  - Medial pterygoid.
  - Lateral surface of temporomandibular joint.

- Terminal branches of facial nerve.
- *Posteromedial surface:*
  - Mastoid process.
  - Sternocleidomastoid muscle.
  - Posterior belly of digastric muscle.
  - Styloid process and muscles attached to it.
  - Facial nerve enters the gland through this surface.
  - External carotid artery is lodged in a groove in its lower part.

> Styloid process separates the gland from internal carotid artery, internal jugular vein and last four (IX, X, XI and XII) cranial nerves.

Three borders – anterior, posterior and medial.

- *Anterior border:* Structures emerging along the border (from above downwards are):
  - Zygomatic branch of facial nerve.
  - Transverse facial artery.
  - Upper buccal branch of facial nerve.
  - Parotid duct.
  - Lower buccal branch of facial nerve.
  - Marginal mandibular branch of facial nerve.
- *Posterior border:* Structures emerging along the border are:
  - Posterior auricular branch of facial nerve.
  - Posterior auricular vessels.
- *Medial border:* Is related to the lateral wall of pharynx.

b. **Capsules of parotid gland:** Parotid gland is surrounded by two capsules:

- ***True capsule:*** Form by condensation of the fibrous stroma of the gland.
- ***False capsule (parotid fascia):***
  - Is formed by splitting of investing layer of deep cervical fascia.
  - Its superficial lamina passés superficial to the gland, is thick and attached to inferior border of zygomatic arch.
  - Its deep lamina passes deep to the gland, is thin and is attached to styloid process and tympanic plate. It also forms stylomandibular ligament (from tip of styloid process to angle of mandible) which separates parotid gland from submandibular gland.

> Inflammatory parotid swelling are very painful due to unyielding nature of parotid fascia.

3. **Draw labeled diagram of the following:**
   a. **Structures emerging from the periphery of the parotid gland**
   b. **Transverse section through the parotid gland showing its relations**

Ans. a. **Structures emerging from the periphery of the parotid gland (Fig. 60.1).**

b. **Transverse section through the parotid gland showing its relations (Fig. 60.2).**

4. **Name the structures passing through the parotid gland.**

Ans. Structures passing through the parotid gland from superficial to deep are:

a. Facial nerve.
b. Retromandibular vein.
c. External carotid artery.

a. **Facial nerve:** Enters the gland through posterior medial surface and divides into five terminal (temporal, zygomatic, buccal, marginal mandibular and cervical) branches. The terminal branches leave the gland through the anteromedial surface and emerge along its anterior border.

> - The parotid gland is divided into a superficial and deep parts which are connected by isthmus. Branches of facial nerve pass forward through the isthmus (the plane between the superficial and deep part), this plane helps surgeons to remove parotid tumor without damaging the nerve.
> - Parotid abscess is drained by horizontal incision (parallel to the branches of facial nerve) in the parotid fascia to avoid injury to the branches of facial nerve.

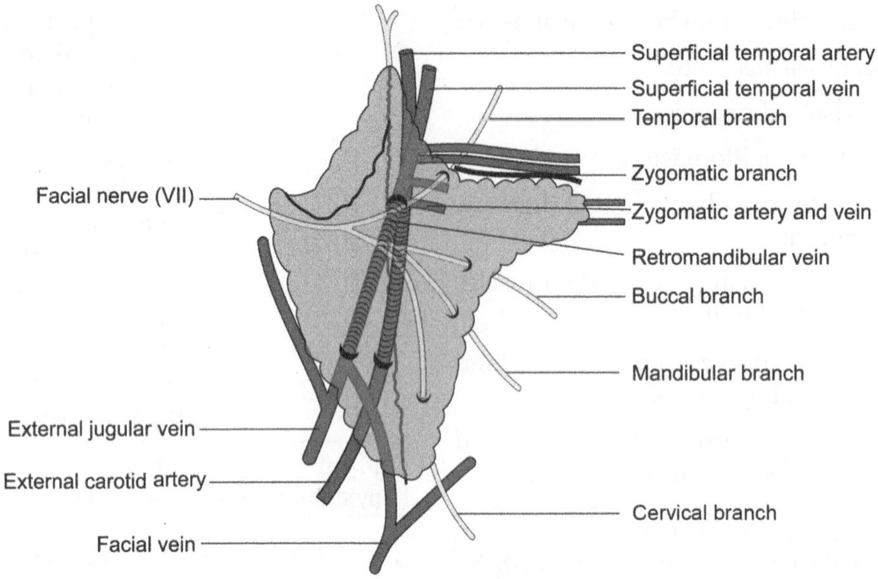

Fig. 60.1: Structures emerging from the periphery of the parotid gland

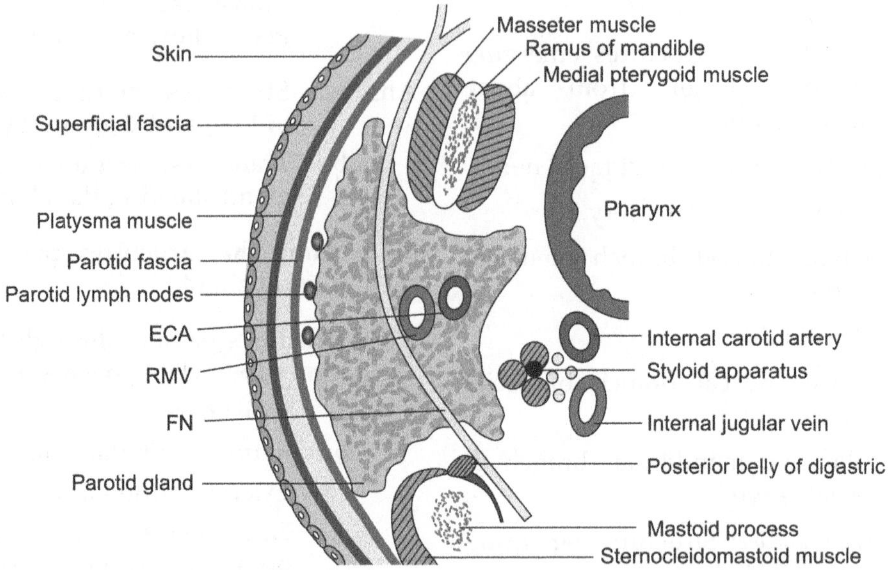

Fig. 60.2: Transverse section through the parotid gland showing its relations

b. **Retromandibular vein:**

- Is formed within the gland by union of superficial temporal and maxillary veins.
- It is divided into anterior and posterior divisions in the lower part of the gland.
- Anterior division joins facial vein to form the common facial vein.
- Posterior division joins posterior auricular vein to form external jugular vein.

c. **External carotid artery:**

- Enters the gland through the postero-medial surface.
- Divides into terminal branches – maxillary and superficial temporal.

5. **Describe briefly:**

a. **Formation, course and opening of parotid duct**

b. **Nerve supply of parotid gland**

Ans. a. **Parotid duct (Stensen's duct):**

- Is thick walled, 5 cm long and 3 mm wide.
- Is formed within the gland by joining of smaller ducts, emerges from the gland at the middle of its anterior border on the surface of masseter (a finger breadth below the zygomatic arch).
- Runs forward and slightly downwards on the masseter.
- At the anterior border of masseter turns medially and pierces:
  - Buccal pad of fat.
  - Buccopharyngeal fascia.
  - Buccinators muscle.
  - Buccal mucosa.
- It runs obliquely between the buccinators and oral mucosa (for 1 cm) before piercing the mucosa to open into the vestibule of mouth opposite to the crown of 2nd upper molar tooth.

b. Nerve supply of parotid gland (Fig. 60.3):

Parotid gland is supplied by:

- Parasympathetic fibers – secretomotor.

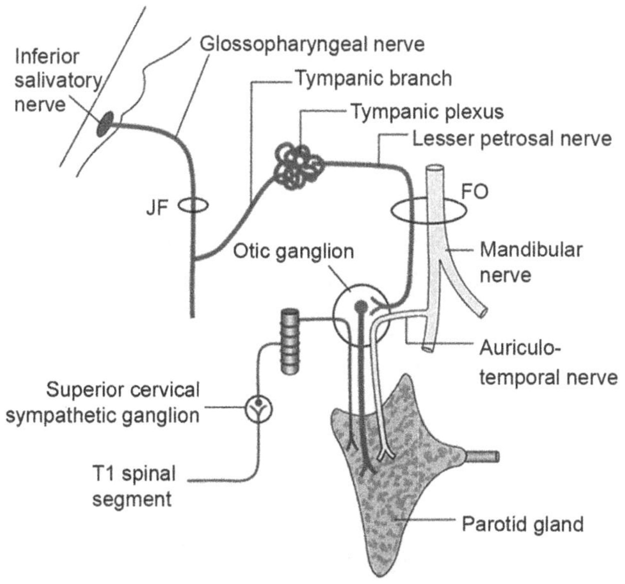

Fig. 60.3: Nerve supply of parotid gland

- Sympathetic fibers – mainly vasomotor.
- Sensory fibers.
- ***Parasympathetic fibers (secretomotor fibers):*** Stimulation of parasympathetic innervations produces watery secretion (rich in enzymes).

Preganglionic fibers arise from inferior salivatory nucleus (in medulla oblongata)

↓

Glossopharyngeal nerve (leaves through jugular foramen)

↓

Tympanic branch of glossopharyngeal nerve

↓

Tympanic plexus (in middle ear cavity)

↓

Lesser petrosal nerve (leaves through foramen ovale)

[Glossopharyngeal nerve to lesser petrosal nerve: Preganglionic fibers pass through]

↓

Synapse in otic ganglion

↓

Postganglionic fibers pass through auriculotemoral branch of mandibular nerve

↓

Supply parotid gland

- ***Sympathetic fibers:*** Mainly vasomotor, and their stimulation also produces thick sticky secretion.

Preganglionic fibers arise from lateral horn of T1 spinal segment

↓

Synapse in superior cervical ganglion

↓

Postganglionic fibers form plexus around external carotid artery to reach parotid gland

- ***Sensory fibers:*** Carry general sensations. Is derived from auriculotemporal nerve.

> **Frey's Syndrome:** Penetrating wounds of parotid gland may damage the auriculotemporal and great auricular nerves. During the process of regeneration, secretomotor fibers of auriculotemporal nerve may join the great auricular nerve and supply the sweat glands of the skin covering parotid gland. Therefore, when the person eats food, beads of perspiration appear on the skin over parotid gland because the stimulus intended for salivation produces sweat instead.

61 CHAPTER NECK – SUPERFICIAL AND DEEP CERVICAL FASCIA

1. **Enumerate:**
   a. **Structures present in the midline of neck**
   b. **Structures present in the superficial fascia of side of neck**
   c. **Compartments of neck**
   d. **Layers of deep cervical fascia**

Ans. a. **Structures present in the midline of neck:**

- *Fibrous raphe:* Extending from symphysis menti to hyoid bone (mylohyoid muscles insert).
- Hyoid bone.
- Thyrohyoid membrane.
- Laryngeal prominence (angle of thyroid cartilage).
- Median cricothyroid ligament.
- Cricoids cartilage.
- Cervical part of trachea.
- Isthmus of thyroid gland (opposite 2nd–4th tracheal cartilages).
- Levator glandulae thyroideae (remnant of tyroglossal duct).
- Anastomosis between anterior branches of superior thyroid arteries.
- Inferior thyroid veins.
- Thyroid artery anastomosis.
- Remains of thymus.
- Jugular venous arch.

Knowledge of anatomy of midline structures of neck is essential to perform tracheostomy (to make an opening in trachea), a life saving surgical procedure which is done in case of upper respiratory tract obstruction.

Contd.

Contd.

It is most commonly done at the level of 2nd to 4th tracheal rings behind the isthmus of thyroid gland. Isthmus of thyroid gland is retracted upwards.

b. **Structures present in the superficial fascia of side of neck:**

- *Muscle:* Platysma.
- *Cutaneous nerves of the neck:* Branches of cervical plexus:
  - Lesser occipital nerve (C2).
  - Greater auricular nerve (C2,C3).
  - Transverse nerves of neck (C2, C3).
  - Supraclavicular nerves (C3, C4).
- *Motor nerve:* Cervical branch of facial nerve.
- *Superficial vein:*
  - Anterior jugular vein.
  - External jugular vein.
- *Superficial cervical lymph nodes.*

c. **Compartments of neck: (Fig. 61.1)**

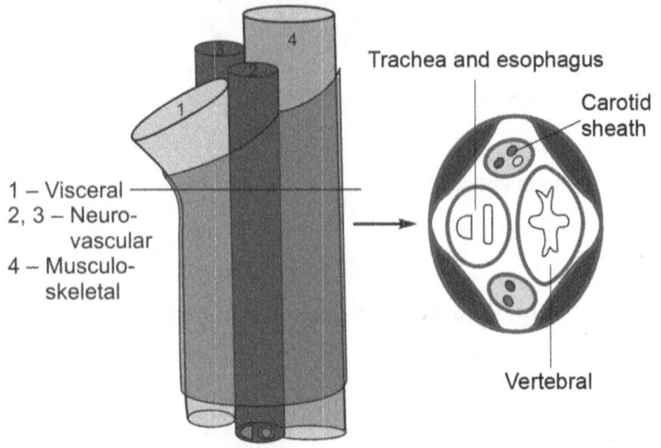

Fig. 61.1: Compartments of neck

- One vertebral – posteriorly.
- Two neurovascular – laterally.
- One visceral – anteriorly.

d. **Layers of deep cervical fascia:**
- Investing layer.
- Pretracheal layer.
- Prevertebral layer.
- Carotid sheath.

2. **Draw labeled diagram showing horizontal and vertical disposition of deep cervical fascia.**

Ans. a. **Horizontal disposition of deep cervical fascia (Fig. 61.2).**

b. **Vertical disposition of deep cervical fascia (Fig. 61.3).**

3. **Describe external jugular vein under the following headings:**
   a. **Formation**
   b. **Course and termination**
   c. **Tributaries**
   d. **Applied anatomy**

Ans. External jugular vein drains blood from the greater part of face and scalp.

a. **Formation:** Begins below the angle of mandible by union of posterior division of retromandibular vein and posterior auricular vein.

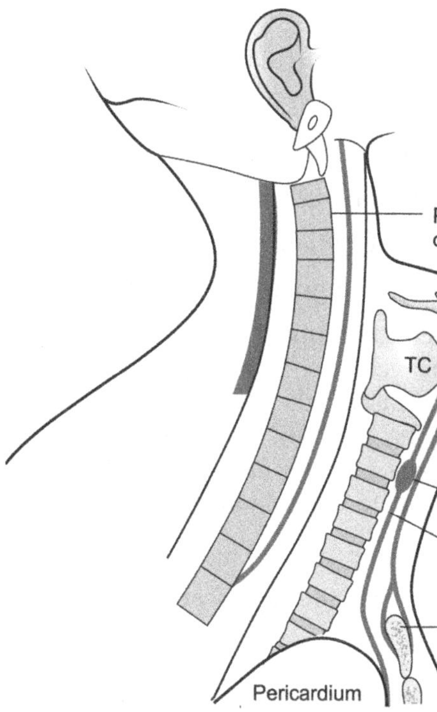

Fig. 61.3: Vertical disposition of deep cervical fascia

b. **Course and termination:** It runs vertically downwards across the sternocleidomastoid muscle and deep to platysma. It pierces the investing layer of deep cervical fascia about 2.5 cm above the clavicle and terminates in subclavian vein.

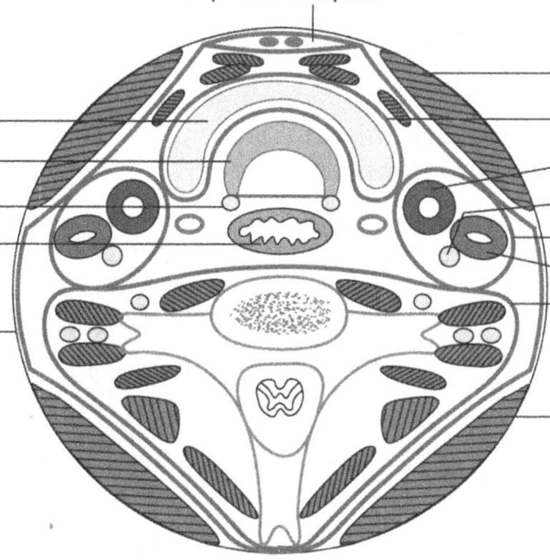

Fig. 61.2: Horizontal disposition of deep cervical fascia

c. **Tributaries:**
   - Posterior auricular.
   - Posterior division of retromandibular.
   - Posterior external jugular.
   - Transverse cervical.
   - Suprascapular.
   - Anterior jugular.

d. **Applied anatomy:** Walls of the external jugular vein are adherent to the deep cervical fascia where it pierces it (2.5 cm above the clavicle). Therefore, if it is cut at this site, its walls cannot collapse which may lead to air embolism which can be fatal.

4. **Describe in brief the layers of deep cervical fascia.**

Ans. a. **Investing layer of deep cervical fascia:** It encircles the neck like a collar deep to superficial fascia. It encloses:
   - *Two muscles:* Sternocleidomastoid and trapezius.
   - *Two glands:* Parotid and submandibular.
   - *Two spaces:* Suprasternal and supraclavicular.

   Attachments:
   - *Superiorly:* External occipital protuberance, superior nuchal line, mastoid process, base of mandible (between angle of mandible and mastoid process it enclose parotid gland).
   - *Inferiorly:* Spine of scapula, acromian process, clavicle, manubrium sterni.
   - *Posteriorly:* Ligamentum nuchae and spine of seventh cervical vertebra.
   - *Anteriorly:* Symphysis menti, hyoid bone.
   - Is continuous with the fascia of the opposite side.

b. **Pretracheal fascia:** It encloses and suspends thyroid gland.

   Attachments:
   - *Superiorly:* Hyoid bone, oblique line of thyroid cartilage, cricoids cartilage.
   - *Inferiorly:* Blends with the adventitia of arch of aorta and pericardium.
   - *Laterally:* Merges with the carotid sheath.

> Is thickened posteriorly to form the suspensory ligament of Berry. The ligament connects the medial surface of the lateral lobes of thyroid gland to cricoids cartilage. Therefore, the gland moves up and down with larynx during deglutition.

c. **Prevertebral fascia:** It lies in front of the cervical and upper three thoracic vertebrae and prevertebral muscles. It forms the floor of posterior triangle.

   Attachments:
   - *Superiorly:* Base of skull in front of foramen magnum.
   - *Inferiorly:* Anterior longitudinal ligament and body of T3 vertebra.
   - It covers the muscles forming floor of the posterior triangle.
   - Cervical and brachial plexus lie deep to it.
   - The trunks of brachial plexus and the subclavian artery emerge between the scalaneus anterior and medius muscles and carry a sheath (axillary sheath) of the fascia along with them to the axilla.
   - The space behind it and in front of vertebrae is prevertebral space.
   - The space in front of it and behind the pharynx is retropharyngeal space. It contains loose areolar tissue and retropharyngeal lymph nodes.

> - The pus collected in the prevertebral space usually arise from the caries of cervical vertebrae. It may project/travel:
>   - Forward and cause midline buldge in the posterior pharyngeal wall.
>   - Laterally first into the posterior triangle and then along axillary sheath into the axilla.
>   - Downwards into superior mediastinum limited by fusion of prevertebral fascia to the T3 vertebra.

Contd.

Contd.

- Pus from the neck infections in front of the prevertebral fascia, i.e., in the retropharyngeal space (from suppuration of the retropharyngeal lymph nodes) project/travel:
  - Forward in the paramedian position (due to fusion of buccopharyngeal fascia to prevertebral fascia in the median plane).
  - May extend down into the superior mediastinum to posterior mediastinum.

d. **Carotid sheath:**

- Is tubular condensation of deep cervical fascia around common and internal carotid arteries, internal jugular vein and vagus nerve.
- Extends from the base of skull to the arch of aorta.
- Is thick around the common and internal carotid arteries and thin around internal jugular vein.
- Ansa cervicalis is embedded in the anterior wall of the carotid sheath.
- Cervical part of sympathetic chain lies behind the carotid sheath and in front of prevertebral fascia.
- ***Contents:***
  - Common carotid artery till the upper border of thyroid cartilage and internal carotid artery above this level.
  - Internal jugular vein in the entire extent.
  - Vagus nerve in the entire extent (is posterior to the carotid arteries and internal jugular vein. The superior and inferior cervical cardiac branches, pharyngeal and superior laryngeal branches of vagus arise inside the carotid sheath.

62 CHAPTER POSTERIOR TRIANGLE OF NECK

1. **Enumerate:**
   a. **Structures forming the boundaries of posterior triangle**
   b. **Structures forming roof of posterior triangle**
   c. **Muscles forming floor of posterior triangle**
   d. **Subdivisions of posterior triangle**
   e. **Contents of occipital and subclavian triangles**

Ans. a. **Structures forming the boundaries of posterior triangle:**
- *Anteriorly:* Posterior border of sternocleidomastoid.
- *Posteriorly:* Anterior border of trapezius.
- *Base:* Intermediate 1/3rd of clavicle.
- *Apex:* On superior nuchal line where trapezius meets sternocleidomastoid.

b. **Structures forming roof of posterior triangle:**
- Skin.
- Superficial fascia with platysma.
- Investing layer of deep cervical fascia.

c. **Floor of the posterior triangle is formed by the prevertebral fascia covering the following muscles (from above downwards):**
- Semispinalis capitis.
- Splenius capitis.
- Levator scapulae.
- Scalenus medius.

d. **Subdivisions of posterior triangle:** Inferior belly of posterior triangle divides the posterior triangle into:
- Larger upper occipital triangle.
- Smaller lower supraclavicular (subclavian) triangle.

e. **Contents of occipital and supraclavicular (subclavian) triangles:**

	Occipital triangle	*Subclavian (supraclavicular) triangle*
Nerves	• Spinal accessory nerve • 3rd and 4th cervical nerves supplying levator scapulae and trapezius • Dorsal scapular nerve (C5) • Initial parts of four cutaneous branches of cervical plexus (great auricular, lesser occipital, transverse cervical and supraclavicular) • Upper trunk of brachial plexus (C5, C6)	• Trunks of brachial plexus • Branches of brachial plexus – Long thoracic nerve – Nerve to subclavius – Suprascapular nerve
Blood vessels	• Occipital artery • Transverse cervical artery	• Third part of subclavian artery • Transverse cervical artery • Suprascapular artery • Dorsal scapular artery
Lymph nodes		• Supraclavicular lymph nodes

Clinical Importance of Supraclavicular Triangle:

- Trunks of the brachial plexus lie are present in this region.
  - ***Brachial plexus block:*** Anaesthetic agent is injected around the trunks of brachial plexus just above the midpoint of clavicle.
  - Injury to trunks of brachial plexus may occur due to trauma at birth or motorbike accidents or stab injuries. Injury to upper trunk causes Erb's palsy and to the lower trunk results in Klumpke's palsy (refer upper limb).
- Supraclavicular lymph nodes (Virchow's nodes) can be palpated here. The nodes are enlarged in cancer of:
  - Stomach
  - Colon
  - Testis
  - Lung
  - Mammary gland
- Bleeding due to severe lacerations of axillary or brachial artery can be controlled by compressing the subclavian artery downward and backward against upper surface of 1st rib in this area.

2. Draw labeled diagram showing:

a. Boundaries and muscles forming floor of posterior triangle

b. Contents of posterior triangle

Ans. a. Boundaries and muscles forming floor of posterior triangle (Fig. 62.1).

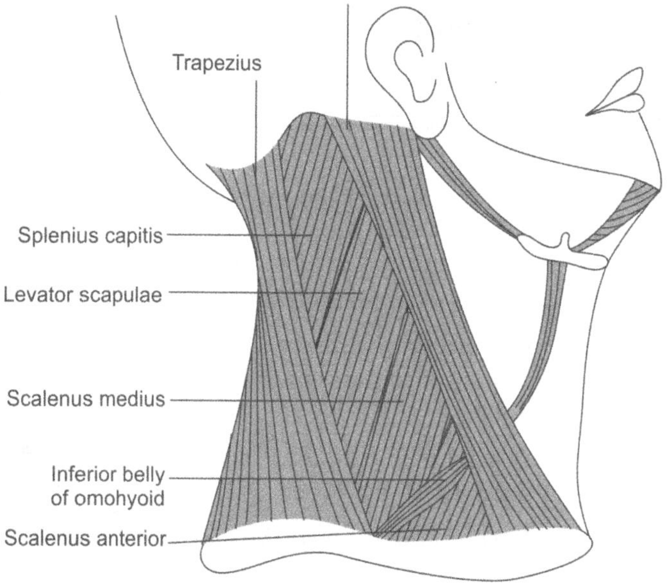

Fig. 62.1: Boundaries and muscles forming floor of posterior triangle

b. Contents of posterior triangle (Fig. 62.2a and Fig. 62.2b).

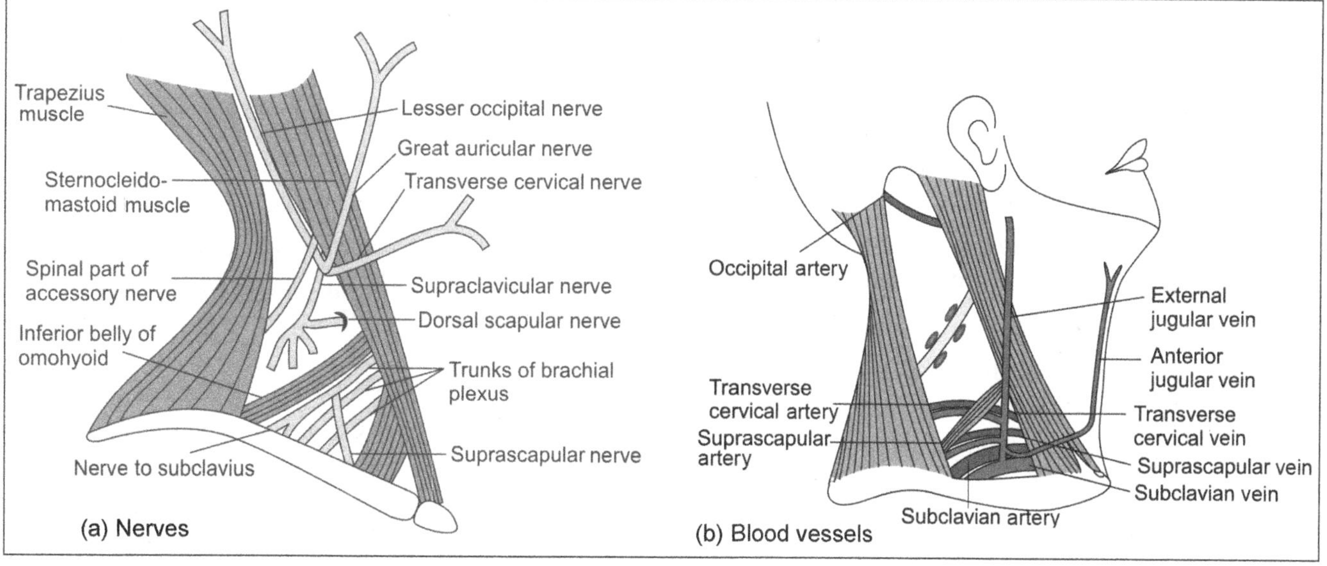

Fig. 62.2: Contents of posterior triangle

CHAPTER 63 ANTERIOR TRIANGLE

1. What are the boundaries of anterior triangle of neck?

Ans. Boundaries of anterior triangle:

- ***Anteriorly:*** Midline of neck extending from symphysis menti to suprasternal notch.
- ***Posteriorly:*** Anterior border of sternocleidomastoid muscle.
- ***Base (above):*** Lower border of mandible and an imaginary line extending from angle of mandible to mastoid process.
- ***Apex (below):*** Where anterior border of sternocleidomastoid meets anterior midline of neck (at suprasternal notch).

2. Name the subdivisions of anterior triangle and write their boundaries and contents.

Ans. Subdivisions of anterior triangle: The superior belly of omohyoid and digastric muscle divide the anterior triangle into the following subdivisions:

- ***Submental triangle:*** Single midline triangle in suprahyoid region.
  - *Boundaries:*
    - On each side: Anterior belly of digastric.
    - Apex: Symphysis menti.
    - Base: Hyoid bone.
  - *Contents:*
    - Submental lymph nodes.
    - Beginning of anterior jugular veins.
- ***Muscular triangle:***
  - *Boundaries:*
    - Anterior: Midline of neck.
    - Posterosuperior: Superior belly of omohyoid.
    - Posteroinferior: Anterior border of sternocleidomastoid.
  - *Contents:*
    - Sternothyroid muscle.
    - Sternohyoid muscle.
- ***Carotid triangle:***
  - *Boundaries:*
    - Superior: Posterior belly of digastric.
    - Anteroinferior: Superior belly of omohyoid.
    - Posterior: Anterior border of sternocleidomastoid.
  - *Muscles forming floor:*
    - Thyrohyoid.
    - Hyoglossus.
    - Inferior constrictor of pharynx.
    - Middle constrictor of pharynx.
  - *Contents:*
    - Arteries:
      - o Common external and internal carotid arteries.
      - o Five branches of external carotid artery – superior thyroid, lingual, facial, ascending pharyngeal, occipital.
    - Veins: Internal jugular vein and its tributaries (common facial, lingual, pharyngeal, superior thyroid).

- Nerves:
  - Glossopharyngeal.
  - Vagus.
  - Hypoglossal.
  - Ansa cervicalis.
  - Cervical part of sympathetic chain.
- Lymph nodes: Deep cervical lymph nodes.
- Others: Carotid body and carotid sinus.

- ***Digastric triangle:***
  - *Boundaries:*
    - Superior: Lower border of mandible and imaginary line joining angle of mandible to mastoid process.
    - Anteroinferior: Anterior belly of digastric.
    - Posteroinferior: Posterior belly of digastric.
  - *Contents:* The triangle is divided into anterior and posterior parts by stylomandibular ligament (from styloid process to angle of mandible).
    - Anterior part:
      - Mylohyoid nerve and vessels.
      - Submental artery.
      - Facial artery and vein.
      - Submandibular lymph nodes.
      - Submandibular gland.
      - Hypoglossal nerve.
    - Posterior part:
      - External carotid artery.
      - Carotid sheath and its contents (internal carotid artery, internal jugular vein and vagus nerve).
      - Structures passing between external and internal carotid arteries:
        - Styloid process.
        - Styloglossus muscle.
        - Stylopharyngeus muscle.
        - Glossopharyngeal nerve.
        - Pharyngeal branch of vagus nerve.
        - Part of parotid gland.

3. Enumerate the infrahyoid and suprahyoid muscles. Write their action and nerve supply.

Ans. See the following Table.

Table: Infrahyoid and suprahyoid muscles

Muscles		*Action*	*Nerve supply*
Infrahyoid muscles	Sternohyoid	Depresses hyoid bone	Ansa cervicalis (C1,C2,C3)
	Sternothyroid	Depresses larynx	Ansa cervicalis
	Thyrohyoid	Depresses hyoid bone Elevates larynx	A branch of hypoglossal nerve carrying C1 fibers
	Omohyoid	Depresses hyoid bone	Superior belly – superior root of ansa cervicalis Inferior belly – ansa cervicalis
Suprahyoid muscles	Digastric*	Depress the mandible (open the mouth) Elevate the hyoid bone	Anterior belly – nerve to mylohyoid (branch of mandibular) Posterior belly – facial nerve
	Geniohyoid	Elevate the hyoid bone	C1 fibers through branch of hypoglossal nerve
	Mylohyoid	Elevates hyoid bone and pulls it forward Depress the mandible	Nerve to mylohyoid (branch of mandibular nerve)
	Stylohyoid	Pulls the hyoid bone upwards and backwards	Facial nerve
Infrahyoid muscles move hyoid bone and larynx during speech and swallowing. Suprahyoid muscles move hyoid bone and mandible during speech and swallowing.			

* Anterior belly of digastric develops from 1st pharyngeal arch, therefore, supplied by branch of mandibular nerve (nerve of 1st pharyngeal arch). Posterior belly is derived from 2nd pharyngeal arch therefore supplied by facial nerve (nerve of 2nd pharyngeal arch).

64 CHAPTER

NERVES AND VESSELS OF NECK

1. **Describe in brief:**
   a. **Cervical plexus**
   b. **Ansa cervicalis**

Ans. a. **Cervical plexus: (Fig. 64.1)**
- Lies in the upper part of the neck behind the prevertebral fascia.
- Is formed by the ventral rami of C1–C4 spinal nerves.
- Each ventral ramus except C1 divides into ascending and descending parts which unite to form three loops.
- Majority of the branches arise from 2nd and 3rd loop.
- It supplies the skin and muscles of the neck and thoracoabdominal diaphragm.
- Its branches are divided into two groups:
  - Superficial (cutaneous) branches.
  - Deep (muscular) branches.
- *Cutaneous branches:*
  - Lesser occipital (C2).
  - Great auricular (C2, C3).
  - Transverse cutaneous nerve of neck (C2, C3).
  - Medial, intermediate and lateral supraclavicular (C3, C4).
- *Muscular branches:*
  - Rectus capitis anterior and lateralis.
  - Longus capitis and longus colli.
  - Scalenus anterior, medius and posterior.
  - Infrahyoid muscles (sternohyoid, sternothyroid, thyrohyoid and omohyoid).
  - Proprioceptive fibers to levator scapulae, trapezius and sterno-cleidomastoid.
  - Diaphragm via phrenic (C3, C4, C5).

b. **Ansa cervicalis: (Fig. 64.2)**

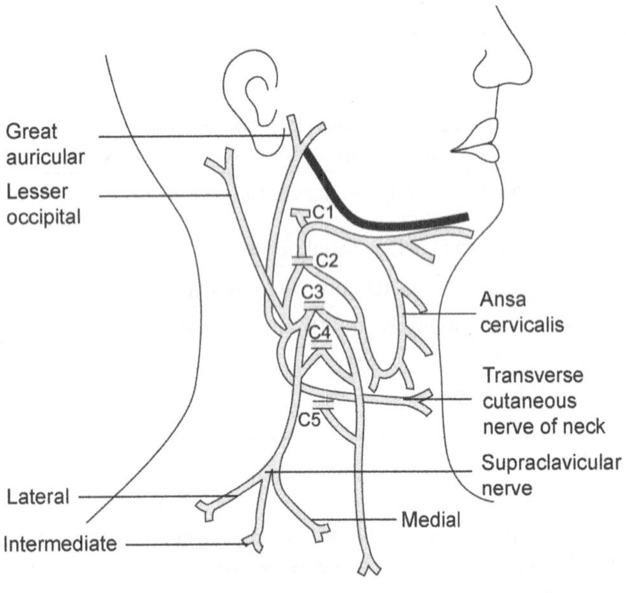

Fig. 64.1: Cervical plexus

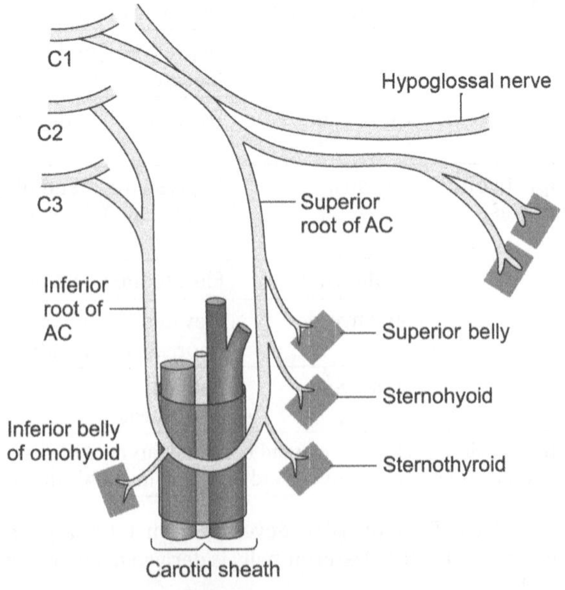

Fig. 64.2: Ansa cervicalis

- Is a U-shaped nerve loop embedded in the anterior wall of carotid sheath.
- Is formed by ventral rami of C1, C2 and C3 spinal nerves.
- It has two roots – superior and inferior which unite to form U-shaped loop.
- *Superior root (descendens hypoglossi):*
  - C1 ventral rami join hypoglossal nerve and few C1 fibers leave hypoglossal nerve to form superior root.
- *Inferior root (descendens cervicalis):*
  - Fibers of ventral rami of C2 and C3 form inferior root.
- Superior root supplies superior belly of omohyoid.
- Branches from the loop supply sterno-hyoid, sternothyroid and inferior belly of omohyoid.

2. **Enumerate:**
   a. **Branches of external carotid artery**
   b. **Branches of internal carotid artery**
   c. **Branches of subclavian artery**
   d. **Tributaries of internal jugular vein**

Ans. a. **External carotid artery: (Fig. 64.3)**

- Is one of the terminal branches of common carotid artery.
- Extends from upper border of lamina of thyroid cartilage to the back of the neck of the mandible.
- Distributes blood to the anterior part of the neck, face, scalp, side of the head, ear and dura mater.

Branches: Total 8 branches:

- *3 anterior branches:*
  - Superior thyroid.
  - Lingual.
  - Facial.
- *2 posterior branches:*
  - Occipital.
  - Posterior auricular.

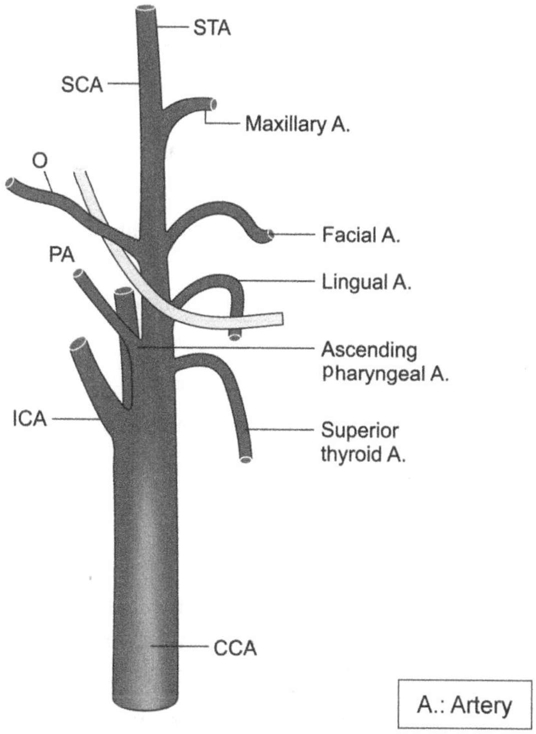

Fig. 64.3: External carotid artery

- *1 medial branch:*
  - Ascending pharyngeal.
- *2 terminal branches:*
  - Maxillary.
  - Superficial temporal.

b. **Internal carotid artery:**

- Is one of the terminal branches of common carotid artery.
- Extends from upper border of thyroid cartilage and enters cranial cavity by passing through the carotid canal.
- Supplies brain, eye, part of scalp.
- *Is divided into four parts:*
  - *Cervical part:* Ascends in the neck from upper border of thyroid cartilage to lower end of carotid canal.
  - *Petrous part:* Passes through carotid canal in the petrous part of temporal bone.
  - *Cavernous part:* Passes through cavernous sinus.
  - *Cerebral part:* Lies at the base of brain.

- ***Branches:***

Part	*Branches*
Cervical part	No branches
Petrous part	• Caroticotympanic branches • Pterygoid branch
Cavernous part	• Superior and inferior hypophyseal arteries • Cavernous branches
Cerebral part	• Anterior cerebral • Middle cerebral • Posterior communicating • Anterior choroidal • Ophthalmic

c. **Subclavian artery:**

- Right subclavian artery is a branch of brachiocephalic trunk and left is direct branch of arch of aorta.
- Supplies upper limb, part of neck, part of thoracic and abdominal walls, parts of brain and spinal cord.
- ***It is divided into three parts by scalenus anterior muscle:***
  - *First part* – From sternoclavicular joint to medial margin of scalenus anterior muscle.
  - *Second part* – Behind the scalenus anterior.
  - *Third part* – From lateral margin of scalenus anterior to the outer border of 1st rib.
- ***Branches:*** See Table at the bottom.

d. **Internal jugular vein:**

- Begins as the continuation of sigmoid sinus at the posterior part of jugular foramen.
- It descends downwards in the carotid sheath to end behind the sternal end of the clavicle by joining subclavian vein to form the brachiocephalic vein.
- Collects the blood from the brain the superficial parts of the face and the neck.
- ***Tributaries:***
  - Inferior petrosal vein.
  - Pharyngeal veins.
  - Common facial vein.
  - Lingual vein.
  - Superior thyroid vein.
  - Middle thyroid vein.
  - Occipital vein (sometimes).

	1st part	*2nd part*	*3rd part*
Branches of subclavian artery	• Internal thoracic (mammary) • Vertebral • Thyrocervical trunk (branches are inferior thyroid, superficial cervical and suprascapular) • Costocervical trunk (only on left side)	• Costocervical trunk (only on right side) – branches are deep cervical and superior intercostals	• Usually no branches but sometimes dorsal scapular artery arises (takes place of deep branch of transverse cervical artery)

65 CHAPTER THYROID GLAND

1. **Describe thyroid gland under the following headings:**
   a. **Location**
   b. **Parts and dimensions**
   c. **Capsules**
   d. **External features and relations**
   e. **Applied**

Ans. a. Location: Thyroid gland is an endocrine gland located in the lower part of front of neck opposite to C5-T1 vertebrae.

b. Parts:

- The gland is H-shaped and consists of two lateral lobes joined by isthmus.
- Each lateral lobe extends upwards up to the oblique line of thyroid cartilage and downwards till 5th/6th tracheal ring.
- Isthmus lies in front of 2nd–4th tracheal rings.
- A small pyramidal lobe may extend upwards from the isthmus and sometimes it is connected to the hyoid bone by a fibromuscular band called levator glandulae thyroideae (remnant of thyroglossal duct).

Dimensions: It weighs approx. 25 gms. Each lobe is 5 cm long, 3 cm wide and 2 cm thick.

c. Capsules: Thyroid gland is enclosed in two capsules:

- ***True capsule:*** Formed by condensation of fibrous stroma of the gland.
- ***False capsule:*** Formed by pretracheal layer of deep cervical fascia.

Venous plexus draining thyroid gland lies deep to true capsule. Therefore, in thyroidectomy, to avoid hemorrhage the gland is removed along with the true capsule (Fig. 65.1).

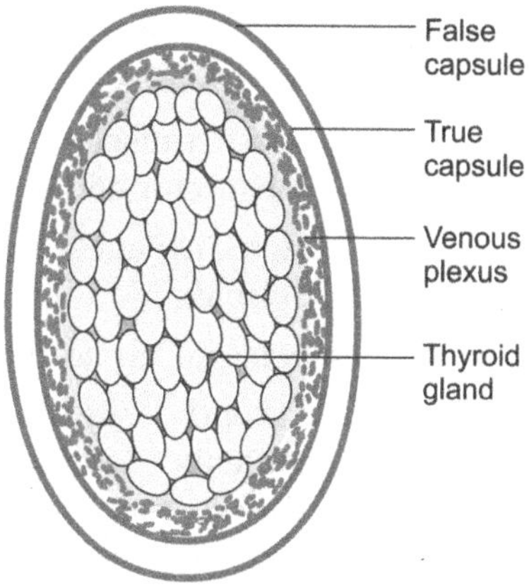

Fig. 65.1: Capsules and location of venous plexus of thyroid gland

d. External features and relations (Fig. 65.2): Each lobe of thyroid gland is pyramidal in shape and has:

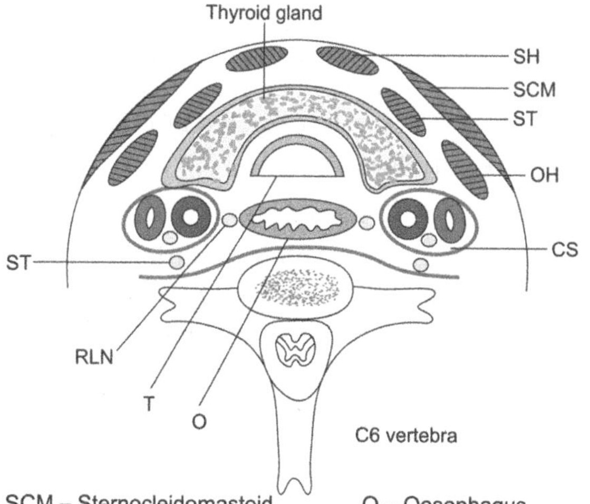

SCM – Sternocleidomastoid
SH – Sternohyoid
ST – Sternothyroid
OH – Omohyoid
CS – Carotid sheath
O – Oesophagus
T – Trachea
RLN – Recurrent laryngeal nerve
ST – Sympathetic trunk

Fig. 65.2: T.S. of neck at the level of thyroid gland

- *Apex:* Extends up to the oblique line of thyroid cartilage and is limited by attachment of sternothyroid muscle.
- *Base:* Extends up to 5th or 6th tracheal ring. Is related to inferior thyroid artery and recurrent laryngeal nerve.
- *Surfaces (3):*
  - *Lateral (superficial) surface:* Is related to the following muscles:
    - Sternohyoid, sternothyroid, superior belly of omohyoid and anterior border of sternocleidomastoid.
  - *Medial surface is related to:*
    - Two tubes – trachea and oesophagus.
    - Two muscles – inferior constrictor and cricothyroid.
    - Two cartilages – cricoids and thyroid.
  - *Posterolateral surface is related to:*
    - Carotid sheath and its contents (common carotid artery, internal jugular vein and vagus nerve).
- *Borders (2):*
  - *Anterior border:* Is thin and is related to anterior branch of superior thyroid artery.
  - *Posterior border:* Is thick and rounded and is related to parathyroid glands and anastomosis between superior and inferior thyroid arteries.
- *Isthmus has:*
  - *Two surfaces:*
    - Anterior surface – related to sternothyroid and sternohyoid muscles and anterior jugular veins.
    - Posterior surface – related to 2nd - 4th tracheal rings.
  - *Two borders:*
    - Superior border – related to anastomosis between anterior branches of superior thyroid arteries.
    - Inferior border – inferior thyroid veins leave isthmus along this border.

Enlarged thyroid gland may compress the structures that form its anatomical relations.

Structure compressed	Effect
• Recurrent laryngeal nerve	Hoarseness of voice
• Trachea	Dyspnea
• Oesophagus	Dysphagia

e. **Applied:**

- The enlargement of thyroid gland is termed as 'goiter'.
  - Endemic goiter occurs due to deficiency of iodine in the diet (decreased levels of T3 and T4). Such goiters present symptoms and signs of hypothyroidism.
  - Toxic goiters/thyrotoxicosis occurs due to excess secretion of T3 and T4 and clinically presents as – increased BMR, tremors, tachycardia.
- Thyroid swellings are usually confined to midline and move up and down with deglutition.
- Hypofunction of thyroid in infants and children is called cretinism and in adults, is called myxedema.
- In partial thyroidectomy the posterior part of thyroid lobes are left behind to avoid removal of parathyroids which otherwise may result in tetany.

2. **Describe briefly the blood supply of thyroid gland.**

Ans. Thyroid gland is highly vascular and is supplied by the following arteries (Fig. 65.3):

- **Superior thyroid artery:**
  - Is a branch of external carotid artery.
  - Descends down to the upper pole of lateral lobe accompanied by external laryngeal nerve (the nerve leaves the artery near the upper pole).
  - At the apex of lateral lobe it divides into anterior and posterior branches.

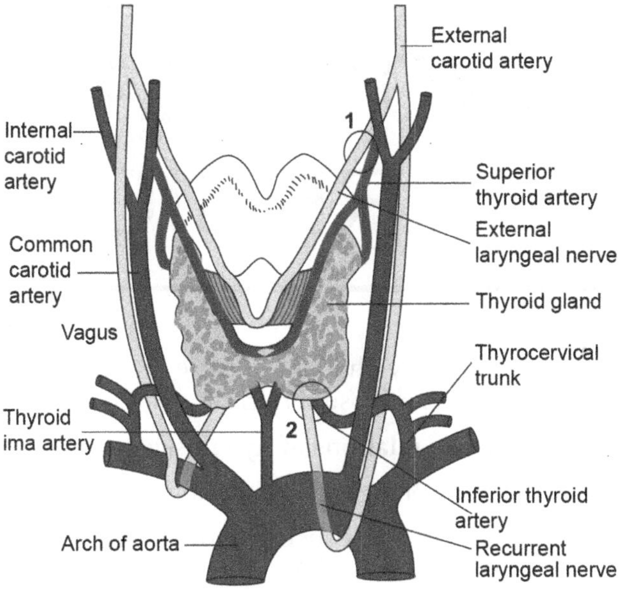

Fig. 65.3: Arterial supply of thyroid gland

- Anterior branch descends along anterior border anastomoses with its fellow of opposite side.
- Posterior branch descends along posterior border and anastomoses with the ascending branch of inferior thyroid artery.
- It supplies upper 1/3rd of the lobe and upper ½ of the isthmus.

- **Inferior thyroid artery:**
  - Is a branch of thyrocervical trunk.
  - It first runs upwards, then passes behind the carotid sheath and descends to reach the base of thyroid gland (forms a loop with convexity upwards).
  - Near the base (lower pole) the artery is very close to recurrent laryngeal nerve.
  - It supplies the lower 2/3rd of the lobe and lower half of the isthmus.
- **Thyroid IMA artery:**
  - Is a branch of brachiocephalic trunk or arch of aorta.
  - Ascends in front of trachea to enter the isthmus.
  - It is not always present.
- **Accessory thyroid arteries:** From tracheal and oesophageal branches of inferior thyroid arteries.

> - Superior thyroid artery lies close to the external laryngeal nerve in its proximal part and they diverge near the apex of lateral lobe (artery is superficial and the nerve is deep to the apex). Therefore, during thyroidectomy the superior thyroid artery should be ligated close to the apex to avoid injury to the external laryngeal nerve.
> - Inferior thyroid artery is very close to the recurrent laryngeal nerve near the base of the thyroid gland. Therefore, during thyroidectomy it should be ligated away from the base to avoid injury to the recurrent laryngeal nerve.

Venous drainage (Fig. 65.4):

- Thyroid veins do not accompany arteries.
- Three pairs of veins arise from the venous plexus present deep to the true capsule.
  - ***Superior thyroid veins*** emerge at the upper pole of thyroid gland and terminates in internal jugular vein.
  - ***Middle thyroid veins:*** Is a short vein, emerges at the middle of the lobe of thyroid gland and drains in internal jugular vein.
  - ***Inferior thyroid veins:*** Emerge at the lower border of isthmus, descend in front of trachea (right and left vein communicate and form plexus in front of trachea) to drain into left brachiocephalic vein.
  - ***Sometimes a fourth vein (vein of Kocher)*** emerges between the middle and inferior thyroid veins which drains into internal jugular vein.

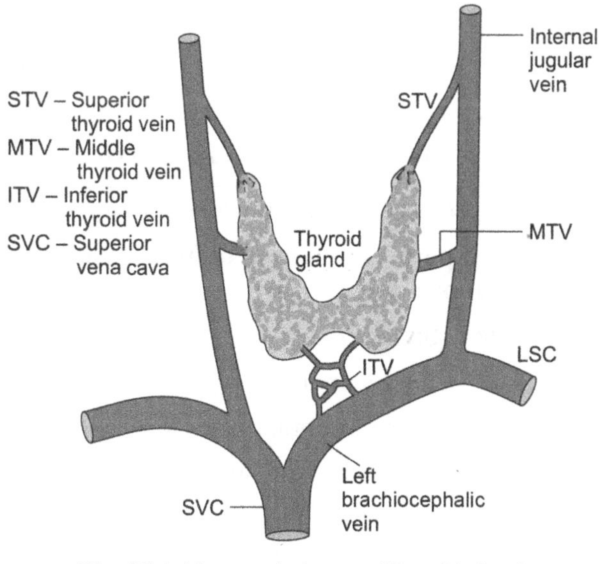

Fig. 65.4: Venous drainage of thyroid gland

66 CHAPTER

SUBMANDIBULAR REGION

1. **What is the extent of submandibular region?**

Ans. Submandibular region is located between the body of mandible (below mylohyoid line) and hyoid bone. It can be divided into superficial and deep parts.

- **Superficial part:** Includes submental and digastric triangles.
- **Deep part:** Includes floor of mouth and root of tongue.

2. **Enumerate:**
   a. **Muscles of submandibular region**
   b. **Superficial relations of hyoglossus**
   c. **Deep relations of hyoglossus**
   d. **Structures passing deep to the posterior border of hyoglossus**

Ans. a. **Muscles of submandibular region are arranged in four layers/planes:**

- *1st layer:* Digastric and stylohyoid.
- *2nd layer:* Mylohyoid.
- *3rd layer:* Geniohyoid, hyoglossus, styloglossus.
- *4th layer:* Geniohyoglossus and middle constrictor of pharynx.

Hyoglossus is the key muscle of this region.

b. **Superficial relations of hyoglossus (from above downwards):**

- Styloglossus.
- Lingual nerve.
- Submandibular ganglion.
- Deep part of submandibular gland with its duct.
- Hypoglossal nerve.

* Mylohyoid muscle overlaps it anterosuperiorly.

c. **Deep relations of hyoglossus:**

- Genioglossus (anteriorly).
- Middle constrictor of pharynx (posteriorly).
- Glossopharyngeal nerve.
- Stylohyoid ligament.
- Lingual artery.

d. **Structures passing deep to posterior border of hyoglossus (from above downwards):**

- Glossopharyngeal nerve.
- Stylohyoid ligament.
- Lingual artery.

3. **Draw labeled diagram of the following:**
   a. **Superficial relations of hyoglossus**
   b. **Connection of submandibular ganglion**

Ans. a. **Superficial relations of hyoglossus (Fig. 66.1).**

b. **Connection of submandibular ganglion (Fig. 66.2).**

4. **Describe submandibular gland under the following headings:**
   a. **Location**
   b. **Parts**
   c. **External features and relations**
   d. **Submandibular duct**
   e. **Nerve supply**
   f. **Applied anatomy**

Ans. Submandibular gland is a mixed type of gland

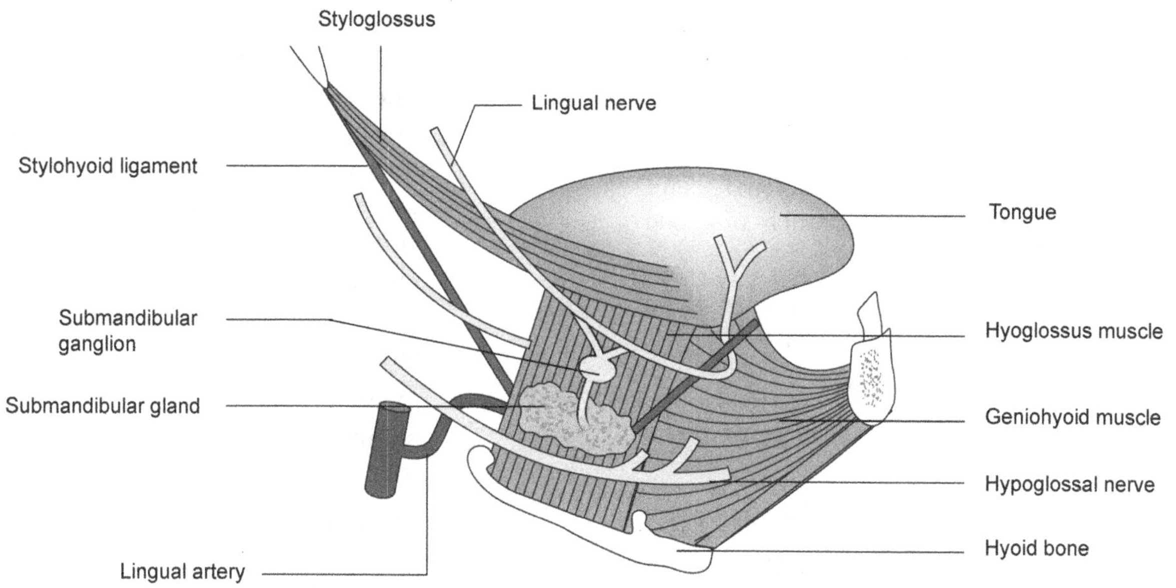

Fig. 66.1: Superficial relations of hyoglossus

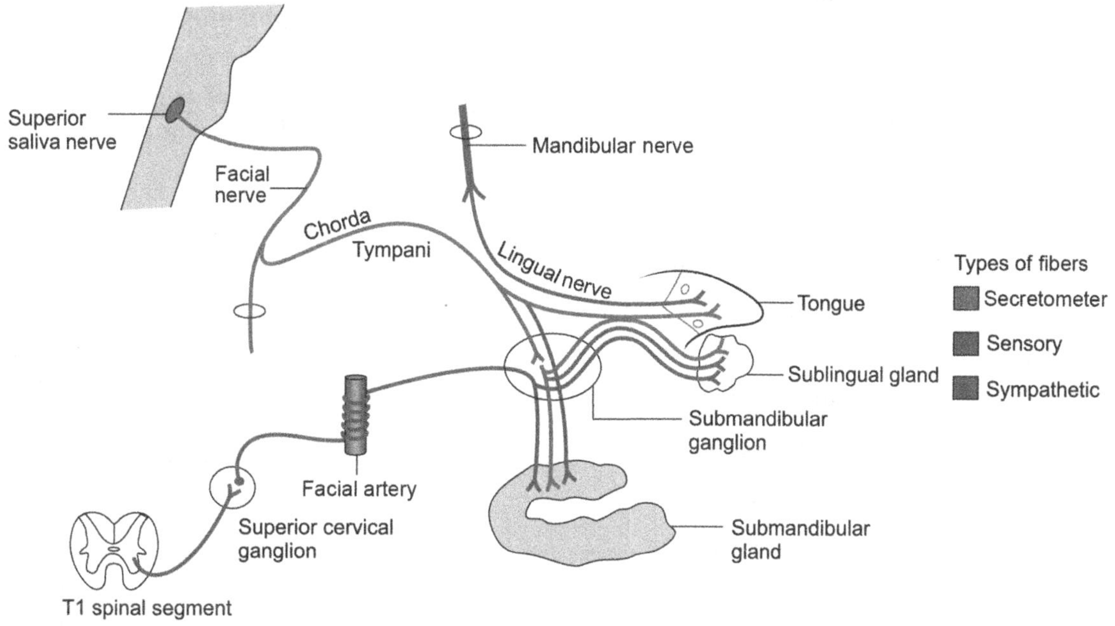

Fig. 66.2: Connection of submandibular ganglion

(contains both mucous and serous acini) but is predominantly serous in nature.

a. **Location:** Is located partly deep to submandibular fossa of mandible and partly below the mandible. Is of the size of a walnut and weighs approx. 10-20 gms.

b. **Parts:** It consists of two parts:
   - ***Large superficial part:*** Fills the anterior part of digastric triangle and lies superficial to mylohyoid muscle.
   - ***Smaller deep part:*** Lies on hyoglossus muscle deep to mylohyoid.

c. **External features and relations:**
   - ***Superficial part*** presents:
     - Two end – anterior and posterior.
     - Three surfaces – inferior (superficial), lateral and medial.
       - *Superficial (inferior) surface* is related to following

structures (from superficial to deep):

- o Skin.
- o Superficial fascia containing platysma and cervical branch of facial nerve.
- o Investing layer of deep cervical fascia.
- o Facial vein.
- o Submandibular lymph nodes.

- *Lateral surface:* Is related to:
  - o Submandibular fossa of mandible.
  - o Medial pterygoid muscle.
  - o Facial artery.
- *Medial surface:* Its relations are divided into three parts:
  - o Anterior part is related to:
    - Mylohyoid muscle.
    - Mylohyoid nerve and vessels.
    - Submental artery.
  - o Middle part is related to:
    - Hyoglossus muscle.
    - Lingual nerve.
    - Submandibular ganglion.
    - Hypoglossal nerve.
  - o Posterior part is related to:
    - Styloglossus muscle.
    - Glossopharyngeal nerve.
    - Stylohyoid ligament.
    - Middle constrictor of pharynx.

d. Submandibular (Wharton's) duct:

- Is 5 cm long and begins on the medial surface of superficial part (at the posterior border of mylohyoid).
- Enters deep part and emerges from the anterior end of deep part and runs forward on hyoglossus (is crossed by lingual nerve from lateral to medial side).
- Continues forwards and upwards between the genioglossus and sublingual gland.
- Opens in the floor of mouth at the summit of sublingual papilla lateral to frenulum of tongue.

e. Nerve supply: Is supplied by branches from submandibular ganglion carrying parasympathetic (secretomotor), sympathetic and sensory fibers.

- ***Parasympathetic (Secretomotor) fibers:***

Preganglionic fibers originate from superior salivatory nucleus in pons

↓

Pass through facial nerve

↓

Pass through chorda tympani branch of facial nerve which joins lingual nerve

↓

Synapse in submandibular ganglion

↓

Postganglionic fibers from submandibular ganglion directly supply submandibular gland

- ***Sympathetic fibers:***

Preganglionic fibers originate from the lateral horn of t1 spinal segment

↓

Relay in superior cervical sympathetic ganglion

↓

Postganglionic fibers form plexus around facial artery and supply submandibular gland

- *Sensory fibers:* From the lingual branch of mandibular nerve.

f. **Applied anatomy:**

- The formation of calculi is more common in submandibular duct than in parotid duct because the submandibular duct ascends to open into the floor of mouth (against gravity) which affects drainage. Secondly, its secretion is more viscous.
- In case of excision of submandibular gland the skin incision should be given 4-5 cm below the angle of mandible parallel to lower border of mandible to save marginal mandibular and cervical branches of facial nerve.
- Swellings of submandibular gland can be palpated bimanually by putting index finger in the floor of mouth and thumb below the lower jaw in front of angle of mandible because deep part is palpable from oral cavity and superficial part from outside.

CHAPTER 67

INFRATEMPORAL FOSSA

1. **Enumerate:**
   a. **Bony boundaries of infratemporal fossa**
   b. **Communications of infratemporal fossa**
   c. **Contents of infratemporal fossa**

Ans. a. **Bony boundaries of infratemporal fossa:**

- *Roof:* Medially – Infratemporal surface of greater wing of sphenoid.
  Laterally – Deficient.
- *Floor:* Open.
- *Medial wall:* Lateral pterygoid plate of sphenoid.
- *Lateral wall:* Ramus of mandible.
- *Anterior wall:* Infratemporal surface of maxilla.
- *Posterior wall:* Tympanic plate and styloid process.

b. **Communications of infratemporal fossa:** Infratemporal fossa communicates:

- *Superiorly:*
  - *Medially* – With middle cranial fossa through foramen ovale and foramen spinosum.
  - *Laterally* – With temporal fossa.
- *Anteromedially:* With pterygopalatine fossa through pterygomaxillary fissure.
- *Anterosuperiorly:* With orbit through inferior orbital fissure.

c. **Contents of infratemporal fossa:**

- *Muscles:* Lateral pterygoid, medial pterygoid and tendon of temporalis.
- *Nerves:* Mandibular nerve and its branches, chorda tympani, otic ganglion.
- *Blood vessels:* 1st and 2nd part of maxillary artery and its branches, maxillary vein and pterygoid plexus of veins.

2. **Write in a tabulated form origin, insertion, action and nerve supply of muscles of mastication.**

Ans. See Table on the next page.

Muscles of mastication and their action: (Fig. 67.1)

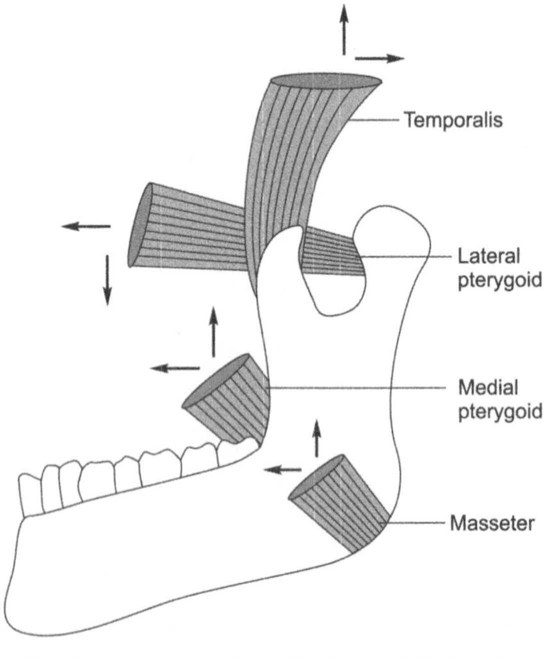

Fig. 67.1: Muscles of mastication and their action

Muscle	*Origin*	*Insertion*	*Action*	*Nerve supply*
Temporalis	Temporal fossa and temporal fascia	Margins and deep surface of coronoid process and anterior border of ramus of mandible	Anterior fibers – Elevation of mandible Posterior fibers – Retraction of mandible	Deep temporal branches from anterior division of mandibular nerve
Lateral pterygoid	Upper head – infratemporal surface of greater wing of sphenoid Lower head – lateral surface of lateral pterygoid plate	Pterygoid fovea on the anterior surface of neck of mandible	Depression of mandible (opening of mouth) Protrusion of mandible Side to side (grinding) movement	Branch from anterior division of mandibular nerve
Medial pterygoid	Superficial head – maxillary tuberosity Deep head – medial surface of lateral pterygoid muscle	Roughened area on the medial surface of angle and adjoining part of ramus of mandible	Elevation, protrusion of mandible Side to side movement	Nerve to medial pterygoid from the trunk of mandibular nerve
Masseter	Lower margin and deep surface of zygomatic arch	Lateral surface of ramus of mandible	Elevation of mandible	Masseteric branch from anterior division of mandibular nerve
• Lateral pterygoid muscle is the key muscle of infratemporal region.				

3. **Describe maxillary artery under the following headings:**
   a. **Origin**
   b. **Subdivisions/parts**
   c. **Branches**
   d. **Distribution**

Ans. Maxillary artery (Fig. 67.2) is the larger of the two terminal branches of external carotid artery.

a. **Origin:** Arises behind the neck of the mandible.

b. **Subdivisions/parts:** Is subdivided into three parts:

- ***1st part (mandibular part):*** Extends from the neck of the mandible to the sphenomandibular ligament. Runs along the lower border of lateral pterygoid muscle. It gives following five branches:
  - Deep auricular.
  - Anterior tympanic.
  - Middle meningeal.

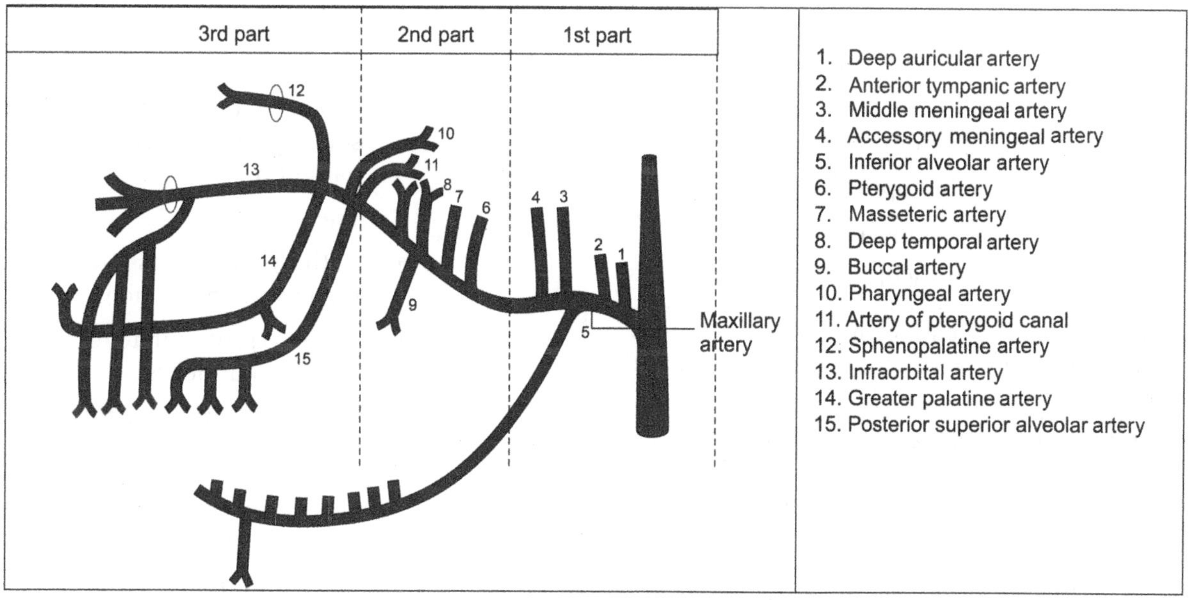

Fig. 67.2: Maxillary artery

– Accessory middle meningeal.
– Inferior alveolar.

- **Middle meningeal artery** is clinically the most important branch. The artery enters the cranial cavity through foramen ovale and divides into anterior and posterior branches. The anterior branch passes upward and forward to pterion and then turns backward and ascends (over precentral gyrus) towards the vertex. The artery and its branches are extradural.
- Following a blow on the pterion region the anterior branch of middle meningeal artery is often torn resulting in formation of extradural hematoma which may compress the motor area (precentral gyrus) of cerebral cortex leading to paralysis of opposite half of the body.

- *2nd part (pterygoid part):* Runs upwards and forwards either superficial or deep to the lower head of the lateral pterygoid muscle. It gives following four branches:
  – Deep temporal.
  – Pterygoid branch.
  – Masseteric artery.
  – Buccal artery.
- *3rd part (pterygopalatine part):* Passes between the two heads of lateral pterygoid muscle and enters pterygopalatine fossa by passing through the pterygomaxillary fissure. It gives following six branches:
  – Posterior superior alveolar.
  – Infraorbital.
  – Greater palatine.
  – Sphenopalatine.
  – Pharyngeal.
  – Artery of pterygoid canal.

- The 1st and 2nd part of maxillary artery lies in infratemporal fossa and 3rd part in pterygopalatine fossa.
- Branches of 1st and 2nd part of maxillary artery follow the branches of mandibular nerve and those of 3rd part follow the branches of maxillary nerve.

c. **Branches:** Described above.

d. **Distribution:** The maxillary artery supplies:
- Upper and lower jaw with teeth.
- Muscles of mastication (temporalis, medial and lateral pterygoid and masseter).
- Nasal cavity.
- Maxillary air sinus.
- Palate.
- Nasopharynx.
- External and middle ear.
- Auditory tube.
- Dura mater.

4. Describe mandibular nerve under the following headings:

a. **Origin and course**
b. **Branches and distribution**
c. **Applied anatomy**

Ans. Mandibular nerve: (Fig. 67.3)

- Is the largest of the three divisions of trigeminal nerve.
- Is a mixed nerve containing both sensory and motor fibers.
- Is the nerve of 1st pharyngeal arch and supplies all structures derived from this arch.

a. **Origin:**
- It begins in the middle cranial fossa.
- It has two roots–large sensory and smaller motor.
- Motor root is attached to the pons. And sensory root arises from trigeminal ganglion.

Course:
- Both the roots pass through the foramen ovale to infratemporal fossa.
- The two roots join to form trunk of the mandibular nerve.
- *The trunk divides into:*
  – Anterior division (mainly motor).
  – Posterior division (mainly sensory).

b. **Branches and distribution**
- *From the trunk:*

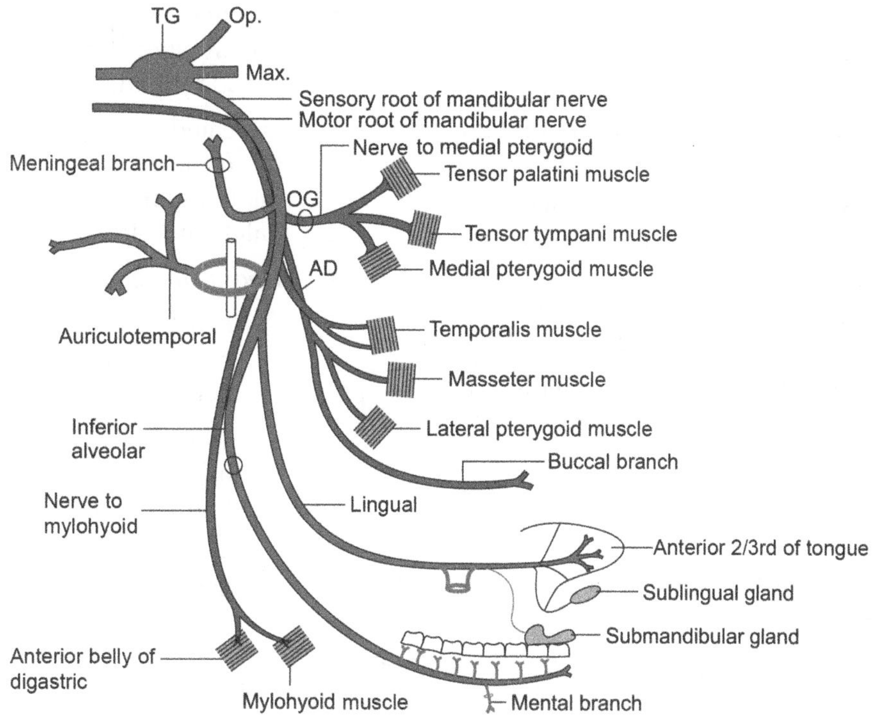

Fig. 67.3: Mandibular nerve

- *Meningeal branch (sensory)* – Supplies dura mater of middle cranial fossa.
- *Nerve to medial pterygoid (motor)* – Supplies 3 muscles (medial pterygoid, tensor veli palatini and tensor tympani).

- ***From the anterior division:*** Anterior division is mainly motor and supplies all the muscles of mastication except medial pterygoid. The branches are:
  - *Motor branches:*
    - Masseteric – Supplies masseter muscle and temporomandibular joint.
    - Deep temporal nerves (two)– Supply temporalis muscle.
    - Nerve to lateral pterygoid – Supplies lateral pterygoid muscle.
  - *Sensory branch:*
    - Buccal supplies skin and mucus membrane of cheek.
- ***From the posterior division:*** Posterior division is mainly sensory.
  - *Sensory branches:*
    - Auriculotemporal nerve – Supplies skin of temple, lateral surface of auricle, external auditory meatus, outer surface of tympanic membrane, temporomandibular joint, parotid gland.
    - Lingual nerve – Supplies anterior 2/3rd of tongue (general sensations), floor of mouth, lingual surface of gums of lower jaw, submandibular and sublingual glands.
    - Inferior alveolar nerve – Is mixed nerve.
      - Sensory branches to lower teeth, skin of chin and skin of mucous membrane of lower lip.
      - Motor branch – Nerve to mylohyoid supplies anterior belly of digastric and mylohyoid muscles.

c. **Applied anatomy:**

- Pain from an infected lower tooth may be referred to the ear because both are supplied by branches of mandibular nerve.
- For the same reason, in cases of cancer of tongue pain radiates to ear and temporal fossa.
- Lingual nerve may get injured during extraction of lower last molar tooth as it is related to the mandible below and medial to the last molar tooth.

5. **Describe briefly the connections of otic ganglion.**

Ans. Otic ganglion: (Fig. 67.4)

- Is a parasympathetic ganglion which is a relay station for secretomotor fibers to parotid gland.
- Is located in the infratemporal fossa below the foramen ovale between the trunk of mandibular nerve (laterally) and tensor palate muscle (medially).
- ***Roots/connections:***
  - *Parasympathetic root* – Lesser petrosal nerve (branch of glossopharyngeal nerve).
  - *Sympathetic root* – Plexus around middle meningeal artery (T1 spinal segment – superior cervical ganglion).
  - *Sensory root* – Auriculotemporal nerve (branch of mandibular nerve).

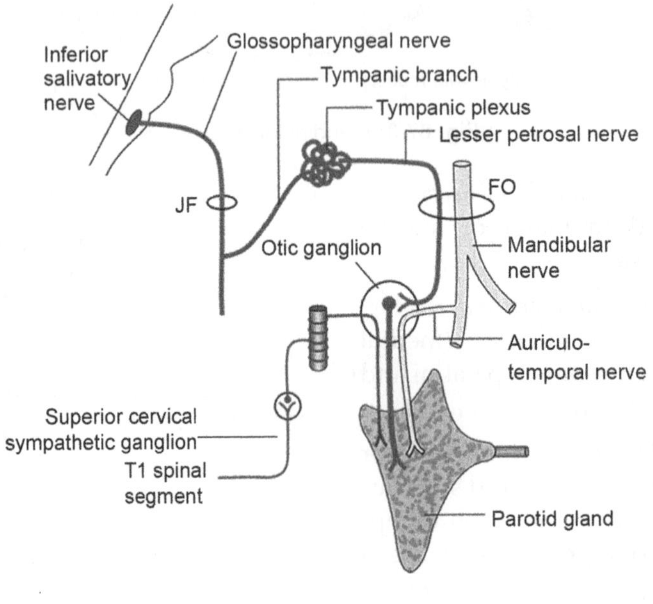

Fig. 67.4: Otic ganglion

68 CHAPTER TEMPOROMANDIBULAR JOINT

1. **Describe temporomandibular joint under the following headings:**
   a. **Type**
   b. **Articular surfaces**
   c. **Fibrous capsule and ligaments**
   d. **Relations and nerve supply**
   e. **Movements**
   f. **Applied anatomy**

Ans. Temporomandibular joint (TMJ) (Fig. 68.1) is between the mandible and right and left temporal bones. The joints help in mastication and opening and closing of mouth.

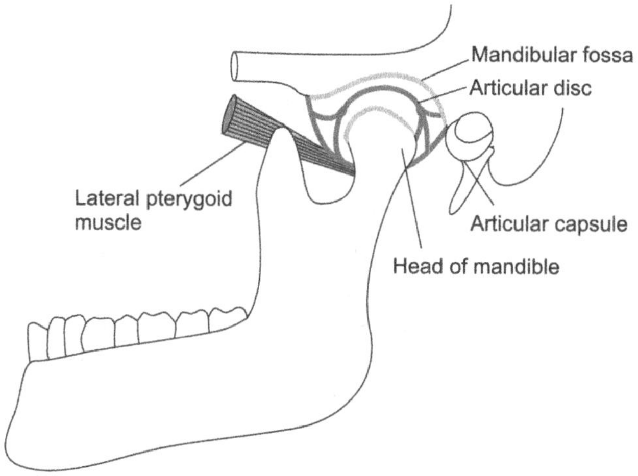

Fig. 68.1: Temporomandibular joint

a. **Type:** TMJ is a bycondylar variety of synovial joint.

b. **Articular surfaces:**
   - ***Superiorly:*** Mandibular fossa on the inferior surface of squamous temporal bone and the articular tubercle in front of mandibular fossa (is concavo-convex from above downwards).
   - ***Inferiorly:*** Head (condyle) of the mandible (is convex).

> - The articular surfaces are covered with fibrocartilage.
> - The joint cavity is divided into two parts by an intra-articular disc of fibrocartilage. It is concavoconvex above and concave below:
>   - Upper meniscotemporal.
>   - Lower menisco mandibular.

c. **Fibrous capsule and ligaments:**
   - ***Fibrous capsule:*** It encloses joint. It is loose above the articular disc and close fitting below it. The fibrous capsule is lined on the inner aspect by synovial membrane. Its attachments are:
     - *Superiorly:* To articular tubercle, margins of mandibular fossa and squamotympanic fissure.
     - *Inferiorly:* To the neck of the mandible.
   - ***Ligaments:***
     - *True ligament:*
       - Lateral/temporomandibular ligament: Extends from the articular tubercle above to the neck of the mandible. The fibers are directed downwards and backwards.

> It is the strongest ligament of the joint and it prevents posterior dislocation of joint.

     - *Accessory ligaments:*
       - Sphenomandibular ligament: Extends from the spine of sphenoid to the lingula of the mandible is located on the medial aspect of the joint.

- Stylomandibular ligament: Extends from the styloid process to the angle of mandible.

  * Both the ligaments become taut when the mandible is protruded.

d. Relations:

- *Anteriorly:* Tendon of lateral pterygoid muscle, masseteric nerve and vessels.
- *Posteriorly:* Parotid gland, superficial temporal vessels, auriculotemporal nerve and external acoustic meatus.
- *Medially:* Maxillary vessels and auriculotemporal nerve.
- *Laterally:* Skin and fascia, parotid gland.

Nerve supply:

- Auriculotemporal nerve.
- Masseteric nerve.

e. Movements: (Fig 68.2)

Movement of mandible	*Muscles responsible*
Elevation	Masseter, medial pterygoid and temporalis (anterior fibers) of both the sides
Depression	Lateral pterygoid of both sides, gravity and infrahyoid muscles
Protraction	Lateral pterygoid and medial pterygoid
Retraction	Posterior fibers of temporalis
Side-to-side (grinding or chewing)	Lateral and medial pterygoids of the two sides act alternately

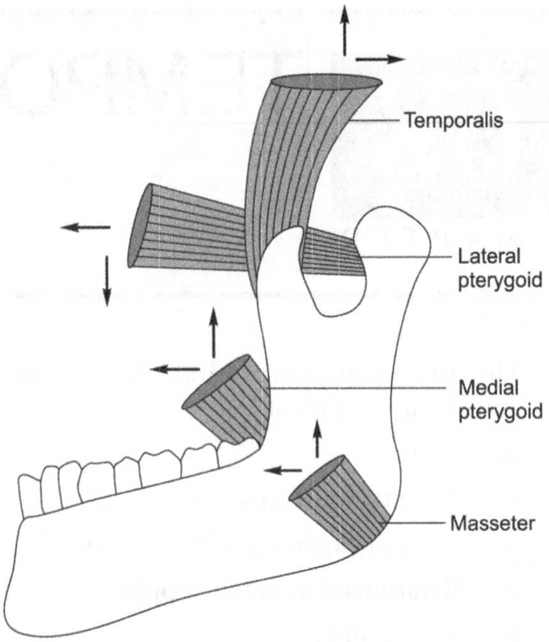

Fig. 68.2: Muscles of mastication and their action

f. Applied anatomy:

- ***Anterior dislocation of mandible:*** When mouth is opened the head of mandible comes to lie beneath the articular tubercle. This is the least stable position of joint. In this position, the anterior dislocation of head of mandible in the infratemporal fossa may occur due to sudden blow on chin or spasm of lateral pterygoid muscles.
- ***Reduction of the anteriorly dislocated mandible*** is done by pressing the last lower molars with thumbs and at the same time elevate the chin (the head of the mandible is lowered and pushed back into the mandibular fossa).

69 CHAPTER PTERYGOPALATINE FOSSA

1. **Enumerate:**
   a. **Bones forming boundaries of pterygopalatine fossa**
   b. **Communications of pterygopalatine fossa**
   c. **Contents of pterygopalatine fossa**

Ans. a. **Pterygopalatine/sphenopalatine fossa** is a pyramidal space below the apex of orbit. Its boundaries are:

- *Anteriorly:* Posterior surface of body of maxilla.
- *Posteriorly:* Pterygoid process and adjoining part of greater wing of sphenoid.
- *Laterally:* Opens into infratemporal fossa through pterygomaxillary fissure.
- *Medially:* Perpendicular plate of palatine bone.
- *Superiorly:* Body of sphenoid bone and orbital process of palatine bone.
- *Inferiorly:* Pyramidal process of palatine bone in the angle between the maxilla and pterygoid process.

b. **Communications of pterygopalatine fossa:** It communicates with the following:

- *Anteriorly:* With orbit through infraorbital fissure.
- *Posteriorly:*
  - With middle cranial fossa through foramen rotundum.
  - With pharynx through palate-vaginal canal.
  - With foramen lacerum through pterygoid canal.
- *Medially:* With nasal cavity through sphenopalatine foramen.
- *Laterally:* With infratemporal fossa through pterygomaxillary fissure.
- *Inferiorly:* With oral cavity through greater and lesser palatine foramina.

c. **Contents of pterygopalatine fossa:**

- Maxillary nerve and its branches.
- Pterygopalatine ganglion and its branches.
- Third part of maxillary artery and its branches.

2. **Describe maxillary nerve under the following headings:**
   a. **Origin and course**
   b. **Branches and distribution**

Ans. Maxillary nerve is the second division of trigeminal nerve. It is purely sensory nerve (Fig. 69.1).

a. **Origin and course:**

- Arises from the anterior aspect of trigeminal ganglion in the middle cranial fossa.
- Enters the lower part of the lateral wall of cavernous sinus.
- Leaves the middle cranial fossa through the foramen rotundum.
- Enters the pterygopalatine fossa.
- Traverse the pterygopalatine fossa and enters the orbit through the inferior orbital fissure as its continuation called *infraorbital nerve.*
- Infraorbital nerve passes through the infraorbital groove and canal (in the floor of orbit) to reach face through the infraorbital foramen.

TG	–	Trigeminal ganglion
PSA	–	Posterior superior alveolar nerve
MSA	–	Middle superior alveolar nerve
ASA	–	Anterior superior alveolar nerve
PG	–	Pterygopalatine ganglion

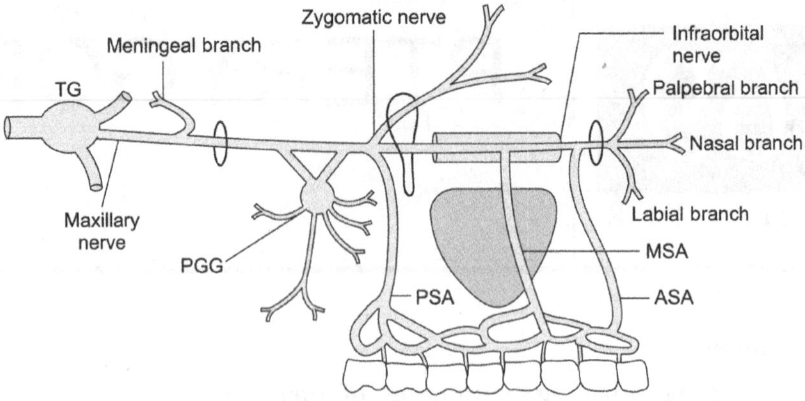

Fig. 69.1: Maxillary nerve

b. **Branches and distribution:**
- ***In the middle cranial fossa:***
  - *Meningeal branch* that supplies the dura mater of middle cranial fossa.
- ***In the pterygopalatine fossa:***
  - *Communicating (ganglionic)* branches pass through pterygopalatine ganglion to supply mucous membrane of palate, nasopharynx and nasal cavity.
  - *Zygomatic branch:* It enters the orbit through the inferior orbital fissure and divides into:
    - Zygomaticotemporal: Supplies skin of temple.
    - Zygomaticofacial: Supplies skin of face.
  - *Posterior superior alveolar nerve:* Supplies upper molar teeth.
- ***In the orbit (branches of infraorbital nerve):***
  - *Middle superior alveolar nerve:* Supplies upper premolar teeth.
  - *Anterior superior alveolar nerve:* Supplies upper canine and incisor teeth.
- ***In the face (terminal branches of infraorbital nerve):***
  - Palpebral branch to lower eyelid.
  - Nasal branch to side of nose.
  - Labial branch to upper lip.

3. **Describe briefly the pterygopalatine ganglion.**

Ans. Pterygopalatine ganglion: (Fig. 69.2)
- Is the largest parasympathetic ganglion.
- Is topographically related to maxillary nerve but functionally to facial nerve (greater petrosal branch).
- Is located in the pterygopalatine fossa.
- Is the size of head of a small pin.
- It has following roots:
  - ***Parasympathetic (secretomotor) root:***
    - Carries preganglionic parasympathetic fibers from superior salivatory nucleus of facial nerve.
    - The fibers reach ganglion via greater petrosal nerve and then through nerve of pterygoid canal (formed by joining of deep petrosal (sympathetic) and greater petrosal (parasympathetic) nerves.
    - Postganglionic fibers from the ganglion supply secretomotor fibers to lacrimal gland and glands of nose, palate and nasopharynx.

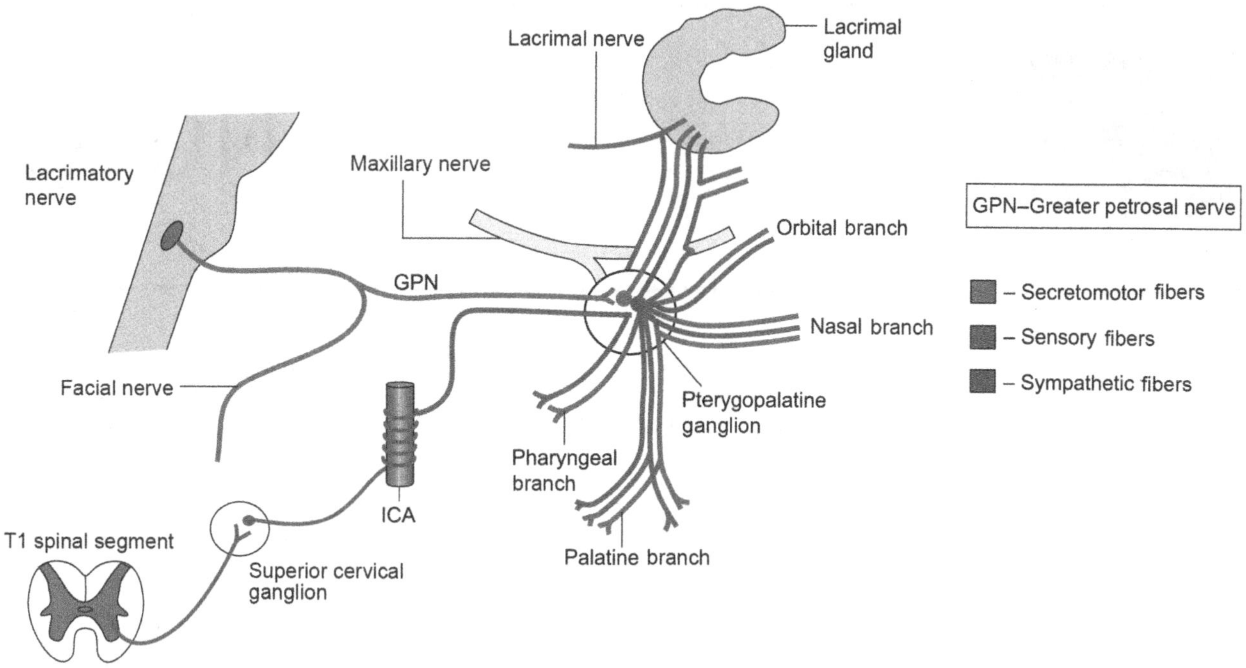

Fig. 69.2: Pterygopalatine ganglion

- *Sympathetic root:*
  - Carries postganglionic sympathetic fibers from superior cervical ganglion (preganglionic fibers arise in T1 spinal segment).
  - The fibers reach via plexus around internal carotid artery and then through the nerve of pterygoid canal.
  - The fibers are vasomotor.
- *Sensory root:*
  - Formed by ganglionic branches of maxillary nerve.
  - Carry general sensations from the palate, orbital periosteum, nasal cavity and nasopharynx.
- ***Branches and distribution:*** The ganglion has following branches:
  - *Orbital:* Pass through inferior orbital fissure and supply orbital periosteum.
  - *Nasal:* Pass through sphenopalatine foramen to supply nasal cavity.
  - *Greater palatine nerve:* Pass through greater palatine foramen to supply palate and nasal cavity. Lesser palatine nerves supply soft palate.
  - *Pharyngeal:* Pass through palatevaginal canal to supply pharynx.

Pterygopalatine ganglion is known as ganglion of 'hay fever' because in allergic conditions viz. hay fever causes irritation of this ganglion which results in running nose and increased secretion from lacrimal gland.

CHAPTER 70
TONGUE

1. Enumerate the functions and parts of tongue.

Ans. Tongue is a muscular organ, essentially made up of skeletal muscle covered by mucous membrane. It is partly located in the oral cavity and partly in oropharynx.

- **Functions of tongue:**
  - Taste, speech, mastication and swallowing.
- **Parts:** Tongue consists of:
  - ***Tip:*** Is directed forward and is in contact with incisors when the mouth is closed.
  - ***Root:*** Lies in the floor of mouth and is attached to mandible and hyoid bone by muscles.
  - ***Body:*** Part between the tip and root. It has two surfaces ventral and dorsal and two lateral borders.
    - *Ventral surface:* Is covered by mucous membrane which is continuous with that of floor of mouth. It shows following features:
      - Frenulum linguae: Midline mucosal fold which connects ventral surface to floor of mouth.
      - Deep lingual vein: Located on either side of frenulum linguae deep to mucosa.
      - Plica fimbriata: Fimbriated mucosal fold lateral to deep lingual veins.
    - *Dorsal surface:* Is divided by V-shaped sulcus into:
      - Anterior 2/3rd (oral part): Mucus membrane is characterized by presence of lingual papillae which give it velvety appearance.
      - Posterior 1/3rd (pharyngeal part): Has large number of lymphoid follicles (lingual tonsil) deep to mucosa.

2. Name the different types of papillae present on the dorsal surface of oral part of tongue.

Ans. Mucus membrane of anterior 2/3rd of tongue has four types of lingual papillae.

Lingual papillae are projections of lamina propria of mucosa covered by stratified squamous epithelium. The four types of papillae are:

- **Filiform papillae:**
  - Are conical in shape.
  - Epithelium covering them is keratinized.
  - Are arranged in rows parallel to sulcus terminalis.
  - Are devoid of taste buds.
- **Fungiform papillae:**
  - Are rounded at top and narrow at base.
  - Are mostly present at tip and margins.
  - Have taste buds.
- **Circumvallate papillae:**
  - Are largest in size (10-12 in number).
  - Are located in front of the sulcus terminalis.
  - Their shape is like truncated cone and are surrounded by a circular sulcus.

Muscles of tongue			
Muscle		*Action*	*Nerve Supply*
Intrinsic	Superior longitudinal	Shorten the tongue and make the dorsal surface concave	All are supplied by hypoglossal (XII cranial) nerve
	Inferior longitudinal	Shorten the tongue and make the dorsal surface convex	
	Transverse	Make the tongue narrow and elongated	
	Vertical	Make the tongue flat and broad	
Extrinsic	Genioglossus	Protrude the tongue (when both the muscles contract)	All the muscles are supplied by hypoglossal nerve except *palatoglossus* which is supplied by *vagoaccessory complex* via pharyngeal plexus
	Hyoglossus	Depress the side of the tongue	
	Styloglossus	Pulls the tongue upwards and backwards	
	Palatoglossus	The two muscles together approximate the palatoglossal arches thereby closing the oropharyngeal isthmus	

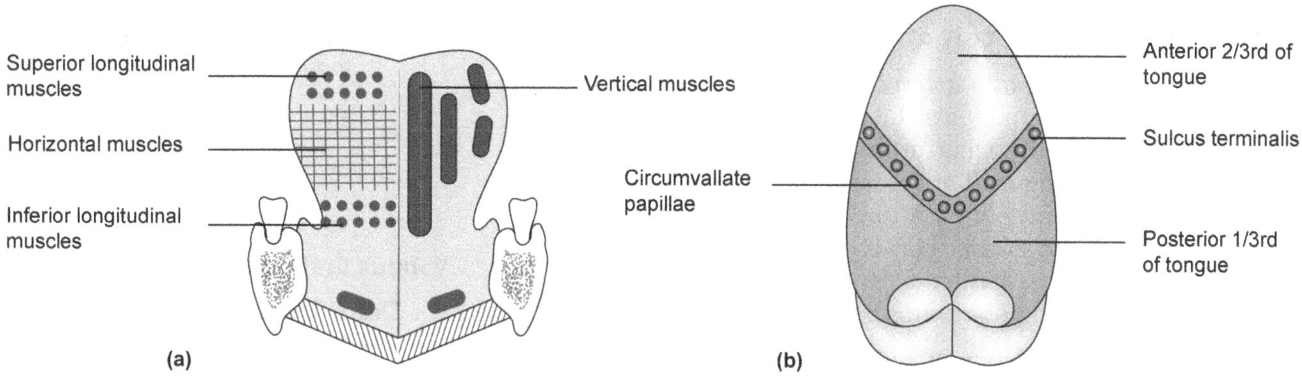

Fig. 70.1: Muscles of tongue (coronal section)

- Have numerous taste buds on the sides.

- **Folliate papillae:**
  - Are leaf like transverse ridges present on the lateral margin in front of sulcus terminalis.
  - They bear taste buds.

3. **Name the muscles of tongue and write their action and nerve supply.**

Ans. The substance of tongue is divided into two halves. Each half of the tongue has four intrinsic and four extrinsic muscles. Intrinsic muscle alter the shape of tongue whereas extrinsic muscles move the tongue (See above Table and Fig. 70.1a and b).

> Genioglossus is known as the 'safety muscle of the tongue' because it protrudes the tongue and prevents it from falling back and thereby blocking airway in an unconscious patient.

4. **Describe briefly:**
   a. **Sensory supply of tongue and correlate it with its development**
   b. **Blood supply of tongue**
   c. **Lymphatic drainage of tongue**

Ans. a. Sensory innervations of tongue and correlation with its development: (Fig. 70.2 and See Table on the next page)

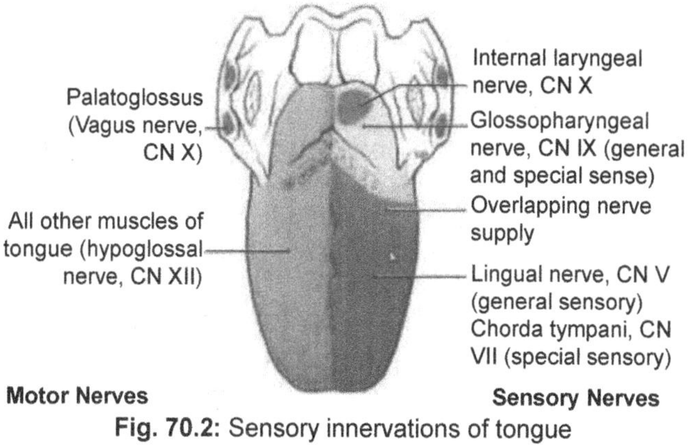

Fig. 70.2: Sensory innervations of tongue

Parts of the tongue	*Nerve carrying general sensation*	*Nerve carrying taste sensation*	*Correlation with development*
Anterior 2/3rd of the tongue (except circumvallate papillae)	Lingual nerve (branch of mandibular nerve)	Chorda tympani (branch of facial nerve)	Mucosa of anterior 2/3rd of tongue develops from 1st pharyngeal arch, therefore, general sensory innervations is by mandibular nerve (nerve of 1st arch). The pretrematic nerve of first arch is facial nerve, therefore taste sensation is carried by chorda tympani, branch of facial nerve
Posterior 1/3rd of the tongue (including circumvallate papillae)	Glossopharyngeal nerve	Glossopharyngeal nerve	Mucosa of the posterior 1/3rd of tongue develops from 3rd pharyngeal arch, therefore supplied by nerve of third arch, i.e., glossopharyngeal nerve
Posterior most part of tongue (including vallecula)	Internal laryngeal nerve (branch of vagus)	Internal laryngeal nerve (branch of vagus)	Mucosa of the vallecula of tongue develops from 4th pharyngeal arch, therefore supplied by nerve of 4th pharyngeal arch, i.e., vagus nerve

b. • **Arterial supply of tongue:**

- ***Lingual artery:*** A branch of external carotid artery (ECA) is the chief artery that supplies tongue. It arises from the anterior aspect of ECA opposite the tip of the greater cornu of hyoid bone. It is divided into three parts by hyoglossus muscle:
    - *1st part:* Lies in the carotid triangle. Forms a loop above the greater cornu.
        - o Branch: Suprahyoid artery.
    - *2nd part:* Passes deep to hyoglossus muscle.
        - o Branch: Dorsal lingual arteries (usually two) supply posterior part of the tongue and tonsil.
    - *3rd part:* Also called deep lingual artery or arteria profunda linguae runs upwards along the anterior border of hyoglossus and then forward on the undersurface of tongue.
        - o Branch: Sublingual artery to sublingual gland and branches to anterior part of tongue.
    - *Other arteries that supply tongue are:*
        - o Tonsillar branch of facial artery.
        - o Ascending pharyngeal artery.

• **Venous drainage:**

- ***Deep lingual veins:*** Drain the dorsum of the tongue run and join the venae comitantes accompanying lingual artery.
- ***Superficial veins of tongue:*** Drain the tip and form the venae comitantes accompanying the hypoglossal nerve.

These veins unite at the posterior border of hyoglossus to form the lingual vein which drains into internal jugular vein.

c. **Lymphatic drainage of tongue (Fig. 70.3):** Lymphatic vessels draining tongue are divided into the following groups:

- ***Apical vessels:*** Drain the tip of the tongue into the submental lymph nodes which may drain into submandibular or jugulo-omohyoid lymph nodes.
- ***Marginal vessels:*** Drain the lateral (marginal) area of anterior 2/3rd of tongue unilaterally into the submandibular lymph nodes which

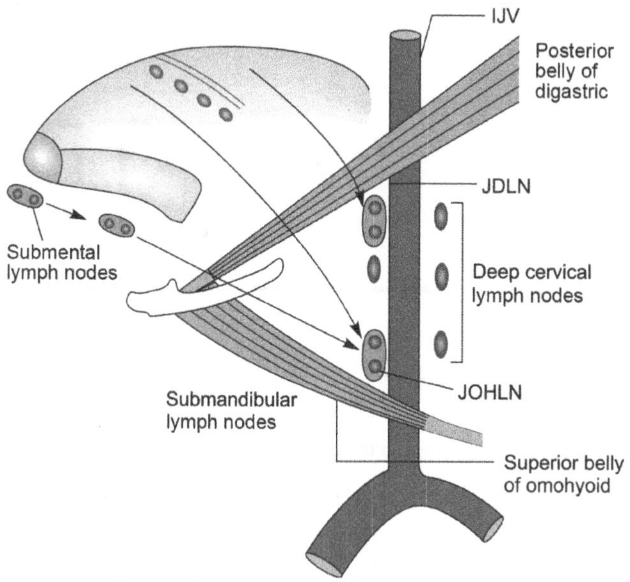

Fig. 70.3: Lymphatic drainage of tongue

then drain into lower group of deep cervical lymph nodes.

- *Central vessels:* Drain the central part of anterior 2/3rd of tongue bilaterally into deep cervical lymph nodes including jugulo-omohyoid lymph nodes.
- *Basal vessels:* Drain posterior 1/3rd of the tongue bilaterally into the jugulodigastric and retropharyngeal lymph nodes.

Malignant tumors of the posterior 1/3rd have poor prognosis.

- There is rich anastomosis across the midline between the lymphatics of posterior 1/3rd of tongue. Therefore tumor of one side readily metastasizes to contralateral side.
- Tumor more than ½ inch from midline do not metastasize to the opposite side till late as there is little cross communication between the lymphatics of the two sides.

71 CHAPTER PALATE

1. **What are the parts of the palate and write their arterial and nerve supply?**

Ans. Palate forms the roof of the proper oral cavity and is divided into two parts:

- **Hard (Bony) palate:** Forms the anterior 4/5th of the palate. Is formed by:
  - Palatine processes of maxillae form the anterior 2/3rd.
  - Horizontal plates of palatine bones form the posterior 1/3rd.
  - *Arterial supply:* Greater palatine arteries (branch of maxillary artery).
  - *Nerve supply:* Is by branches from pterygopalatine ganglion.
    - Greater palatine nerve.
    - Nasopalatine nerve.
- **Soft palate:** Forms the posterior 1/5th of the palate. Is a fibromuscular mobile flap that is attached anteriorly to hard palate. Nasal surface is lined by pseudostratified ciliated columnar epithelium. Oral surface is lined by stratified squamous epithelium.
  - *Arterial supply:*
    - Lesser palatine arteries (branches of maxillary artery).
    - Ascending palatine branch of facial artery.
    - Palatine branches of ascending pharyngeal artery.
  - *Nerve supply:*
    - *Motor:* All the muscles of soft palate are supplied by cranial root of accessory via pharyngeal nerve except tensor veli palatini which is supplied by nerve to medial pterygoid (branch of mandibular nerve).
  - *Sensory:*
    - Lesser palatine (from maxillary nerve via pterygopalatine ganglion).
    - Glossopharyngeal nerve.

2. **Describe soft palate under the following headings:**
   a. **External features**
   b. **Muscles of soft palate**
   c. **Functions of soft palate**

Ans. a. External features: Soft palate has two surfaces and two borders (in resting position).

- *Surfaces:*
  - Anterior (oral) surface.
  - Posterior surface is continuous with the floor of the nasal cavity.
- *Borders:*
  - *Superior:* Is attached to the posterior border of hard palate.
  - *Inferior:* Is free and a small conical projection called uvula hangs down from its middle.
- *Laterally:* Two folds of mucous membrane each containing a muscle extend down to the tongue and pharynx.
- Anterior palatoglossal fold containing palatoglossus muscle reaches the tongue at the junction of its anterior 2/3rd and posterior 1/3rd.

- Posterior palatopharyngeal fold containing palatopharyngeus muscle descends on the lateral wall of the oropharynx.

b. **Muscles of soft palate (Fig. 71.1):** Soft palate consists of following five pairs of muscles (See the following Table):
   - ***Two muscles enter from above (take origin from the base of skull):***
     - Tensor veli palatini.
     - Levator veli palatini.
   - ***Two muscles descend down from the palate:***
     - Palatoglossus.
     - Palatopharyngeus.
   - ***One muscle descends into the uvula in the midline:***
     - Musculus uvulae.

c. **Functions of soft palate:**
   - Separates oropharynx from nasopharynx during swallowing.
   - Isolates oral cavity from oropharynx during chewing so that breathing is not affected.

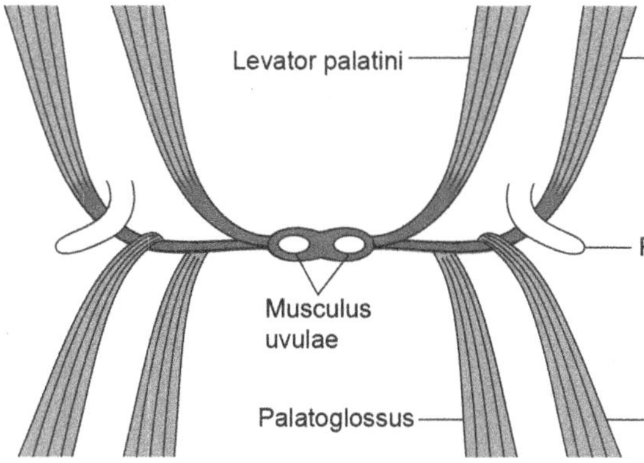

Fig. 71.1: Muscles of soft palate

Attachments and actions of the muscles of soft palate

Muscles	*Origin*	*Insertion*	*Action*
Tensor veli palatini	Lateral aspect auditory tube, spine of sphenoid, scaphoid fossa.	Its tendon hooks around the pterygoid hamulus and forms aponeurosis which is attached to the inferior surface of hard palate behind the palatine crest and posterior border of hard palate.	Tightens the soft palate and helps in opening the auditory tube.
Levator veli palatini	Inferior surface of petrous part of temporal bone near its apex, medial aspect of auditory tube.	Upper surface of palatine aponeurosis.	Elevation of soft palate and helps in opening the auditory tube.
Palatoglossus	Inferior surface of palatine aponeurosis.	Side of tongue at the junction of its oral and pharyngeal part.	Elevation of tongue. Approximation of the two palatoglossal arches to close the oropharyngeal isthmus.
Palatopharyngeus	Superior surface of palatine aponeurosis and posterior border of hard palate (arises by two fascicule which are separated by levator veli palatini).	Posterior border of lamina of thyroid cartilage.	Pulls the pharyngeal and laryngeal walls upwards during swallowing.
Musculus uvulae	Posterior nasal spine and palatine aponeurosis.	Mucosa of uvula.	Shortens and raises the uvula.

- Helps to modify the quality of voice by varying the degree of closure of pharyngeal isthmus.
- Protects nasal mucosa during sneezing by appropriately directing the blast of air through nasal and oral cavity.
- Prevents the entry of sputum into nose during coughing.

- Paralysis of muscles of soft palate produces:

  a. Nasal regurgitation of liquids.

  b. Nasal twang in voice.

  c. Flattening of palatal arch on the side of lesion.

  d. Deviation of uvula, opposite to the side of lesion.

72 CHAPTER TONSIL

1. **What is Waldeyer's tonsillar ring?**

Ans. It is a ring of lymphoid tissue at the oropharyngeal isthmus, formed by:

- Pharyngeal tonsil.
- Tubal tonsils.
- Palatine tonsils.
- Lingual tonsil.

> **Adenoids:** Is hypertrophy/enlargement of pharyngeal tonsil that may block nasopharynx and cause difficulty in nasal breathing and phonation. It may block the pharyngeal orifices of the auditory tube causing hearing impairment. Typical facial appearance is termed adenoid facies characterized by:
>
> - Pinched nose due to airway obstruction (nasopharynx).
> - Open mouth due to mouth breathing.

2. **Describe palatine tonsil under the following headings:**
   a. **Location**
   b. **External features**
   c. **Relations**
   d. **Blood supply and lymphatic drainage**

Ans. a. **Location:** Palatine tonsils are collection of lymphoid tissue present in the submucosa of oropharynx. They are located in the tonsillar fossa, one on each side, in the lateral wall of the oropharynx. Boundaries of tonsillar fossa/sinus are:

- ***Anterior:*** Palatoglossal arch.
- ***Posterior:*** Palatopharyngeal arch.
- ***Superior:*** Where the palatoglossal and palatopharyngeal arches meet.
- ***Inferior:*** Dorsal surface of posterior 1/3rd of the tongue.
- ***Lateral:*** Lateral wall of oropharynx.

b. **External features:** Palatine tonsil is almond shaped. It has:

- ***Two poles:*** Upper and lower.
- ***Two borders:*** Anterior and posterior.
- ***Two surfaces:*** Medial and lateral.

c. **Relations: (Fig. 72.1)**

- ***Upper pole*** is related to soft palate.
- ***Lower pole*** extends upto the dorsum of posterior 1/3rd of tongue.
- ***Anterior border*** is related to palatoglossal arch and *posterior border* to palatopharyngeal arch.
- ***Medial surface:***
  - Is free and faces the oropharynx.
  - Is covered by stratified squamous non-keratinized epithelium.
  - Is pitted due to the presence of 15-20 crypts. The largest of them called intratonsillar cleft/crypta magna (remnant of 2nd pharyngeal pouch).
- ***Lateral surface*** (structure related to this surface form *tonsillar bed).*

  From medial to lateral they are:

  - Fibrous capsule formed by condensation of pharyngobasilar fascia.
  - Loose areolar tissue *(peritonsillar space)* containing paratonsillar vein.

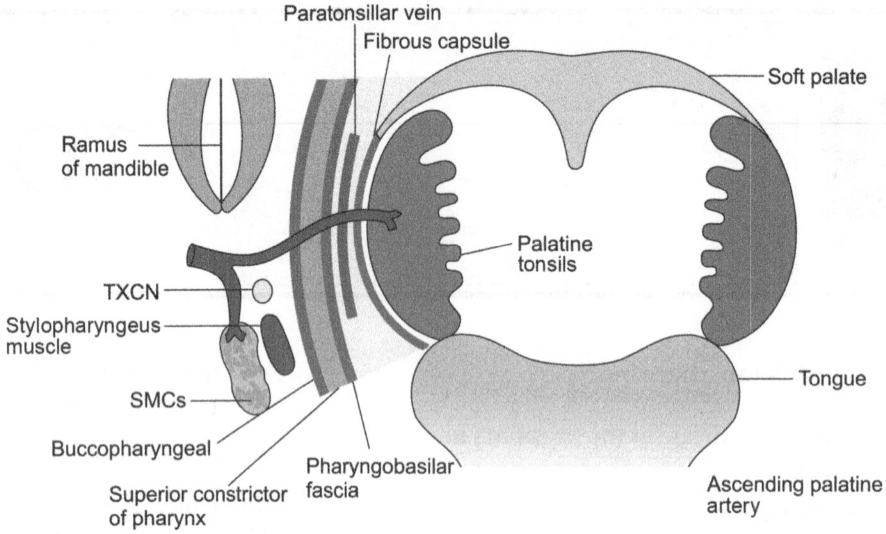

Fig. 72.1: Relations of tonsil

- Superior constrictor muscle of pharynx.

Tonsillar bed is related to the following structures:

- *Arteries:* Loop of facial artery and its ascending palatine branch, ascending pharyngeal artery.
- *Muscles:* Styloglossus and stylo-pharyngeus.
- *Nerve:* Glossopharyngeal nerve.

d. **Blood supply and lymphatic drainage:**

- ***Arterial supply (Fig. 72.2):*** Palatine tonsil is supplied by 5 arteries.
  - Tonsillar branch of facial artery (chief artery).
  - Dorsal lingual branch of lingual artery.
  - Ascending palatine branch of facial artery.
  - Descending palatine branch of ascending pharyngeal artery (branch of external carotid artery).
  - Branch from greater palatine artery (branch of maxillary artery).
- ***Venous drainage:*** Venous plexus around tonsil drains into:
  - Paratonsillar vein which descends from soft palate across the lateral aspect of tonsillar capsule and pieces superior constrictor of pharynx to drain into pharyngeal venous plexus.
  - Tonsillar veins which accompany tonsillar branch of facial artery and drain into common facial vein.
- ***Lymphatic drainage:*** Lymphatics from tonsil drains mainly into jugulodigastric lymph nodes (called

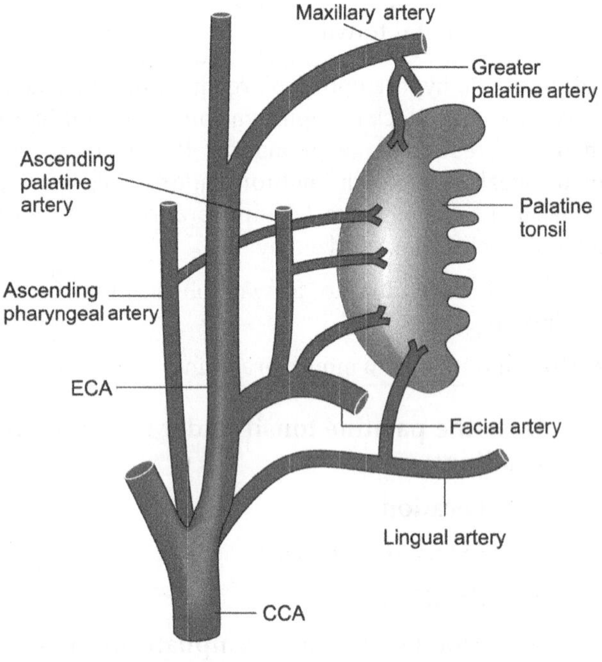

Fig. 72.2: Arterial supply of tonsil

tonsillar nodes as they are enlarged in tonsillitis).

Palatine tonsillectomy is surgical removal of palatine tonsil. During tonsillectomy:

- ***Severe haemorrhage may occur:***
  - From the *paratonsillar veins.*
  - From *tonsillar branch of facial artery.*
- ***Glossopharyngeal nerve*** may be injured causing loss of general and taste sensation from the posterior 1/3rd of the tongue.

Quinsy/Peritonsillar abscess is accumulation of pus in peritonsillar space in chronic tonsillitis.

73 CHAPTER PHARYNX

1. **Describe pharynx under the following headings:**
   a. **Extent**
   b. **Subdivisions and their important features**

Ans. Pharynx is a funnel shaped fibromuscular tube forming the upper part of air and food passage. It is 12-14 cm long. Its width at upper end is 3.5 cm and at lower end 1.5 cm. It is continuous inferiorly with esophagus.

a. **Extent:** From base of skull to the lower border of cricoids cartilage (vertebral level C6).

b. **Subdivisions and their important features:** The anterior wall of pharynx is deficient anteriorly as it opens into nasal cavity, oral cavity and larynx from above downwards. Therefore, the subdivisions of pharynx are:

– *Nasopharynx:*
  - Extends from base of skull to the soft palate.
  - Has roof, posterior wall and lateral wall.
  - *Communicates:*
    - o Anteriorly with nasal cavity.
    - o Inferiorly with oropharynx through *pharyngeal isthmus.*
    - o Laterally thorough auditory tube with middle ear.
  - Pharyngeal tonsil projects in the nasopharynx from the junction of its roof and posterior wall.
  - The medial end of auditory or pharyngotympanic tube opens through tubal orifice into the lateral wall on each side.
    - o Tubal orifice is bounded above and posterioly by tubal elevation. Tubal tonsil is located here.
    - o Two mucosal folds extend from the tubal elevation.
      - ▪ Salpingopalatine fold containing levator palati muscle extends to the soft palate.
      - ▪ Salpingopharyngeal fold containing salpingopharyngeus muscle.

> • Hypertrophy of pharyngeal tonsil is called adenoids.
>
> • A midline pharyngeal bursa present in the pharyngeal tonsil denotes the site of attachment of notochord to the endoderm of primitive pharynx.
>
> • A depression in the mucosa above the pharyngeal tonsil denotes the site of path of Rathke's pouch. Sometimes remnant cells of Rathke's pouch may give rise to pharyngeal hypophysis, which may become malignant.

  - Extends from soft palate to the tip of epiglottis.
  - *Communicates:*
    - o Above: With nasopharynx through pharyngeal isthmus.
    - o Below: With laryngopharynx.
    - o In front: With oral cavity through oropharyngeal isthmus (between the palatoglossal arches).
  - Lateral wall presents palatoglossal and palatopharyngeal arches enclosing tonsillar fossa for the palatine tonsil.

- *Laryngopharynx:*
  - Extends from upper border of epiglottis to their lower border of cricoids cartilage.
  - *Communicates:*
    - o Above: With oropharynx.
    - o Below: With oesophagus.
    - o Anteriorly: With larynx through laryngeal inlet.
  - Lateral wall has recess known as piriform fossa on either side of the laryngeal inlet. The boundaries of piriform fossa are:
    - o Medial: Aryepiglottic fold.
    - o Lateral: Mucosa covering the thyrohyoid membrane and lamina of thyroid cartilage.

Piriform fossa:

- One important feature of piriform fossa is that internal laryngeal nerve and superior laryngeal vessels pierce the thyrohyoid membrane and transverse from lateral to medial beneath the mucosa of the floor of piriform fossa to reach larynx.
- Occasionally, ingested food particles such as fish bone may get impacted in the fossa. If care is not taken while removing the foreign particle, internal laryngeal nerve may be injured causing loss of sensations from the supraglottic part of larynx.

2. **Enumerate:**
   a. **Layers of pharyngeal wall**
   b. **Muscles of pharynx**
   c. **Nerves supplying pharynx**
   d. **Structures passing:**
      - **Above the superior constrictor**
      - **Between superior and middle constrictor**
      - **Between middle and inferior constrictor**
      - **Below the inferior constrictor**

Ans. a. Layers of pharyngeal wall:

- Mucosa.
- Submucosa.
- Pharyngobasilar fascia.
- Muscular coat (inner circular and outer longitudinal muscles).
- Buccopharyngeal fascia.

b. Muscles of pharynx:

- ***Circular layer***
  - Superior, middle and inferior constrictors.
- ***Longitudinal layer***
  - Stylopharyngeus, palatopharyngeus and salpingopharyngeus.

c. Nerves supplying pharynx:

- ***Motor supply:*** All the muscles of pharynx are supplied by vagoaccessory complex via pharyngeal plexus of nerves except stylopharyngeus which is supplied by glossopharyngeal nerve.
- ***Sensory supply:***
  - *Nasopharynx:* By pharyngeal branch of pterygopalatine ganglion (fibers from maxillary nerve).
  - *Oropharynx:* By glossopharyngeal nerve.
  - *Laryngopharynx:* By internal pharyngeal nerve.

d. Structures passing through the gaps between the constrictors of pharynx: (Fig. 73.1)

- ***Above the superior constrictor:***
  - Auditory tube.
  - Levator veli palatini.
  - Ascending palatine artery.
  - Palatine branch of ascending pharyngeal artery.
- ***Between superior and middle constrictor:***
  - Stylopharyngeus muscle.
  - Glossopharyngeal nerve.
- ***Between middle and inferior constrictor:***
  - Internal laryngeal nerve.
  - Superior laryngeal vessels.

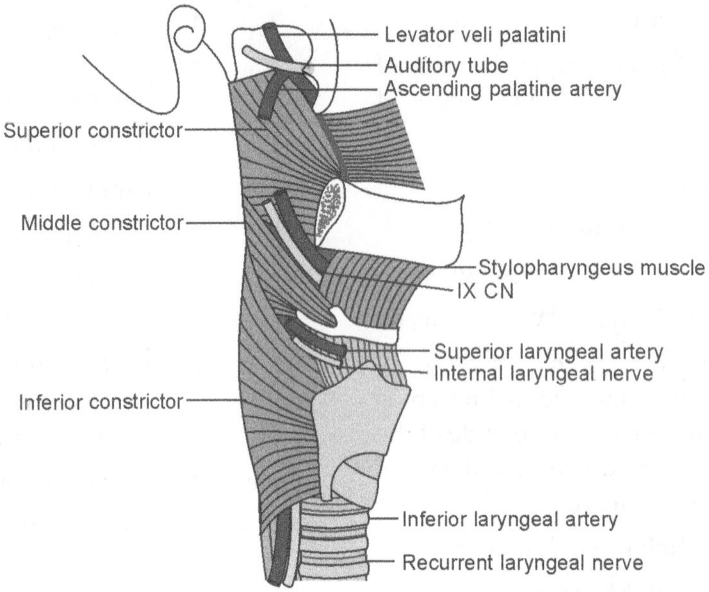

Fig. 73.1: Structures passing through the gaps between the constrictors of pharynx

- *Below the inferior constrictor:*
  - Recurrent laryngeal nerve.
  - Inferior laryngeal vessels.

3. **Describe briefly:**
   a. **Passavant's ridge**
   b. **Killian's dehiscence and pharyngeal diverticulum**

Ans. a. Passavant's ridge: Some fibers of palatopharyngeus muscle pass horizontally backwards from the palatine aponeurosis along the lateral and posterior wall of nasopharyngeal isthmus to blend with superior constrictor muscle. When the soft palate is elevated the muscle forms a ridge (Passavant's ridge). During swallowing the soft palate and Passavant's ridge are approximated to shut off nasopharynx from oropharynx which prevents regurgitation of food into the nasopharynx and nasal cavity.

b. Killian's dehiscence and pharyngeal diverticulum (Fig. 73.2): Inferior constrictor muscle has two parts viz. thyropharyngeus and cricopharyngeus. Fibers of thyropharyngeus pass obliquely to the posterior median raphe, whereas the fibers of cricopharyngeus run horizontally. A potential gap, therefore, exists between the thyropharyngeus and cricopharyngeus muscles which is seen as a dimple in the lining mucosa of this region of pharynx. Pharyngeal diverticulum may develop through this weak area of pharynx in case of neuromuscular incoordination, i.e., if cricopharyngeus fails to relax following contraction of thyropharyneus part. The increased pressure forces the mucosa and submucosa posteriorly through the Killian dehiscence. The diverticulum gradually enlarges in downward direction behind the pharynx.

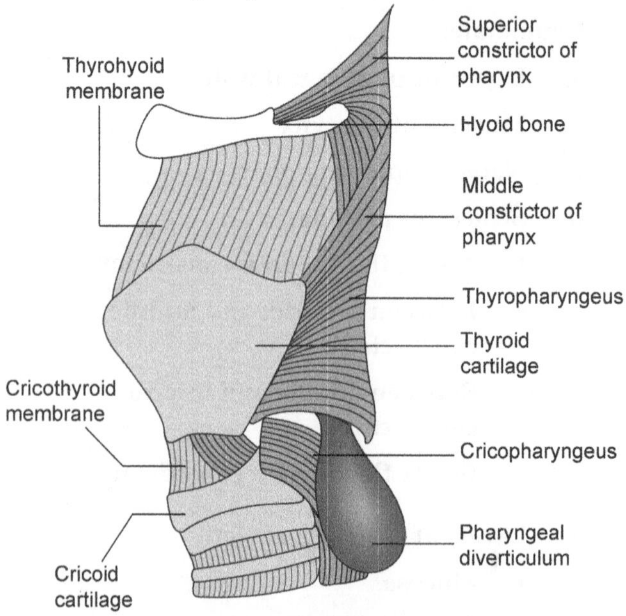

Fig. 73.2: Pharyngeal diverticulum

74

CHAPTER

LARYNX

1. Describe briefly larynx under the following headings:

a. Functions

b. Location

c. Subdivisions of laryngeal cavity

d. True and false vocal cords

Ans. a. **Functions:** Larynx is the organ of voice production (voice box) and part of upper respiratory tract.

b. **Location:** It is located in front of the neck opposite 3rd to 6th cervical vertebrae in adults. It extends from the upper border of epiglottis to the lower border of cricoids cartilage.

c. **Subdivisions of laryngeal cavity:** Laryngeal cavity is sub-divided into three parts by two pairs of mucosal folds, i.e., upper vestibular and lower vocal folds.

- ***Vestibule:*** Extends from the laryngeal inlet to the vestibular fold.
- ***Ventricle/sinus:*** Extends between the vestibular and vocal folds.
- ***Infraglottic part:*** Extends from the vocal fold to the lower border of the cricoids cartilage.

> **Saccule** is a blind diverticulum that extends upwards from the anterior part of sinus/ventricle of larynx. The secretions of the mucous glands of saccule lubricate the vocal folds.
>
> **Laryngocele:** Abnormally enlarged, distended and air filled saccule.

- ***Rima glottidis:*** Is the narrowest part of the laryngeal cavity. It is bounded by:
  - Vocal folds and vocal processes of arytenoids laterally.
  - Thyroid cartilage anteriorly.
  - Interarytenoid mucosal fold posteriorly.

> **Laryngeal obstruction** (choking) is caused by aspirated food particles that are usually lodged at the rima glottidis.

d. **True vocal cords (vocal folds):**

- Are called true vocal cords because their movement is responsible for phonation.
- Each vocal fold contains vocal ligament and vocalis muscle.
- Extend from the angle of thyroid cartilage to the vocal process of arytenoids cartilage.
- Alter the shape and size of rima glottidis during respiration and phonation.
- Are lined by stratified squamous nonkeratinized epithelium.
- Appear pearly white in laryngoscopy due to the absence of blood capillaries, submucosa and the type of covering epithelium.

False vocal cords (vestibular folds):

- Are called so because they do not take part in phonation.
- Each contains vestibular ligament.
- Are covered by pseudostratified ciliated epithelium.
- Have submucosa.
- Appear pink in laryngoscopy due to the presence of blood capillaries in the submucosa.

2. **Enumerate:**
   a. **Cartilages of larynx**
   b. **Ligaments and membranes of larynx**
   c. **Intrinsic muscles of larynx and their action**
   d. **Extrinsic muscles of the larynx and their action**
   e. **Nerves supplying larynx**

Ans. a. **Cartilages of larynx (Fig. 74.1a,b):** The framework of larynx is made up of cartilages and membranes.

- ***Unpaired cartilages:***
  - *Thyroid cartilage:* V-shaped hyaline cartilage with two laminae fused in the median plane that forms a median laryngeal prominence (Adam's apple) particularly apparent in males. An oblique line on the lateral surface of lamina provides attachment to sternothyroid, thyrohyoid and inferior constrictor of pharynx.
  - *Cricoid cartilage:* Signet ring shaped hyaline cartilage. It lies at the level of C6 vertebra and its lower border marks the end of larynx.
  - *Epiglottis:* Leaf shaped elastic cartilage. Its lower end is attached to the back of thyroid cartilage.
- ***Paired cartilages:***
  - *Arytenoid cartilages:* Partly elastic and partly hyaline cartilages. Are pyramid shaped and have two processes:
    - Vocal processes: Provides attachment to vocal cord and vocalis muscle.
    - Muscular process: Provides attachment to thyroarytenoid, lateral and posterior cricoarytenoids.
    - Corniculate cartilages: Elastic cartilages that lie on the apex of arytenoids cartilage within the aryepiglottic folds.
    - Cuneiform cartilages: Elastic cartilages that lie anterior to corniculate cartilages within the aryepiglottic folds.

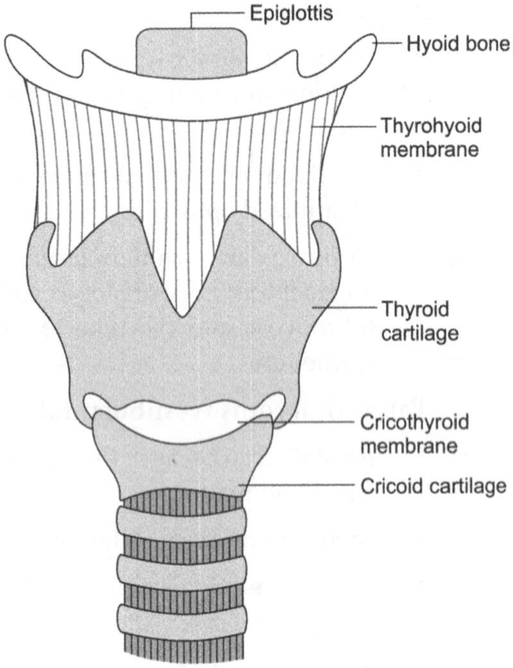

(a) Anterior view

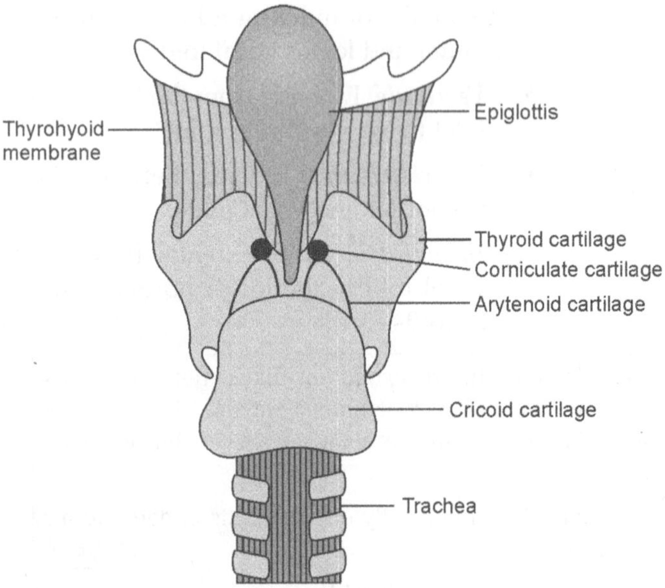

(b) Posterior view

Fig. 74.1: Cartilages of larynx

b. **Membranes and ligaments of larynx:**
- ***Extrinsic membrane:*** Lie external to the laryngeal cavity.
  - *Thyrohyoid membrane:*
    - Extends between the upper border of thyroid cartilage and upper border of body and greater cornu of hyoid bone.
    - Its thick median part forms median thyrohyoid ligament and thickened posterior margins form lateral thyrohyoid ligaments.
    - Is pierced by internal laryngeal nerve and superior laryngeal vessels.
- ***Extrinsic ligaments:***
  - Median cricothyroid ligament.
  - Cricotracheal ligament.
  - Hyoepiglottic ligament.
- ***Intrinsic membranes (Fig. 74.2):*** Are lined on inner aspect by laryngeal mucosa.
  - *Quadrangular/quadrate membrane:*
    - Is a quadrangular shaped fibroelastic membrane in the lateral wall of vestibule of larynx.
    - Its upper free margin is in aryepiglottic fold and free lower margin forms vestibular ligament (false vocal cord).
    - Is attached to epiglottis, thyroid and arytenoids cartilages.
  - *Cricovocal membrane:*
    - Is triangular fibroelastic membrane in the lateral wall of infraglottic part of the larynx.
    - Its upper free margin forms vocal ligament (true vocal cord).
    - Its lower margin is attached to the arch of cricoids cartilage.
    - Is attached to thyroid, cricoids and arytenoids cartilages.
    - Cricovocal membranes are continuous across the midline and form conus elasticus.

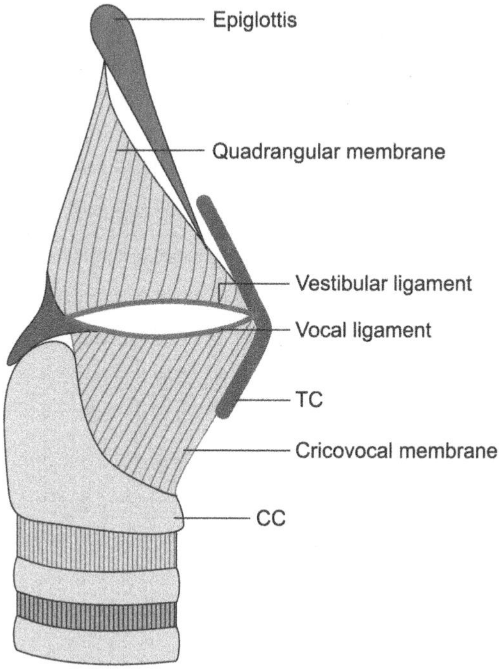

Fig. 74.2: Intrinsic membranes of larynx

c. **Intrinsic muscles of larynx and their action:** Their attachments are confined to the cartilages of larynx.

	Muscle	*Action*
Muscles that close or open the glottis	Posterior cricoarytenoid	Abduct vocal cord
	Lateral cricoarytenoid	Adduct vocal cord
	Transverse arytenoid	
Muscles that tense or relax the vocal cords	Cricothyroid	Tense the vocal cord
	Thyroarytenoid	Relax the vocal cord
	Vocalis	
Muscles that open or close the laryngeal inlet	Thyroepiglotticus	Open the laryngeal orifice
	Aryepiglotticus	Close the laryngeal orifice
	Oblique arytenoids	

Posterior cricoarytenoid muscles are known as safety muscles of the larynx because they are the only muscles which abduct the vocal cords. If they are paralysed the unopposed action of adductors of vocal cord can block the air entry which can be fatal.

d. **Extrinsic muscles of the larynx and their action:** They connect the laryngeal cartilages to the neighbouring structures.

Action	*Muscles*	
Elevators of larynx	Primary elevators (attached to thyroid cartilage)	Stylopharyngeus
		Palatopharyngeus
		Salpingopharyngeus Thyrohyoid
	Secondary elevators (attached to hyoid bone)	Mylohyoid
		Geniohyoid
		Stylohyoid
		Digastric
Depressors oflarynx	Sternohyoid	
	Sternothyroid	
	Omohyoid	

e. **Nerves supplying larynx:**

- *Motor supply:* All the intrinsic muscles of larynx are supplied by the recurrent laryngeal nerve except cricothyroid which is supplied by external laryngeal nerve.
- *Sensory supply:* Mucous membrane of larynx is supplied by branches of vagus nerve:
  - *Above the vocal cords:* Internal laryngeal nerve (branch of superior laryngeal nerve).
  - *Below the vocal cords:* Recurrent laryngeal nerve.

Damage to recurrent laryngeal nerve:

- ***Unilateral injury:***
  - Results in ipsilateral paralysis of all intrinsic muscles except cricothyroid.
  - Paralysed vocal cord lies in paramedian position.
  - Does not give rise to respiratory symptoms but voice changes such as ing hoarseness may occur.
- ***Bilateral injury:***
  - Vocal cords lie in cadaveric position.
  - Result in breathing difficulties and aphonia, i.e., inability to speak.

75 CHAPTER

NASAL CAVITY AND PARANASAL AIR SINUSES

1. **Enumerate:**
   a. **Bones and cartilages forming nasal septum**
   b. **Bones and cartilages forming lateral wall of nose**
   c. **Openings in the lateral wall of nose**
   d. **Functions of paranasal air sinuses**

Ans. a. **Bones and cartilages forming nasal septum: (Fig. 75.1)**

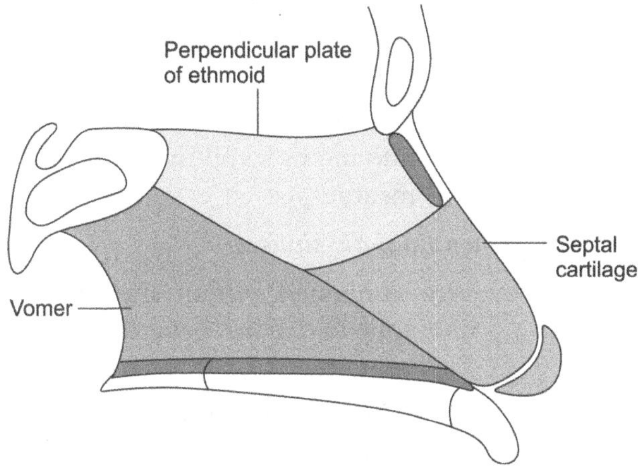

Fig. 75.1: Bones and cartilages forming nasal septum

- *Bones:*
  - Perpendicular plate of ethmoid bone.
  - Vomer.
  - Small contribution from the processes of frontal, maxillary, nasal and palatine bones.
- *Cartilages:*
  - Septal cartilage.
  - Septal processes of major alar cartilages.

b. **Bones and cartilages forming lateral wall of nose:**

- *Bones:*
  - Nasal bone.
  - Frontal process of maxilla.
  - Lacrimal bone.
  - Superior and middle conchae (ethmoid bone).
  - Inferior concha.
  - Perpendicular plate of palatine.
  - Medial pterygoid plate of sphenoid.
- *Cartilages:*
  - Lateral nasal cartilage.
  - Major alar cartilage.
  - Minor alar cartilage.

c. **Openings in the lateral wall of nose: (Fig. 75.2)**

Site		*Opening/s*
Sphenoethmoidal recess		Sphenoidal air sinus
Superior meatus		Posterior ethmoidal sinus
Middle meatus	On bulla ethmoidalis	Middle ethmoidal air sinus
	In hiatus semilunaris	Frontal air sinus Anterior ethmoidal air sinus Maxillary air sinus
Inferior meatus		Nasolacrimal duct

d. **Functions of paranasal air sinuses:**

- Add resonance to the voice.
- Make the skull lighter.
- Humidify and warm the inspired air.

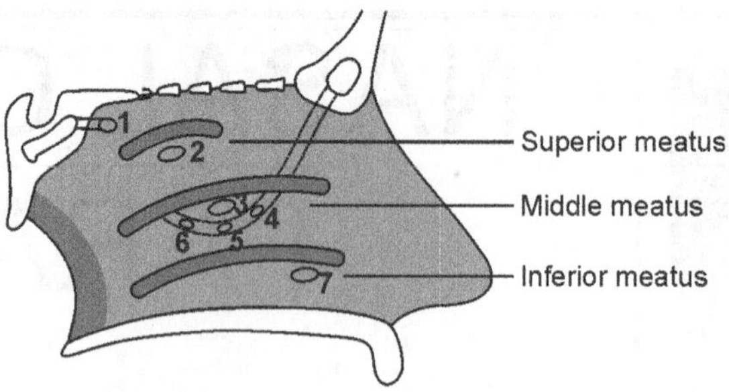

Fig. 75.2: Openings in the lateral wall of nose

2. **Draw labeled diagram to show arteries supplying nasal septum.**

Ans. Arteries supplying nasal septum: (Fig. 75.3)

Little's area or Kiesselbach's area:
- Is the anteroinferior part of nasal septum.
- It is the site of rich anastomoses between the branches of sphenopalatine, anterior ethmoidal, greater palatine and superior labial branch of facial artery.
- Nose picking results in bleeding from this site (epistaxis).

3. **Describe briefly paranasal air sinuses.**

Ans. Paranasal air sinuses: Are air filled spaces present in the bones surrounding the nasal cavity.

- ***Frontal air sinus:***
  - Lies in frontal bone deep to superciliary arches.
  - Opens into hiatus semilunaris of the middle meatus via frontonasal duct.
  - Is supplied by supraorbital branch of ophthalmic nerve.
- ***Ethmoidal air sinuses:***
  - Consist of number of ethmoidal air cells present within the ethmoidal labyrinth between the orbit and nasal cavity.
  - Are innervated by anterior and posterior ethmoidal nerves (branches of ophthalmic nerve).
  - Are divided into following groups:
    - *Posterior ethmoidal air cells:* Drain into superior meatus.
    - *Middle ethmoidal air cells:* Drain on summit of ethmoidal bulla of the middle meatus.
    - *Anterior ethmoidal cells:* Drain into hiatus semilunaris of middle meatus.
- ***Sphenoidal air sinuses:***
  - Are contained within the body of the sphenoid bone behind the nasal cavity.
  - Open into sphenoethmoidal recess of the nasal cavity.

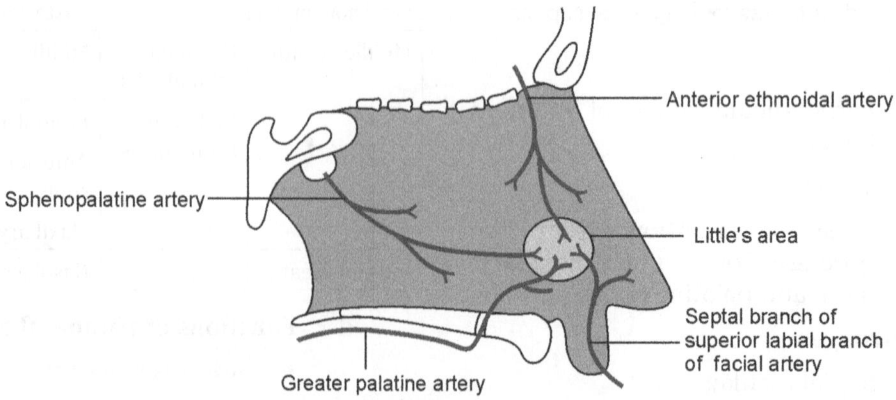

Fig. 75.3: Arteries supplying nasal septum

- Important relations:
  - *Above:* Optic chiasma and pituitary gland.
  - *Laterally:* Cavernous sinus and carotid artery.
- Are innervated by posterior ethmoidal and branches from maxillary nerve via pterygopalatine ganglion.

• *Maxillary air sinuses:*
- Are the largest and the only paranasal sinuses present at the time of birth.
- Are located in the body of maxilla lateral to the nasal cavity and inferior to the floor of orbit.
- Are pyramidal in shape with following boundaries:
  - Apex extends into zygomatic process of maxilla.
  - Base is formed by nasal surface of body of maxilla.
  - Roof is formed by floor of orbit.
  - Anterior wall is formed by anterior surface of maxilla.
  - Posterior wall is related to infratemporal fossa.
  - Floor is formed by alveolar and palatine process of maxilla.
- Drain into posterior part of hiatus semilunaris of middle meatus.
- Are innervated by infraorbital and superior alveolar nerves.

Maxillary air sinus is the most commonly infected air sinus due to:

- High position of its opening which hinders the natural drainage of sinus.
- Pus from infected frontal air sinus may run via hiatus semilunaris the maxillary sinus because of the location of their openings.

Due to anatomical proximity of the sphenoidal sinus and pituitary gland, the sinus is used as a route to approach pituitary gland in transnasal, transsphenoidal hypophysectomy.

CHAPTER 76 PTERYGOPALATINE FOSSA

1. **Enumerate:**
   a. **Structures forming boundaries of pterygopalatine fossa**
   b. **Openings in the pterygopalatine fossa and structures passing through them**
   c. **Contents of pterygopalatine fossa**

Ans. a. **Structures forming boundaries of pterygopalatine fossa:**

It is a pyramidal space located deep to infratemporal fossa and below the apex of orbit. Its boundaries are formed by the following structures:

- *Anterior:* Posterior surface of maxilla.
- *Posterior:* Pterygoid process and greater wing of sphenoid. Three openings are:
  - Foramen rotundum.
  - Pterygoid canal.
  - Palatovaginal canal.
- *Medial:* Perpendicular plate of palatine bone. The opening is:
  - Sphenopalatine foramen.
- *Lateral:* It is open. Pterygomaxillary fissure is present.
- *Inferior:* Anterior and posterior walls meet, i.e., maxilla and pterygoid process.
- *Superior:* Body of sphenoid.

b. **Openings in the pterygopalatine fossa and structures passing through them:**

- *Anterior:* No openings.
- *Posterior:* Three openings are:
  - *Foramen rotundum to middle cranial cavity:* Transmits maxillary nerve.
  - *Pterygoid canal to foramen lacerum:* Transmits nerve to pterygoid canal.
  - *Palatovaginal canal to nasophraynx:* Transmits pharyngeal nerves.
- ***Medial: Sphenopalatine foramen to the nasal cavity:*** Transmits sphenopalatine artery and nasopalatine nerve.
- ***Lateral: Pterygomaxillary fissure to the infratemporal fossa:*** Transmits 3rd part of maxillary artery.
- ***Inferior: Greater and lesser palatine canals to oral cavity:*** Transmit greater and lesser palatine nerve and vessels.
- ***Anterosuperior: Inferior orbital fissure to orbit:*** Transmits infraorbital nerve and vessels.

c. **Contents of pterygopalatine fossa:**

- Maxillary nerve and its branches.
- Pterygopalatine ganglion and its branches.
- Third part of maxillary artery and its branches.

2. **Describe briefly the course, branches and distribution of maxillary nerve.**

Ans. Maxillary nerve:

- Is the 2nd division of trigeminal nerve.
- Is a pure sensory nerve.

Course:

- Commences from the anterior border of trigeminal ganglion.
- Passes along the lateral wall of the cavernous sinus.
- Leaves the cranial cavity via foramen rotundum.

- Enters pterygopalatine fossa.
- Continues as infraorbital nerve by passing through inferior orbital fissure and then infraorbital canal in the floor of orbit.

Branches and distribution:

- ***In the cranial cavity: Meningeal branch:*** Innervates dura mater of the middle cranial fossa.
- ***In the pterygopalatine fossa:***
  - 2-3 ganglionic branches to pterygopalatine ganglion (sensory branches pass through the branches of pterygopalatine ganglion to nasal cavity palate, nasopharynx and orbit).
  - *Posterior superior alveolar nerves:* Supply upper molar teeth and maxillary sinus.
  - *Zygomatic nerve:* Dives into zygomaticotemporal and zygomaticofacial nerves which supply:
    - Skin over the temporal region and over the zygomatic bone.
    - Zygomaticotemporal branch carries postganglionic parasympathetic fibers (secretomotor fibers) from pterygopalatine ganglion to the lacrimal branch of ophthalmic nerve which supplies lacrimal gland.
- ***Infraorbital nerve:***
  - *In the infraorbital canal:*
    - Middle superior alveolar nerve: Innervates upper premolar teeth, gums and maxillary sinus.
    - Anterior superior alveolar nerve: Innervates upper canine and incisors, gums and maxillary sinus.
  - *On the face:*
    - Palpebral branch to lower eyelid.
    - Nasal branch to ala of nose.
    - Labial branch of upper lip.

3. **Draw labeled diagram showing connections of pterygopalatine ganglion.**

Ans. See Figure 76.1.

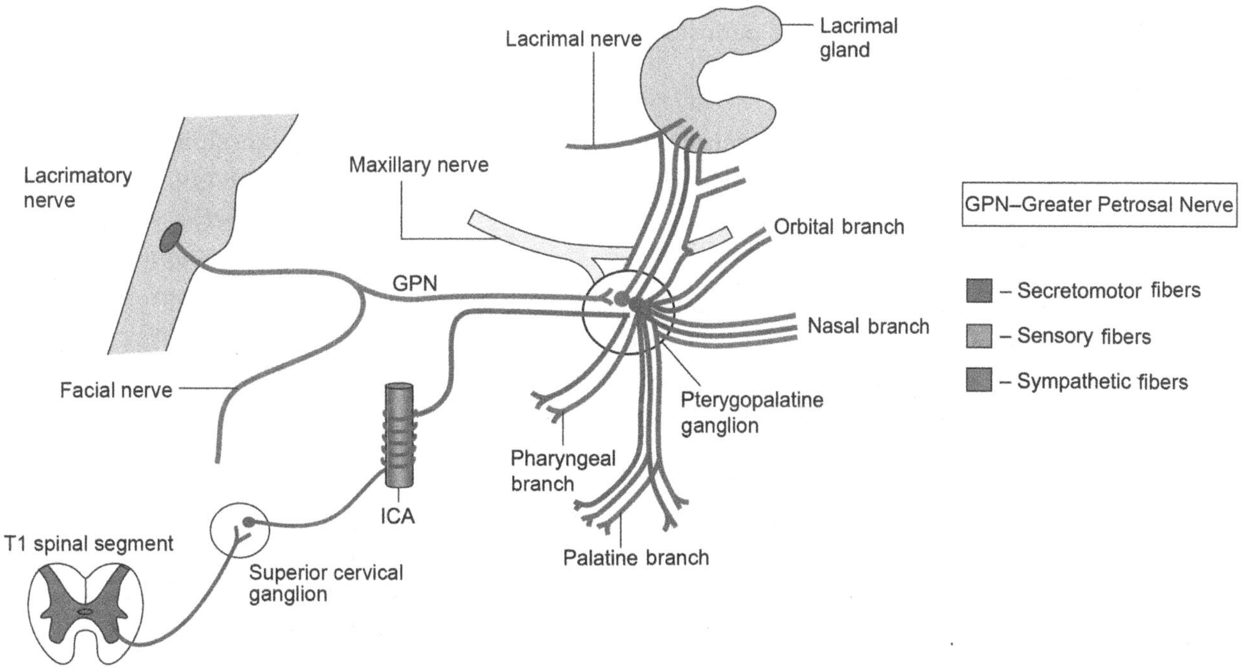

Fig. 76.1: Pterygopalatine ganglion

77 CHAPTER

DURA MATER AND DURAL VENOUS SINUSES

1. **Enumerate:**
   a. **Layers of meninges covering brain**
   b. **Dural folds**
   c. **Dural venous sinuses**

Ans. a. Layers of meninges covering brain:

- *Dura mater:*
  - Is tough, fibrous, outermost layer.
  - Epidural space separates dura mater from skull bones.
  - Subdural space separates it from arachnoid mater.
  - Has two layers – outer periosteal and inner endosteal.
- *Arachnoid mater:*
  - Thin transparent layer connected to pia mater by web like trabeculae.
  - Is separated from pia mater by subarachnoid space which is filled with CSF and contains the main blood vessels supplying brain.
  - Forms arachnoid villi that project into dural venous sinuses and help in drainage of CSF.
- *Pia mater:*
  - Closely applied to the brain and dips into the sulci.

> **Subdural hematoma:** It is due to rupture of cerebral veins as they pass from brain to dural venous sinuses.
>
> **Epidural hematoma:** Due to rupture of middle meningeal artery or vein.
>
> **Subarachnoid hemorrhage:** It results usually from the rupture of aneurysm of an artery at the base of brain. The diagnosis is confirmed by presence of blood in the CSF.

b. Dural folds:

- *Falx cerebri:*
  - Is sickle shaped of dura mater lying between the two cerebral hemispheres.
  - Extends from crista galli to the tentorium cerebelli.
  - Its upper margin encloses superior sagittal sinus.
  - Its free lower margin contains inferior sagittal sinus.
- *Falx cerebelli:*
  - Small sickle shaped fold between the two cerebellar hemispheres.
  - Encloses occipital sinus along its posterior margin.
- *Tentorium cerebelli:*
  - Is a crescentic fold that separates cerebellum from the occipital lobes of cerebrum.
  - Its free anterior concave border bounds tentorial notch and is attached to anterior clinoid process.
  - Its attached posterolateral margin encloses transverse and sigmoid sinuses on either side.
- *Diaphragma sellae:*
  - Is a horizontal fold that forms roof of hypophyseal fossa and covers pituitary gland.
  - It has a central aperture for the infundibulum (hypophyseal stalk).

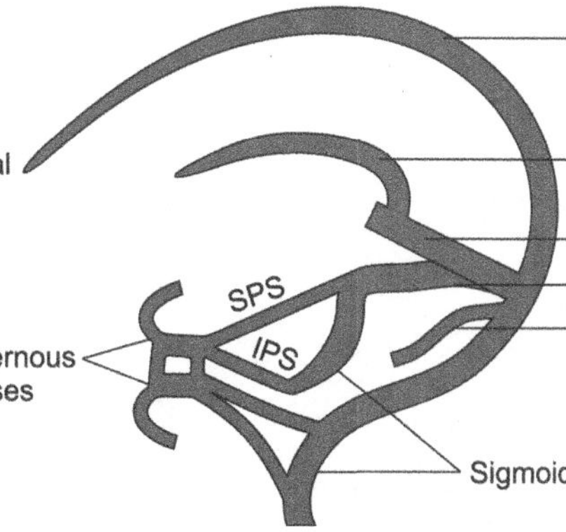

Fig. 77.1: Dural venous sinuses

c. **Dural venous sinuses: (Fig. 77.1)**

- Venous channels present usually between the two layers of dura mater.
- Are lined by endothelium.
- Have no muscle tissue in their walls.
- Have no valves.
- *Drain blood from:*
  - Superior sagittal sinus.
  - Brain.
  - Meninges.
  - Cranial bones.
- Also drains CSF.
- Communicate with veins outside the cranial cavity via emissary veins.
- ***Are total 20 in number:*** 6 unpaired and 7 paired.
- ***Unpaired dural venous sinuses:***
  - Superior sagittal sinus.
  - Inferior sagittal sinus.
  - Straight sinus.
  - Occipital sinus.
  - Anterior intercavernous sinus.
  - Posterior intercavernous sinus.
- ***Paired dural venous sinuses:***
  - Cavernous sinuses.
  - Superior petrosal sinuses.
  - Inferior petrosal sinuses.
  - Transverse sinuses.
  - Sigmoid sinuses.
  - Sphenoparietal sinuses.
  - Petrosquamous sinuses.
  - Superior sagittal sinuses.

Venous channels other than dural venous sinuses that drain blood from the cranial cavity are:

Basilar plexus of veins:

- Are interconnecting venous channels present on the basilar part of occipital bone.
- Are connected to the inferior petrosal sinuses.
- Communicate inferiorly with the intervertebral venous plexuses.

Diploic veins:

- Are located in the diploe of the skull bones (venous spaces between the outer and inner tables of the flat skull bones.
- Are valveless.
- Are connected to the dural venous sinuses via emissary veins.

Emissary veins:

- Small veins that connect dural venous sinuses to the extracranial and diploic veins.
- Do not have valves.
- Their function is to equalize the venous pressure within and outside the cranium.

* As they are valveless they may carry extracranial infections to the intracranial venous sinuses leading to venous thrombosis/meningitis/encephalitis.

2. **Describe briefly the location, relations, tributaries, draining channels and communications of cavernous sinuses.**

Ans. Cavernous sinuses: (Fig. 77.2)

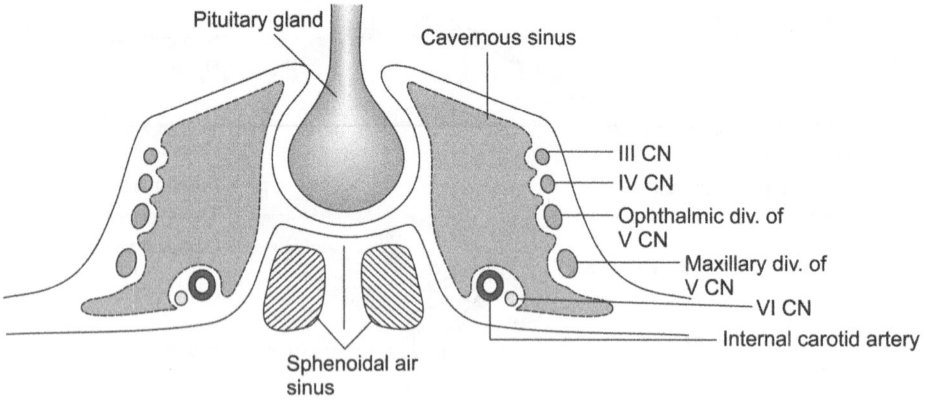

Fig. 77.2: Cavernous sinuses and their relations

- ***Location:***
  - Are the paired venous sinuses located between the endosteal and periosteal layers of dura mater in the middle cranial fossa on either side of the body of sphenoid bone.
  - Extend from the medial end of superior orbital fissure to the apex of petrous temporal bone (2 cm long and 1 cm wide).
- ***Relations:***
  - *With the structures outside the sinus:*
    - Superior: Optic chiasma, internal carotid artery.
    - Inferior: Foramen lacerum.
    - Medial: Pituitary gland, sphenoidal air sinus.
    - Lateral: Temporal lobe and uncus.
  - *Structures in the lateral wall of the sinus:* Four cranial nerves pass along the lateral wall of the sinus. From above downwards they are:
    - Oculomotor nerve (III CN).
    - Trochlear nerve (IV CN) enter orbit through superior orbital fissure.
    - Ophthalmic division of trigeminal nerve.
    - Maxillary division of trigeminal nerve–enters pterygopalatine fossa via foramen rotundum.
  - *Structures passing through the sinus:*
    - Internal carotid artery surrounded by sympathetic plexus.
    - Abducent nerve (VI CN) – is inferolateral to the artery.

  * All the structures, i.e., those in the lateral wall and those passing through the sinus are separated from the venous blood by endothelial lining.
- ***Tributaries:***
  - Superior ophthalmic vein. } From the orbit
  - Inferior ophthalmic vein. } From the orbit
  - Central vein of retina. } From the orbit
  - Middle meningeal vein.
  - Sphenoparietal sinus. } From the brain
  - Superficial middle cerebral vein. } From the brain
  - Inferior cerebral veins.
  - Hypophyseal veins.
- ***Draining channels:*** Venous blood from cavernous sinus drains into:
  - Junction of transverse and sigmoid sinuses via superior petrosal sinus.
  - Internal jugular vein via inferior petrosal sinus.
- ***Communications:*** Cavernous sinus communicates with:
  - Facial vein via superior ophthalmic vein.
  - Pterygoid plexus of veins via emissary veins passing through foramen ovale.

- Opposite cavernous sinus via anterior and posterior intercavernous sinuses.
- Internal vertebral venous plexuses via basilar plexus of veins.

Cavernous sinus thrombosis: The most common cause is spread of infection from the dangerous area of face (squeezing a pimple or boil). The signs and symptoms (due to involvement of closely related structures) are:

- ***Papilledema (edema of optic disc):*** Due to engorgement of central vein of retina.

Contd.

Contd.

- ***Exophthalmos/proptosis:*** Due to engorgement of ophthalmic veins.
- ***Ophthalmoplegia (paralysis of extraocular muscles):*** Due to involvement of III, IV and VI cranial nerves which supply extraocular muscles.
- ***Dilated and fixed pupil and ptosis:*** Due to involvement of oculomotor nerve (parasympathetic fibers).

Pulsating exophthalmos: Due to abnormal communication between cavernous sinus and internal carotid artery.

78 CHAPTER ORBIT AND EYEBALL

1. **Enumerate:**
   - a. **Contents of orbit**
   - b. **Extraocular muscles, their nerve supply and action**
   - c. **Branches of ophthalmic artery**
   - d. **Branches of ophthalmic nerve**

Ans. a. Contents of orbit:

- Eyeball.
- Extraocular muscles.
- *Nerves:* Oculomotor, trochlear, abducent and lacrimal, frontal and nasocilliary branches of trigeminal nerve.
- *Blood vessels:* Ophthalmic artery and its branches, superior and inferior ophthalmic veins.
- Lacrimal gland.
- Fat.

b. Extraocular muscles, their nerve supply and action: (Fig. 78.1)

Muscle	*Action*	*Nerve supply*
Superior rectus	Elevation, adduction and intorsion	Oculomotor
Inferior rectus	Depression, adduction and extorsion	Oculomotor
Lateral rectus	Abduction	Abducent
Medial rectus	Adduction	Oculomotor
Superior oblique	Depression, abduction and intorsion	Trochlear
Inferior oblique	Elevation, abduction and extorsion	Oculomotor

Strabismus/squint: Unilateral paralysis of lateral or medial rectus muscle results in deviation of eye to the opposite side.

- ***Internal or medial squint:*** Paralysis of lateral rectus muscle.
- ***External or lateral squint:*** Paralysis of medial rectus muscle.

Paralysis of superior oblique muscle: Causes diplopia on looking down as in walking down the stairs.

c. Branches of ophthalmic artery: Ophthalmic artery is a branch of internal carotid

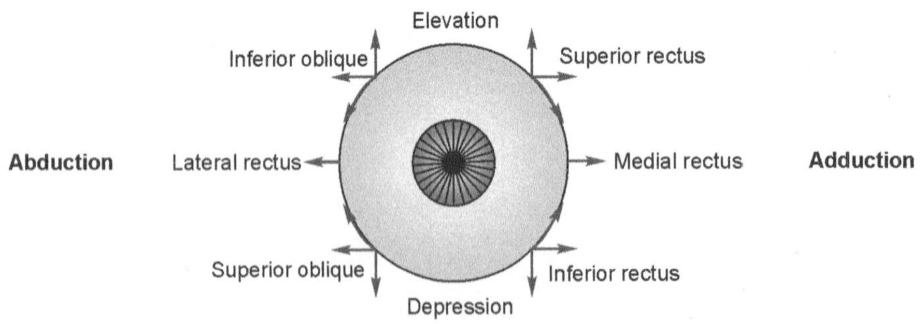

Fig. 78.1: Extraocular muscles and their action

artery and enters orbit through optic canal. Its branches are:

- ***Central artery of retina:*** Supplies optic nerve and retina.
- ***Muscular branches:*** Supply extra-ocular muscles. They also give rise to anterior ciliary branches which supply anterior part of eyeball.
- ***Long and short posterior ciliary branches:*** Pierce the sclera to supply eyeball.
- ***Lacrimal artery:*** Supplies lacrimal glands and via lateral palpebral branches supplies eyelids.
- ***Supraorbital artery:*** Reaches face by passing through the supraorbital foramen and supplies forehead and scalp.
- ***Posterior ethmoidal artery:*** Passes through the posterior ethmoidal foremen and supply posterior ethmoidal air cells.
- ***Anterior ethmoidal artery:*** Passes through anterior ethmoidal foramen and supplies anterior and middle ethmoidal air cells, frontal sinus, nasal cavity and external nose.
- ***Medial palpebral branches:*** Supply eyelids.
- ***Terminal branches:***
  - *Supratrochlear:* Leaves orbit and supplies forehead and scalp.
  - *Dorsal nasal artery:* Supplies side of nose and anastomoses with facial artery (anastomosis between branches of internal and external carotid arteries).

> Central artery of retina is an end artery and therefore, its occlusion results in blindness.

d. **Branches of ophthalmic nerve: (Fig. 78.2)**

- Is pure sensory nerve.
- Is divided into three branches which enter the orbit through the superior orbital fissure.
- ***Lacrimal nerve:*** Supplies lacrimal gland, conjunctiva and upper eyelid.

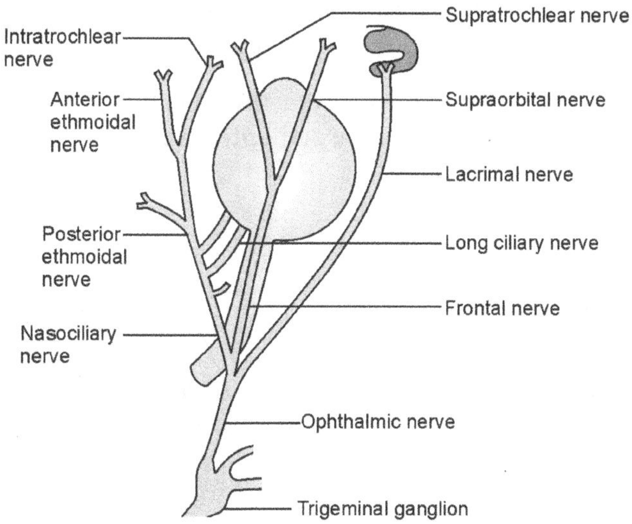

Fig. 78.2: Branches of ophthalmic nerve

- ***Frontal nerve:*** Divides into:
  - *Supraorbital nerve:* Supplies forehead, scalp, upper eyelid and frontal air sinus.
  - *Supratrochlear nerve:* Supplies forehead, scalp and upper eyelid.
- ***Nasociliary nerve:*** Gives following branches:
  - A *communicating branch to ciliary ganglion.*
  - 2-3 *long ciliary branches* which carry postganglionic sympathetic fibers to dilator papillae.
  - *Posterior ethmoidal nerve:* Supplies ethmoidal and sphenoidal air sinuses.
  - *Anterior ethmoidal nerve:* Divides into:
    - Internal nasal nerve: Divides into medial nasal and lateral nasal branches which supply nasal septum and lateral wall of nasal cavity respectively.
    - External nasal nerve: Supplies skin of nose.
  - *Infratrochlear nerve:* Supplies eyelids, conjunctiva, lacrimal sac and skin of nose.

2. **Draw schematic diagram to show:**
   a. **Structure of the eyeball**
   b. **Structure passing through the superior orbital fissure and optic canal**

Ans. a. **Structure of the eyeball (Fig. 78.3).**
b. **Structure passing through the superior orbital fissure and optic canal (Fig. 78.4).**

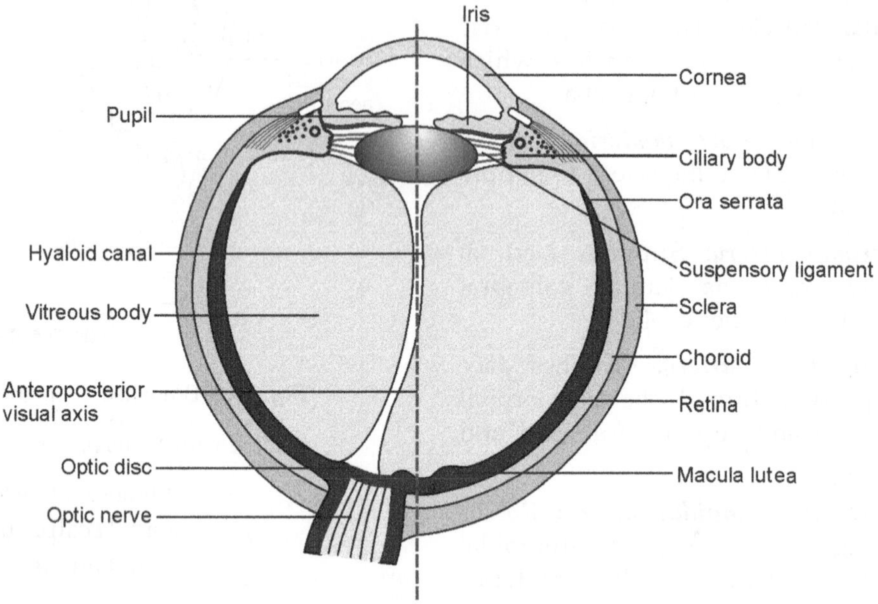

Fig. 78.3: Structure of the eyeball

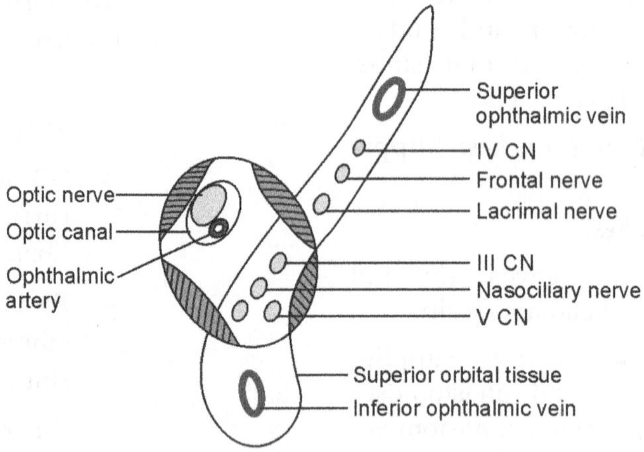

Fig. 78.4: Structure passing through the superior orbital fissure and optic canal

79 CHAPTER EAR

1. **Describe briefly:**
   a. **Sensory innervations of auricle**
   b. **Contents of middle ear/tympanic cavity**
   c. **Boundaries and relations of middle ear cavity**
   d. **Parts of internal ear**

Ans. a. Sensory innervations of auricle: The following nerves supply the skin of auricle:

- *Great auricular nerve (ventral ramii of C2, C3):* Supplies lower 1/3rd of the auricle/pinna on both the sides.
- *Auriculotemporal nerve:* Supplies upper 2/3rd of the lateral surface of auricle.
- *Lesser occipital (ventral ramus of C2):* Supplies upper 2/3rd of the medial/cranial surface of auricle.
- *Auricular branch of vagus:* Supplies the root of auricle (near external acoustic meatus).

* Few fibers of facial nerve accompany the auricular branch of vagus.

b. Contents of middle ear/tympanic cavity:

- *Three ear ossicles:* Malleus, incus and stapes.
- *Two muscles:* Tensor tympani and stapedius.
- *Nerves:* Chorda tympani (branch of facial nerve) and tympanic plexus (formed by branch of glossopharyngeal nerve and caroticotympanic nerves from sympathetic plexus around internal carotid artery).
- Blood vessels of middle ear.
- Air.

c. Boundaries and relations of middle ear cavity: (Fig. 79.1)

- Middle ear cavity is an air filled biconcave space in the petrous part of temporal nerve.
- ***It is bounded by the following six walls:***
  – *Roof/tegmental wall:* Is formed by tegmen tympani which separates its middle ear from middle

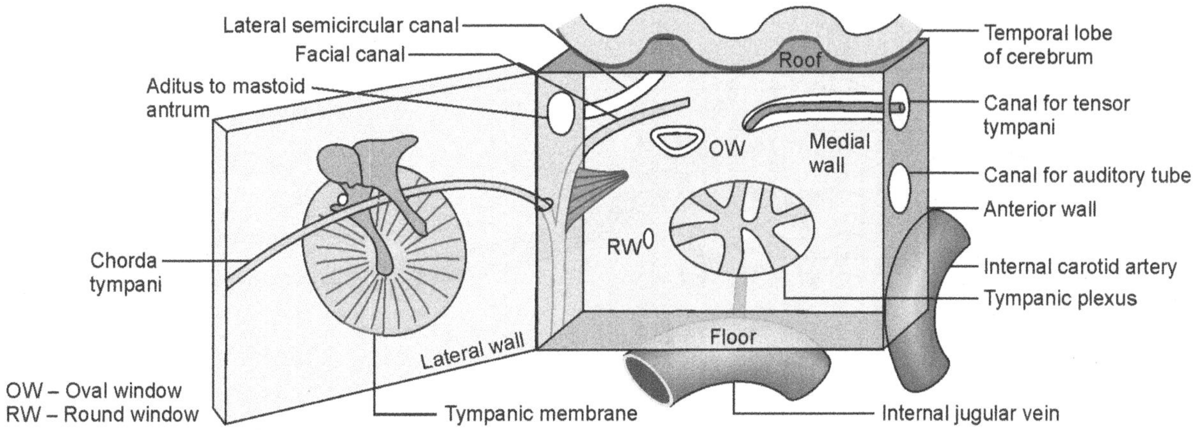

Fig. 79.1: Boundaries and relations of middle ear cavity

cranial fossa and temporal lobe of cerebrum.

- *Floor/jugular wall:* Formed by jugular fossa which separates middle ear from internal jugular vein.
- *Anterior/carotid wall:* Is narrow and has three openings. From above downwards they are:
  - Anterior canaliculus for chorda tympani nerve.
  - Canal for tensor tympani.
  - Opening of auditory tube.

* Below the auditory tube a thin bony lamina separates middle ear from the carotid canal and internal carotid artery.

- *Posterior/mastoid wall:* Aditus to mastoid antrum leads to mastoid air cells. Facial nerve runs in facial canal along the medial part of posterior wall.
- *Lateral/tympanic wall:* Is formed by tympanic membrane. Chorda tympani a branch of facial nerve passes across the tympanic membrane.
- *Medial/labyrinthine wall:* Separates middle ear from the internal ear. It presents following features:
  - Promontory formed by basal turn of the cochlea.
  - Fenestra vestibule (oval window).
  - Fenestra cochlea (round window).
  - Prominence of facial canal.

d. **Parts of internal ear: (Fig. 79.2)**

- ***Consists of two parts:***
  - Outer bony labyrinth.
  - Inner membranous labyrinth.
- Membranous labyrinth houses receptors for hearing and equilibrium.
- ***Bony labyrinth*** consists of three parts:
  - Vestibule.
  - Cochlea.
  - 3 Semicircular canals.

* All contain *perilymph,* in which the membranous labyrinth is suspended.

- ***Membranous labyrinth*** contains *endolymph* and has following parts:
  - *Utricle and saccule* are present in the vestibule and they contain sense organs called *maculae* which detect linear acceleration of the head.
  - *3 semicircular ducts* are present in the 3 semicircular canals, their dilated ends are called *ampullae cristae* which detect rotational acceleration.
  - *Cochlear duct* is present within the cochlea which contains *organ of corti* responsible for sense of hearing.

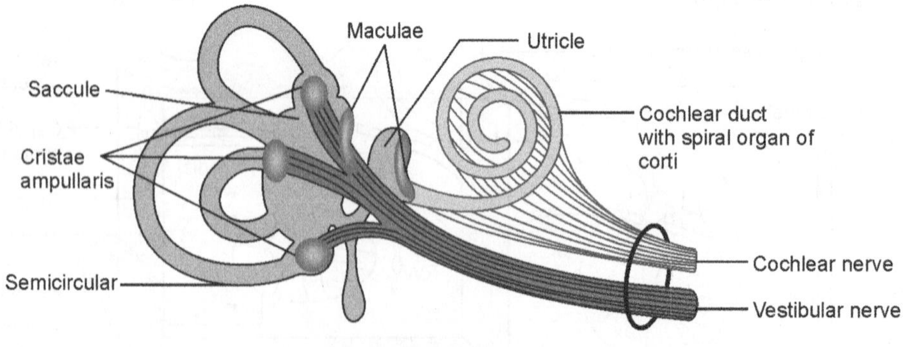

Fig. 79.2: Parts of internal ear

2. **Write short notes on:**
   a. **Tympanic membrane**
   b. **Auditory/pharyngotympanic tube**

Ans. a. Tympanic membrane: (Fig. 79.3)

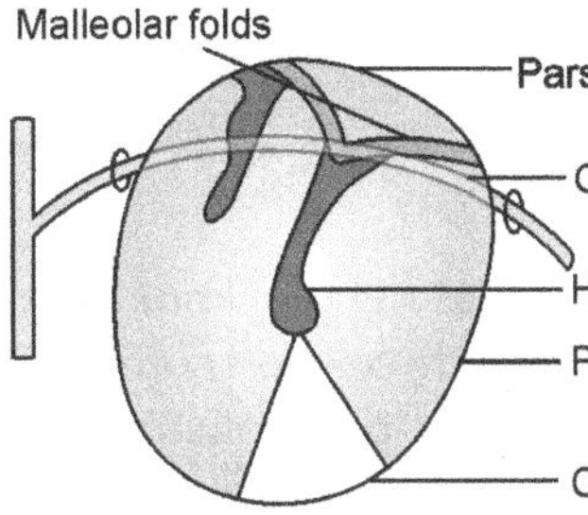

Fig. 79.3: Tympanic membrane

- Lies obliquely at the medial end of external auditory meatus.
- Separates external ear from the middle ear.
- ***Consists of three layers (derived from three germ layers):***
  - Outer layer – skin.
  - Middle layer – fibrous.
  - Inner layer – mucous membrane.
- ***Is divided into two parts:***
  - *Pars flaccida:* Small triangular area between the malleolar folds. This part is lax due to the absence of fibrous layer.
  - *Pars tensa:* Larger part that is tense.
- Medial surface is convex, maximum convexity is where handle of malleus is attached, it is called umbo.
- When examined, a bright cone of light is seen in the anteroinferior quadrant.
- ***Nerve supply:***
  - *Lateral surface* is supplied by auriculotemporal nerve and auricular branch of vagus.
  - *Medial surface* is supplied by glossopharyngeal nerve through the tympanic plexus.

> In myringotomy the surgical incision is placed in the posteroinferior quadrant to avoid injury to chorda tympani nerve.

b. **Auditory/pharyngotympanic tube:**

- Is a trumpet shaped tube which connects middle ear with nasopharynx.
- Is 3.5-4 cm long.
- Is directed downwards, forwards and medially.
- ***Is divided into two parts:***
  - *Cartilaginous part*–Anterior 2/3rd.
  - *Bony part* – Posterior 1/3rd, lies in petrous part of temporal part.
- It balances the air pressure in the middle ear with the atmospheric pressure, thus allowing free movement of tympanic membrane.
- Muscles attached to the cartilaginous part of auditory tube are–tensor tympani, levator palatini, tensor palate and salpingopharyngeus. Most of them help in opening of the tube.
- ***Nerve supply:***
  - Lateral part of the tube is supplied by glossopharyngeal nerve via tympanic plexus.
  - Medial part is supplied by pharyngeal branch of pterygopalatine ganglion carrying sensory fibers from maxillary nerve.

> In infants the auditory tube is shorter and is less oblique as compared to adults and therefore it is easier for the infection to spread from the nasopharynx to the middle ear cavity.

CHAPTER 80

CRANIAL NERVES

1. **Enumerate:**
   a. **The cranial nerves**
   b. **Functional components of cranial nerves**

Ans. a. **The cranial nerves are:**

I. Olfactory.
II. Optic.
III. Oculomotor.
IV. Trochlear.
V. Trigeminal.
VI. Abducens.
VII. Facial.
VIII. Vestibulocochlear.
IX. Glossopharyngeal.
X. Vagus.
XI. Accessory.
XII. Hypoglossal.

b. **Functional components of cranial nerves:** A total of seven functional columns are present in the brainstem for the location of nuclei of cranial nerves. Four are sensory (afferent) and three are motor (efferent). The functions, components and the structures innervated are as follows: (See the following Table)

2. **Write in a tabulated form the functional components, branches and distribution of III to XII cranial nerves. Draw labeled diagram to illustrate their branches.**

Ans. a. **Oculomotor nerve: (Fig. 80.1)**

- It is the 3rd cranial nerve.
- Is purely motor nerve.
- Its nuclei lie in midbrain at the level of superior colliculus.
- It emerges from the ventral aspect of midbrain (in the interpeduncular fossa) between posterior cerebral and superior cerebellar arteries.
- Runs forward in the lateral wall of the cavernous sinus.
- Passes through the superior orbital fissure to enter the orbit.

Functional component		*Structures innervated (in the head and neck region)*
Motor	General somatic efferent (GSE)	Skeletal muscles of somatic origin (muscles of tongue, extraocular muscles)
	Special visceral efferent (SVE)	Skeletal muscles derived from branchial arches (I, II, III, IV and VI branchial arch)
	General visceral efferent (GVE)	Smooth muscle and glands (preganglionic parasympathetic fibers in III, VII, IX and X CNs.)
Functional component		*Type of sensation/s received*
Sensory	General visceral afferent (GVA)	General sensations from the viscera
	Special visceral afferent (SVA)	Taste sensation
	General somatic afferent (GSA)	Exteroceptive (touch, pain, temperature) and proprioceptive sensations
	Special somatic afferent (SSA)	Special senses (olfaction, vision, hearing)

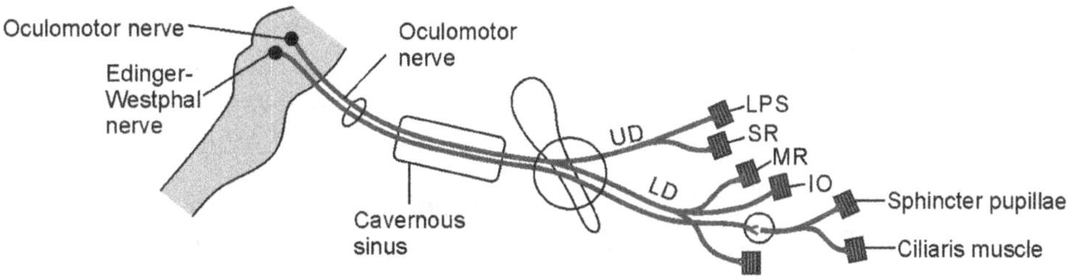

Fig. 80.1: Oculomotor nerve

Functional component	*Nucleus*	*Structures innervated*
GSE	Oculomotor nucleus (in midbrain)	Supplies following extraocular muscles: • Superior rectus • Inferior rectus • Medial rectus • Inferior oblique • Levator palpebrae superioris
GVE	Edinger-Westphal nucleus (in midbrain)	Sphincter papillae and ciliaris muscles

Lesion of oculomotor nerve–The symptoms are:

- Lateral strabismus - due to paralysis of medial rectus unopposed action of lateral rectus muscle.
- Ptosis - due to paralysis of levator palpebrae superioris.
- Dilated pupil - paralysis of sphincter papillae.
- Loss of accommodation–due to paralysis of medial rectus, sphincter papillae and ciliaris muscles.
- Diplopia on looking medially and superiorly.

b. **Trochlear nerve: (Fig. 80.2)**

- Is the IV cranial nerve (smallest CN).
- Is purely motor nerve.
- Its nucleus is located in the midbrain at the level of inferior colliculus.
- Emerges on the dorsal surface below the inferior colliculi (is the only cranial nerve to emerge on the dorsal surface of brainstem).

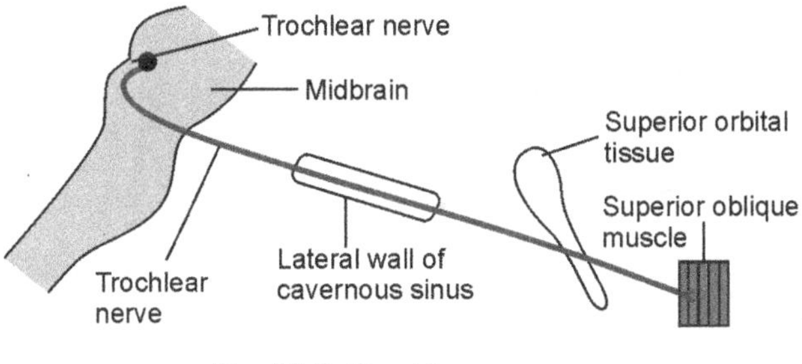

Fig. 80.2: Trochlear nerve

- The two nerves decussate and wind around the cerebral peduncles to reach the ventral aspect of midbrain.
- Run in the lateral wall of the cavernous sinus below the oculomotor nerve.
- Enter the orbit by passing through the superior orbital fissure.

Functional component	*Nucleus*	*Structures innervated*
GSE	Trochlear nucleus (in midbrain)	Superior oblique muscle of eyeball

Trochlear nerve lesion: The symptoms are:

- Diplopia on looking downward–due to paralysis of superior oblique muscle.
- Patient faces difficulty while going downstairs or reading a book.

c. **Abducens nerve (so named because it abducts the eye): (Fig. 80.3)**

- Is the 6th cranial nerve.
- Is purely motor nerve.
- Its nucleus is located in the lower part of pons in the floor of IV ventricle, deep to facial colliculus.

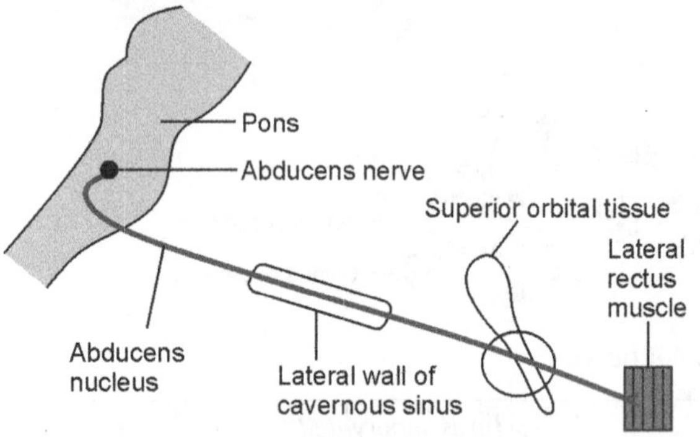

Fig. 80.3: Abducens nerve

- Emerges at the lower border of pons above the pyramids of medulla oblongata.
- Passes through the cavernous sinus inferolateral to the internal carotid artery.
- Enters the orbit by passing through the superior orbital fissure.
- It has the longest intracranial course and is most susceptible to damage due to increased intracranial pressure.

Functional component	*Nucleus*	*Structures innervated*
GSE	Abducens nucleus (in lower pons)	Lateral rectus muscle

Abducens nerve lesion: The symptoms are:
- ***Medial strabismus:*** Due to paralysis of lateral rectus and unopposed action of medial rectus muscle.
- Diplopia on looking towards the paralysed side.

d. Trigeminal nerve: (Fig. 80.4)

- It is the 5th cranial nerve.
- It is mixed (sensory and motor) nerve.
- It emerges from the ventral surface of pons at its junction with the middle cerebellar peduncle.
- ***It has two roots:***
  - Smaller medial motor root.
  - Larger lateral sensory root.
- ***It has three divisions:***
  - Ophthalmic.
  - Maxillary.
  - Mandibular.

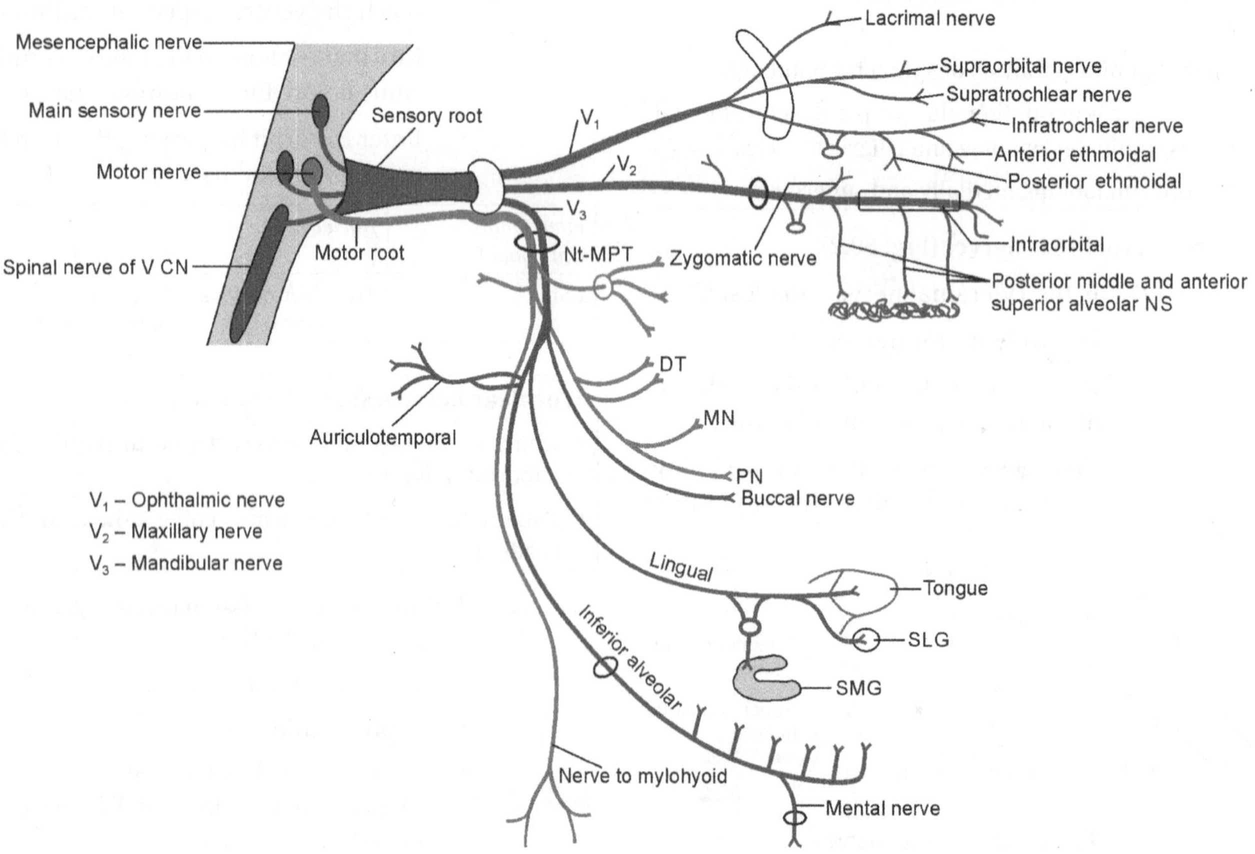

Fig. 80.4: Trigeminal nerve

Functional component	*Nucleus*	*Structures innervated*
SVE	Motor nucleus of trigeminal nerve	All the muscles derived from 1st branchial arch: Temporalis Masseter Lateral pterygoid Medial pterygoid Tensor tympani Tensor palatini (Masseter to Tensor palatini: Muscles of mastication) Anterior belly of digastric mylohyoid
GSA	Main sensory nucleus of V CN	Carry touch and pressure sensations from the anterior part of scalp, face, gums, teeth, mucous membrane of mouth, nasal cavity, paranasal air sinuses, maxillary sinus, nasopharynx, hard palate, dura mater of anterior and middle cranial fossa.
	Spinal nerve of V CN	Carry pain and temperature sensations from the anterior part of scalp, face, gums, teeth, mucous membrane of mouth, nasal cavity, paranasal air sinuses, maxillary sinus, nasopharynx, hard palate dura mater of anterior and middle cranial fossa.
	Mesencephalic nerve	Carries proprioceptive sensations from muscles of mastication and temporomandibular joint.

e. **Facial nerve: (Fig. 80.5)**
- It is the seventh cranial nerve.
- It is a mixed (sensory and motor) nerve.
- Its nuclei lie in the lower part of the pons.
- It emerges at the lower border of pons as two roots, large medial motor

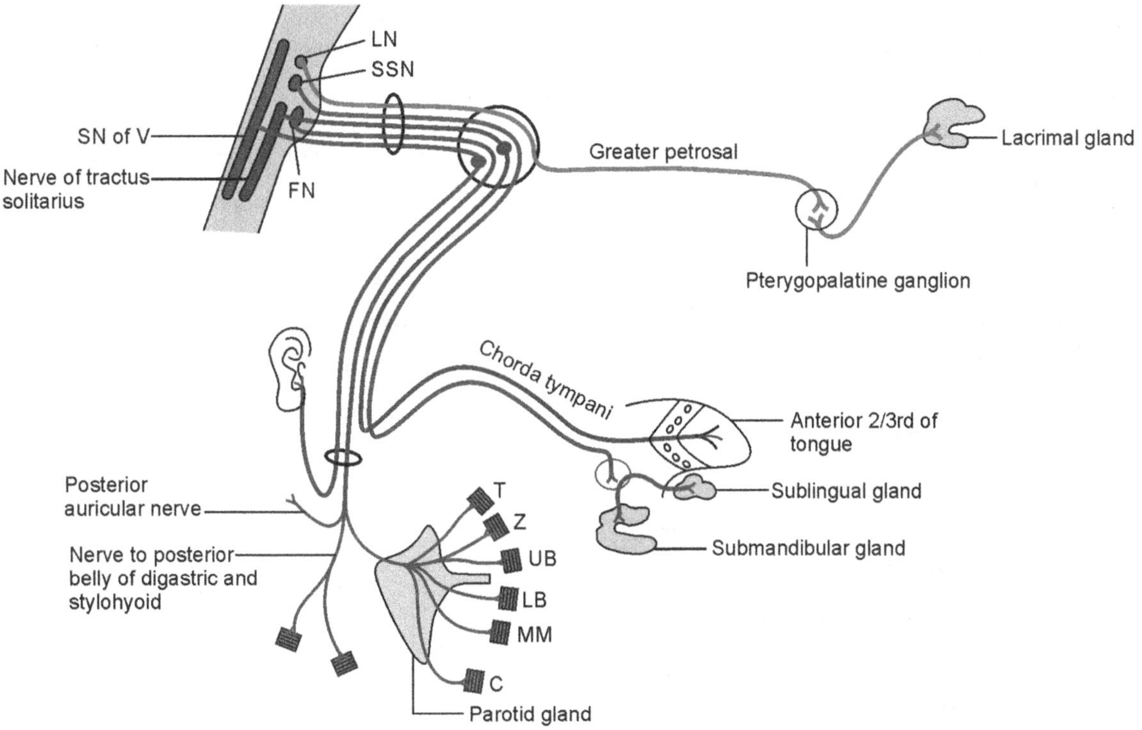

Fig. 80.5: Facial nerve

root and a small lateral sensory root (nervus intermedius).

- Leaves the cranial cavity by passing through the internal acoustic meatus.
- It then enters the facial canal which is divided into three segments viz. labyrinthine, tympanic and mastoid.
  - Labyrinthine segment of facial canal lies above the vestibule of internal ear. The facial nerve passes through this part to reach the medial wall of middle ear where it bends (external genu–location of geniculate ganglion) sharply backwards.
  - The nerve then passes through the tympanic segment of facial canal which runs horizontally backward in the medial wall of the middle ear till it reaches the junction of medial and posterior wall of middle ear.
  - It passes vertically downward in the mastoid part of facial canal in the posterior wall of middle ear to reach the stylomastoid foramen.
- After emerging from the stylomastoid foramen it runs forwards, crosses the styloid process and enters the posteromedial surface of parotid gland.
- Within the gland it lies lateral to retromandibular vein and external carotid artery and divides into 5 terminal branches.
- ***Branches of facial nerve:***
  - *In the facial canal:*
    - Greater petrosal nerve (from geniculate ganglion).
    - Nerve to stapedius.
    - Chorda tympani nerve.
  - *Branches below the stylomastoid foramen:*
    - Posterior auricular nerve.
    - Nerve to posterior belly of digastric and stylohyoid muscles.
  - *Branches on face:*
    - Temporal nerve.
    - Zygomatic nerve.
    - Buccal nerves – upper and lower.
    - Marginal mandibular.
    - Cervical.

Facial nerve lesion:

- ***Supranuclear lesion:***
  - Muscles of the lower part of face of opposite side are paralysed.
  - Muscles of upper part of face are spared because they are contolled by both the cerebral hemispheres.
- ***Infranuclear lesion:*** Symptoms depend on the site of lesion:
  - *At the stylomastoid foramen (Bell's palsy):* Paralysis of all the muscles of facial expression on the same side (see Page No. 214).
  - *Above the origin of chorda tympani:* All the symptoms of lesion (i) and decreased salivation and loss of taste sensation from anterior 2/3rd of the tongue.
  - *Above the origin of nerve to stapedius:* All the symptoms of lesion (i) and (ii) and hyperacusis.
  - *At the geniculate ganglion:* All the symptoms of lesion (i) and (ii) and (iii) and loss of lacrimation.

f. **Vestibulocochlear nerve:**

- Is the eighth cranial nerve.
- Is purely sensory nerve.
- ***Has two components:***
  - *Cochlear component:* Concerned with hearing.
  - *Vestibular component:* Concerned with maintenance of equilibrium.
- Emerges at the cerebellopontine angle.
- Leave the cranial cavity by passing through the internal acoustic meatus.

Functional component	*Nucleus*	*Structures innervated*
SVE	Motor nucleus of facial nerve	All the muscles derived from *2nd branchial arch* Occipitofrontalis Muscles of face Platysma Stapedius Posterior belly of digastric Stylohyoid muscle
GVE	Superior salivatory nucleus	Secretomotor fibers to submandibular and sublingual gland
	Lacrimatory nucleus	Secretomotor fibers to lacrimal gland
SVA	Nucleus of tractus solitarius	Carry taste sensation from anterior 2/3rd of tongue (except circumvallate papillae)
GSA	Spinal nucleus of trigeminal nerve	Few cutaneous fibers from external ear
SSA	Ventral and dorsal nuclei	Innervate sensory receptors of hearing - organ of corti
	Superior, inferior, medial and lateral vestibular nuclei	Innervate sensory receptors for equilibrium - maculae and cristae ampullaris

Lesion of vestibulocochlear nerve – Symptoms are:

- Tinnitus (buzzing or ringing sensation), deafness vertigo, nausea.

g. **Glossopharyngeal nerve: (Fig. 80.6)**

- Is the ninth cranial nerve.
- Is a mixed (sensory and motor) nerve.
- Emerges from the ventral surface of medulla posterior to the olive.
- Leaves the cranial cavity through the jugular foramen.
- In the neck it lies medial to styloid process and descends between the internal jugular vein and internal carotid artery and then between external and internal carotid arteries.
- It then passes along with stylopharyngeus muscle through the gap between superior and middle constrictors of pharynx and divides into terminal branches.
- ***Branches:***
  - *Tympanic branch* – carry preganglionic parasympathetic fibers to parotid gland.
  - *Carotid branches* – supply carotid body and sinus.
  - *Pharyngeal branches* – join pharyngeal plexus.
  - *Tonsillar branch* – supplies palatine tonsil and soft palate.
  - *Lingual branch* – supplies posterior 1/3rd of tongue.
  - *Muscular branch* to stylopharyngeus.

Functional component	*Nucleus*	*Structures innervated*
SVE	Nucleus ambiguus	Muscle derived from *3rd branchial arch* Stylopharyngeus muscle
GVE	Inferior salivatory nucleus	Secretomotor fibers to parotid gland
GVA	Nucleus of tractus solitarius	Carry general sensations from middle ear, auditory tube, soft palate, oropharynx, tonsil and posterior 1/3rd of tongue
SVA	Nucleus of tractus solitarius	Carry taste sensation from posterior 1/3rd of tongue (including circumvallate papillae)

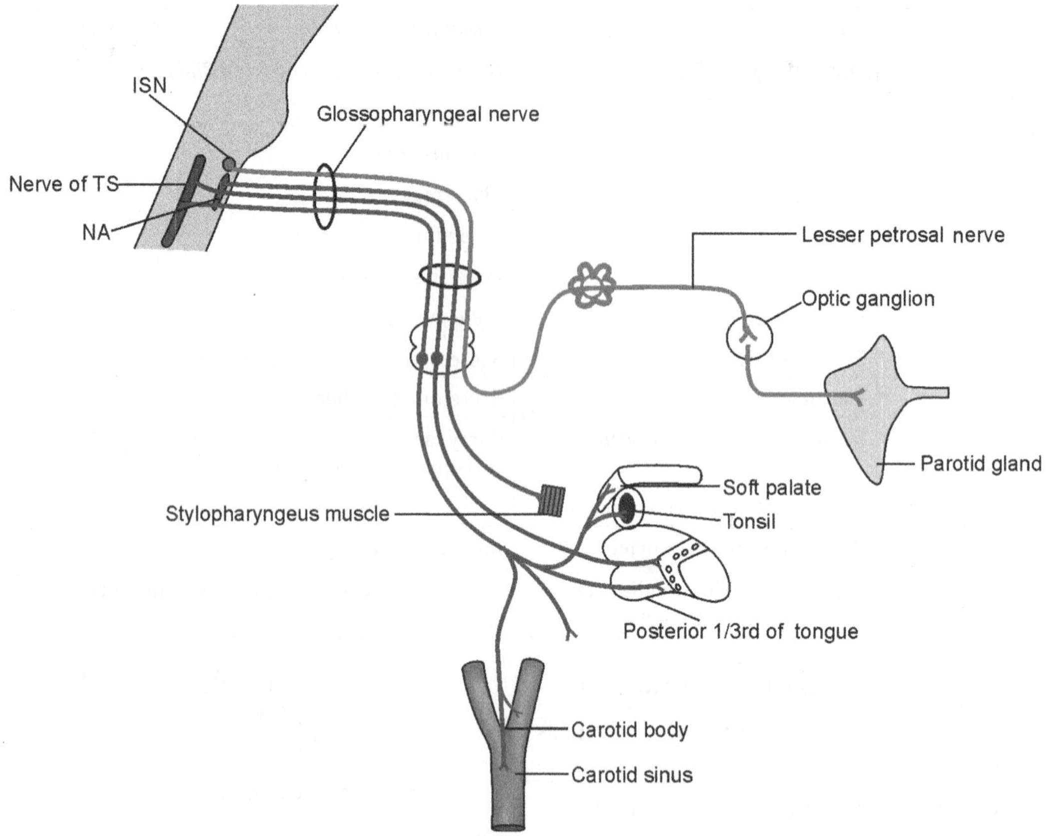

Fig. 80.6: Glossopharyngeal nerve

Lesion of glossopharyngeal nerve leads to:

- Loss of general and taste sensation from posterior 1/3rd of the tongue.
- Loss of salivation from parotid gland.
- Ipsilateral loss of gag reflex:
  - *Gag reflex:* On touching the posterior part of tongue or soft palate or pharynx there is reflex contraction of pharyngeal muscles causing gagging and retching.
  - The afferent fibers for gag reflex pass in glossopharyngeal nerve.
  - The efferent fibers for gag reflex pass in vagus nerve.

h. **Vagus nerve:**

- It is the 10th cranial nerve.
- Is a mixed (sensory and motor) nerve.
- Emerges from the ventral surface of medulla oblongata posterior to olive below the glossopharyngeal nerve.
- Leaves the cranial cavity through the jugular foramen.
- Descends in the neck within the carotid sheath.
- Enters the thorax by passing through the thoracic inlet.
- ***Branches in the neck:***
  - *Auricular branch* – to external ear.
  - *Pharyngeal branch* – to pharyngeal plexus.
  - *Superior laryngeal nerve which divides into:*
    - External laryngeal nerve – Supplies cricothyroid muscle.
    - Internal laryngeal nerve – Innervates mucosa of larynx above the vocal folds, posterior most part of tongue and epiglottis.

Functional component	*Nucleus*	*Structures innervated*
SVE	Nucleus ambiguus	Muscle derived from 4th and *6th branchial arches.* Muscles of palate (except tensor palatini), pharynx (except stylopharyngeus) and larynx (except cricothyroid).
GVE	Dorsal motor nerve of vagus	Parasympathetic fibers to heart, bronchial tree and GIT (till the junction of right 2/3rd and left 1/3rd of transverse colon).
GVA	Dorsal motor nerve of vagus	Carry general sensations from mucus membrane of pharynx, larynx, trachea, GIT (till the junction of right 2/3rd and left 1/3rd of transverse colon).
SVA	Nucleus of tractus solitarius	Carry taste sensation from posterior most part of tongue and epiglottis.
GSA	Spinal nucleus of trigeminal	General sensations from the skin of auricle.
GSE	Spinal nucleus of accessory nerve in upper 4-5 cervical segments of spinal cord	Sternocleidomastoid and tapezius muscles.

- *Recurrent laryngeal nerve:* All the muscles of larynx except cricothyroid and mucosa of larynx below the vocal fold.
- *Superior and inferior cervical cardiac branches* that supply heart through cardiac plexus.

Lesion of vagus nerve leads to:
- Nasal regurgitation of swallowed liquids and nasal twang of voice - due to ipsilateral paralysis of muscles of palate.
- Hoarseness of voice and cadaveric position of vocal cord (on the affected side) - due to paralysis of laryngeal muscle.
- Loss of ipsilateral gag reflex – vagus nerve forms the efferent limb of the gag reflex.
- Dysphagia.

i. **Accessory nerve: (Fig. 80.7)**
- It is the 11th cranial nerve.
- ***It has two parts:***
  - *Spinal:* Emerges from the upper 4-5 cervical segments of spinal cord.
  - *Cranial:* Emerges from the ventral surface of medulla oblongata.
- Spinal and cranial part leave the cranial cavity through jugular foramen.
- Cranial part joins vagus.
- Spinal part innervates two muscles – sternocleidomastoid and trapezius.

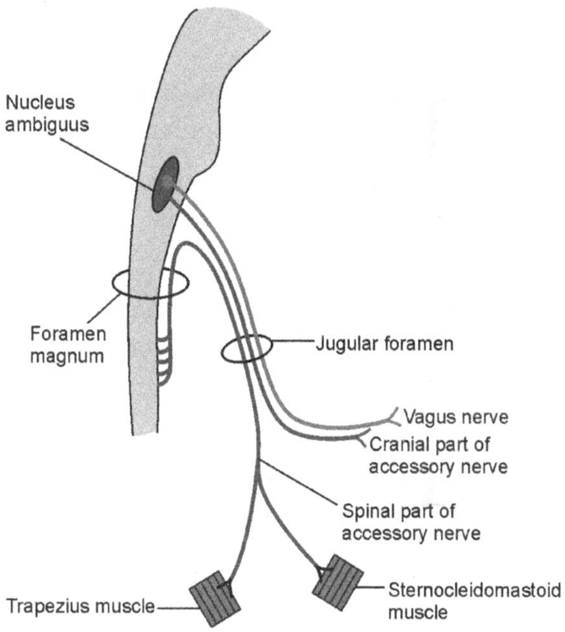

Fig. 80.7: Accessory nerve

Lesion of spinal part of accessory nerve leads to:
- ***Drooping of shoulder:*** Due to paralysis of tapezius muscle.
- ***Inability to tilt the head towards the shoulder on the same side and turn the chin to the opposite side:*** Due to paralysis of sternocleidomastoid muscle.

j. **Hypoglossal nerve: (Fig. 80.8)**
- Is the 12th cranial nerve.
- Is purely motor nerve.
- Its nucleus is located in the medulla in the lower part of the floor of the IV ventricle.

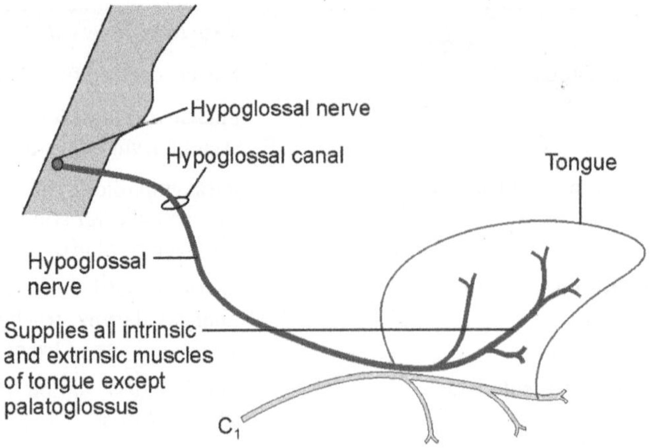

Fig. 80.8: Hypoglossal nerve

- Emerges from the ventral surface of medulla between the pyramid and olive.
- Leaves the cranial cavity by passing through the hypoglossal canal.
- Descends in the neck between the internal jugular vein and internal carotid artery.
- Passes deep to posterior belly of digastric and stylohyoid muscle to reach the carotid triangle.
- It passes forwards by passing superficial to internal carotid, external carotid and lingual arteries.
- It runs superficial to hyoglossus muscle and then deep to mylohyoid.
- It supplies all the muscles of tongue except palatoglossus.

Functional component	*Nucleus*	*Structures innervated*
GSE	Hypoglossal nucleus in medulla oblongata	All the intrinsic and extrinsic muscles of tongue except palaloglossus

Lesion of hypoglossal nerve results in:
- Tongue deviates towards the paralysed side when the patient tries to protrude the tongue due to unopposed action of genioglossus of normal side.